16th Workshop Conference Hoechst

Regulation of Secondary Metabolite Formation

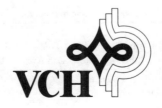

© VCH Verlagsgesellschaft mbH, D-6940 Weinheim (Federal Republic of Germany), 1986

Distribution:
VCH Verlagsgesellschaft, Postfach 12 60/12 80, D-6940 Weinheim (Federal Republic of Germany)
USA und Canada: VCH Publishers, 303 N.W. 12th Avenue, Deerfield Beach FL 33442-1705 (USA)

ISBN 3-527-26475-2 (VCH Verlagsgesellschaft)
ISBN 0-89573-499-0 (VCH Publishers)

Regulation of Secondary Metabolite Formation

Proceedings of the Sixteenth
Workshop Conference Hoechst,
Gracht Castle, 12–16 May 1985

Edited by
Horst Kleinkauf, Hans von Döhren,
Horst Dornauer, and Georg Nesemann

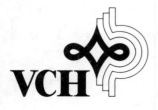

VCH

Horst Kleinkauf
ordentlicher Professor für Biochemie
Technische Universität Berlin
Institut für Biochemie und
Molekulare Biologie
D-1000 Berlin (West)

Hans von Döhren
Privat-Dozent
Technische Universität Berlin
Institut für Biochemie und
Molekulare Biologie
D-1000 Berlin (West)

Horst Dornauer
Leiter der Abteilung
Pharma Forschung Mikrobiologie
Hoechst AG
D-6000 Frankfurt
Federal Republic of Germany

Georg Nesemann
ehem. Leiter der Abteilung
Pharma Forschung Mikrobiologie
Hoechst AG
D-6000 Frankfurt
Federal Republic of Germany

Deutsche Bibliothek Cataloguing-in-Publication Data

Regulation of secondary metabolite formation: Gracht Castle,
12–16 May 1985 / ed. by Horst Kleinkauf ... –
Weinheim; Deerfield Beach, Fl.: VCH, 1986.
   (Proceeding of the ... workshop conference Hoechst; 16)
   ISBN 3-527-26475-2 (Weinheim)
   ISBN 0-89573-499-0 (Deerfield Beach, Fl.)
NE: Kleinkauf, Horst [Hrsg.]; Hoechst-Aktiengesellschaft: Proceedings of the ...

Printing: betz-druck gmbh, D-6100 Darmstadt
Bindung: Georg Kränkl, D-6148 Heppenheim
Printed in the Federal Republic of Germany

Preface

Horst Kleinkauf

Technical University of Berlin, Institute of Biochemistry and Molecular Biology,
Franklinstr. 29, D-1000 Berlin 10 (West)

The conference "Regulation of Secondary Metabolite Formation" held at Gracht Castle has been sponsored by Hoechst AG in a series of workshop meetings with the intention of promoting communication among scientists.

The research on secondary metabolism is now in a progressive phase for a number of reasons. Genetic studies have been extended to industrial organisms. Molecular genetic techniques have entered the antibiotic fields. Many *in vitro* enzyme systems have been established in transformation and synthesis of secondary metabolites. Our aim at this meeting has been to present the state of research, to reflect its directions, and to direct and combine efforts in the near future.

The field of secondary metabolites, which is presented here almost exclusively at the microbial level, only slowly finds its way into cellular biochemistry. There have been severe obstacles in selection and complementation of strains, or the elucidation of regulatory events. There are still only slight improvements in this respect, but many recent results have added new excitement and new experimental strategies.

Non-producer strains of both procaryotic and eucaryotic types may contain the complete structural information of an enzyme or pathway without expressing it. Complementation by specific DNA sequences then leads to an expression. Regulatory DNA regions can be approached by genetic engineering techniques, and the regulation of isolated genes can be studied. Genes of enzymes participating in antibiotic formation have been cloned, and permit efficient structural studies. Combinations of sets of genes from different strains may lead to the formation of novel hybrid compounds. On the other hand, only scarce information is available on the biology of the organisms, their metabolism and their regulatory control mechanisms. This should lead us to intensify the general studies on the relevant organisms and to select certain reference strains. In the long run this should enable us to understand the role of many unique compounds that have found their various applications for their producer organisms. And with this knowledge many regulatory mechanisms will be revealed which will be of benefit in future production methods.

On behalf of all participants I would like to thank Dr. Dornauer and Dr. Nesemann especially for their invitation to this conference. A conference such as this can be the ideal ground onto which the seeds of friendship can be thrown so that they grow and develop into a much more lasting and rewarding scientific contact and co-operation.

Berlin, in August 1985 H. Kleinkauf

Opening Address

Horst Dornauer

HOECHST AG, Department of Microbiology, D-6230 Frankfurt am Main 80, FRG

Ladies and Gentlemen,

On behalf of the Management of the Pharmaceutical Research Division of Hoechst AG, Frankfurt, and the Organizing Committee, I have pleasure in welcoming all of you to the 16th Workshop Conference Hoechst at Gracht Castle, entitled "Regulation of Secondary Metabolite Formation".

It is most gratifying to see so many distinguished scientists and renowned experts from all over the world assembled in this room.

My sincere thanks are due to Professor Kleinkauf for having set the scientific scope for this Workshop and for having selected the topmost speakers and participants. I wish to thank all of you for having accepted our invitation.

The idea of having a conference like this was born 14 years ago with the objective of summarizing recent progress in different scientific disciplines important to Drug Research. This year's conference is actually the 16th meeting in a series of workshops sponsored by our company, being however the first one devoted to microbiology. In view of the enormous progress recently achieved in this field, reviewing secondary metabolite formation is more than adequate.

The last decade, ladies and gentlemen, displayed a revival of secondary metabolite research and important discoveries, after a period of satisfaction with the "Antibiotic Golden Era" of the 1940s and 1950s. Microbial secondary metabolites are nowadays a conditio sine qua non in our society. The predominant application of new chemical entities still lies in the field of antibacterial, antifungal and antitumor chemotherapy. However, dramatic progress in the methods by which novel secondary metabolites are discovered and designed has opened new applications including their use against parasites and insects for animals, and for plant growth stimulation as well.

Another sphere of research which has made rapid strides in recent years is that of enzyme inhibition. Catalyzed by the use of simple enzyme assays for screening, a large number of extremely potent enzyme inhibitors have been isolated and identified from microbial broths, some of which being more active than previously known synthetic inhibitors. Compounds of this type include inhibitors of the angiotensin converting enzyme and renin for blood pressure regulation, inhibitors of intestinal glycosidases for control of diabetes, hyper-lipoproteinaemia and obesity, and inhibitors of enkephalinase, just to mention a few.

The last decade, however, has witnessed a breakthrough in recombinant DNA technology. Besides probing the mysteries of life itself, the new techniques lead to unique ways of producing important biological substances. At the moment there is rapid progress in the development of recombinant DNA technology using antibiotic-producing streptomyces and fungi. Methods have been established for cloning of genes using vectors with wide host ranges. Since knowledge about rate-limiting steps in the biosynthesis of antibiotics is available only in a few antibiotic-producing organisms, direct approaches to gene amplification of certain steps to overcome this lack are not yet possible. Advances in this field, however, are beginning to unravel the complex biochemical mechanisms. The further development of genetic methods and optimization of vectors with a wide host range, low copy number and sufficient cloning sites will be of great importance for the improvement of existing antibiotics and for the production of novel "hybrid" compounds as well.

I will conclude my opening remarks now and although being the 13th today, I look forward to an interesting and enjoyable Conference and wish this Workshop every success.

Introductory Remarks

Hans von Döhren

Technical University of Berlin, Institute of Biochemistry and Molecular Biology,
Franklinstr. 29, D-1000 Berlin 10 (West)

In pharmacology especially, secondary metabolites have found numerous applications. Their effective production has always been of considerable economical interest as we well know from the beta-lactam field. The present era of biotechnology, which can partially be characterized as a shift from random mutational improvement to the direct manipulation of genes, is now currently finding its way towards commercial organisms.

It has been the aim of the organizers of this workshop to gather experts of the various aspects related to secondary metabolism and to exchange and discuss the present results. The compounds and events treated include antibiotics (β-lactams, tetracyclines, aminoglycosides, tylosine, peptides), alkaloids (ergotamines), special metabolites (siderophores), hormones or signals (A-factor), developmental events (sporulation, aerial mycelia), and plant fungal infections (phytoalexins).

With the exception of the last mentioned example, the products are of microbial origin with *Streptomyces* being the most prominent host (β-lactams, tetracyclines, aminoglycosides), followed by β-lactam synthesizing fungi *(Penicillium, Cephalosporium)*, related mycotoxins *(Fusarium, Aspergillus)* and ergot alkaloid producers *(Claviceps)*, as well as peptide forming *Bacilli*.

Many of these systems are now being studied at the gene level, and the initial steps towards an understanding of regulatory mechanisms are being made. Recombinant DNA techniques will permit comparative studies of structural genes (like β-lactam forming enzymes in *Streptomyces* and *Cephalosporium*), promoter regions (such as overlapping promoters in *Bacillus subtilis*), functional (sigma factors) and regulatory proteins (A-factors, activators, repressors or perhaps resistance factors). Most of our data concerning the production and overproduction of antibiotics will then enable us presumably to produce more precise questions about the regulatory mechanisms.

Applications of results and procedures in the various production processes of secondary metabolites have been presented, proposed, or can be expected in the near future. Improvement of antibiotic production has been achieved by nutritional manipulations, mutational techniques such as protoplast fusion, or the introduction of additional genes by recombinant DNA techniques. Significant steps are being made in the enzymology of metabolite formation. Biosynthetic steps of many compounds have been unravelled, enzymes and multienzymes combining several steps have been isolated, and structural genes of some of these have been cloned. Directed biosynthesis, utilizing precursor control, has been performed *in vivo*, or with isolated enzymes. New β-lactam compounds have been produced by isopenicillin N-synthetase from synthetic tripeptides. Combination of enzymes of different pathways by genetic techniques has led to the production of hybrid metabolites. Indeed, such compounds suggest the increasing application of the cellular "machinery" in organic synthesis, including the direct use of free and cellular enzymes and their mutational modification, both procedures being significantly enhanced by genetic technology.

These impressive achievements can be retraced in the following contributions, which reflect quite comprehensively our knowledge and the state of the art of experimental biology of secondary metabolism in the middle of 1985.

Acknowledgements

The conference on which this volume is based would not have been possible without the generous sponsorship of Hoechst AG Frankfurt.

Acknowledgements are due to Mrs. C. Day of the Institute of Biochemistry and Molecular Biology, and Ms. C. Frick, of Hoechst AG, for their invaluable secretarial engagement during the organisation of the conference. Special thanks are also due to Mr. H.J. Jakobs and Mr. V. Fürnkranz for maintaining the technical facilities in good order. The editors wish to thank Mrs. C. Day, Mrs. E. Denaro, Mrs. H. Kühnauer and Mrs. R. Schirmer for their excellent assistance in the editorial work involved.

We also wish to express our gratitude to VCH Verlagsgesellschaft (formerly Verlag Chemie) for their good co-operation and especially for the swift publication of these proceedings.

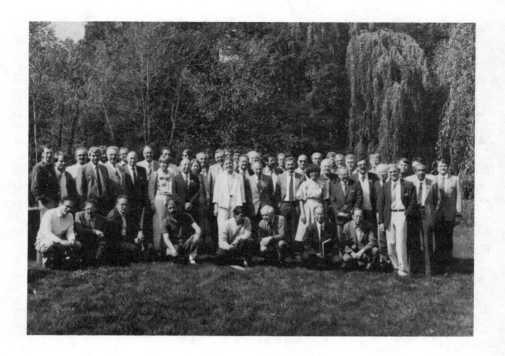

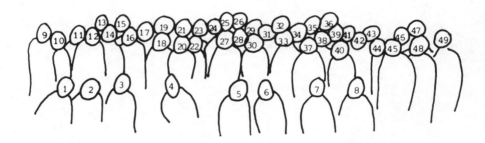

1. R. Losick	14. K. Esser	26. M. Mracek	38. A.L. Demain
2. J. Lengeler	15. J. Scholtholt	27. C. Frick	39. M. Luckner
3. Y. Aharonowitz	16. E. von Wasielewski	28. H.J. Rehm	40. K. Kieslich
4. H. von Döhren	17. H. Grisebach	29. G. Nesemann	41. H. Dornauer
5. M.A. Marahiel	18. S. Grabley	30. Sir E.P. Abraham	42. J.F. Martin
6. L.C. Vining	19. J. Betz	31. R. Bender	43. J.D. Bu'Lock
7. S. Ōmura	20. Y. Okami	32. R. Zocher	44. H. Dellweg
8. D.A. Hopwood	21. S. Goulden	33. P. Schindler	45. H. Kleinkauf
9. A. Braña	22. H. Schrempf	34. H.G. Floss	46. D.A. Sukatsch
10. U. Keller	23. H.G. Schlegel	35. V. Běhal	47. K. Sauber
11. W. Aretz	24. G. Seidl	36. K.-P. Koller	48. B.N. Ganguli
12. A. Pühler	25. G. Rieß	37. C. Day	49. U. Gräfe
13. W. Badziong			

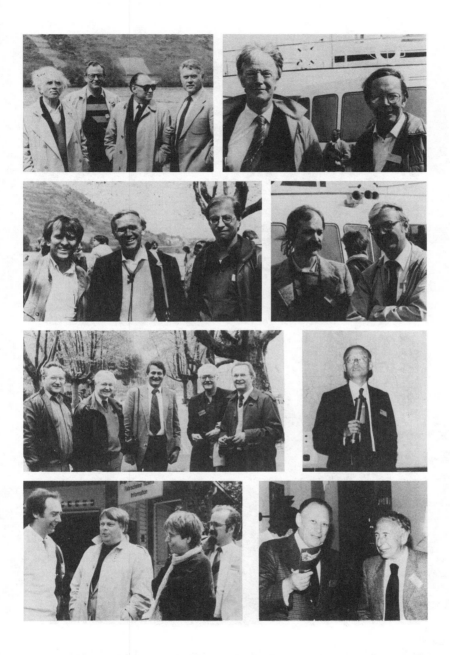

First row: G. Nesemann; J. Scholtholt; E. v. Wasielewski; H. Dornauer; J. Bu'Lock; D.A. Hopwood

Second row: U. Keller; H. Kleinkauf; R. Zocher; H. v. Döhren; M. Luckner

Third row: Y. Aharonowitz; L. Vining; U. Gräfe; A.L. Demain; H.J. Rehm; S. Ōmura

Fourth row: J. Betz; D.A. Sukatsch; S. Grabley; W. Aretz; E. v. Wasielewski; Sir E.P. Abraham

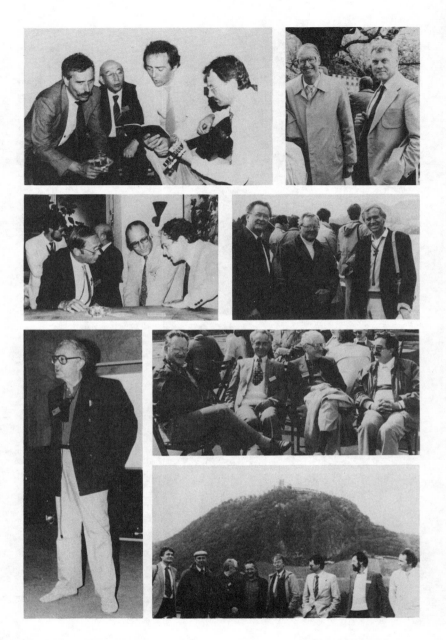

First row: P. Schindler; Y. Okami; J. Betz; K. Sauber; H. Grisebach; H. Dornauer
Second row: K.-P. Koller; D.A. Hopwood; H.G. Floss; R. Losick; H.J. Rehm; K. Kieslich; H. Kleinkauf
Third row: A.L. Demain; Y. Aharonowitz; H.G. Schlegel; A.L. Demain; J.F. Martín
Fourth row: U. Gräfe; V. Běhal; A.L. Demain; Y. Aharonowitz; J.D. Bu'Lock; K. Sauber; R. Bender; J. Betz

Contents

Contributors

Sir Edward P. Abraham
University of Oxford
Sir William Dunn School of Pathology
South Parks Road
Oxford OX1 3RE, England

Yair Aharonowitz
Tel-Aviv University
The George S. Wise Faculty of
  Life Sciences
Department of Microbiology
Ramat-Aviv
69978 Tel-Aviv, Israel

Zia U. Ahmed
Dalhousie University
Department of Biology
Halifax, Nova Scotia
Canada B3H 4J1

Emilio Alvarez
Universidad de León
Departamento de Microbiología
Facultad de Biología
(E.I.T. Agrícolas)
ctr. Circunvalación, s/n.
León, Spain

José L. Barredo
Universidad de León
Departamento de Microbiología
Facultad de Biología
(E.I.T. Agrícolas)
ctr. Circunvalación, s/n.
León, Spain

Vladislav Běhal
Czechoslovak Academy of Sciences
Institute of Microbiology
Vídeňská 1083
14220 Prague 4, Czechoslovakia

Hana Ben-Artzi
Tel-Aviv University
The George S. Wise Faculty of Life
  Sciences
Department of Microbiology
Ramat-Aviv
69978 Tel-Aviv, Israel

Ernst J. Bormann
GDR Academy of Sciences
Central Institute of Microbiology
and Experimental Therapy
DDR-6900 Jena, GDR

Alfredo F. Braña
Universidad de Oviedo
Departamento Interfacultativo de
  Microbiología
Oviedo, Spain

John D. Bu'Lock
Victoria University of Manchester
Weizmann Microbial Chemistry Laboratory
Department of Chemistry
Manchester M13 9PL, England

Jesús M. Cantoral
Universidad de León
Departamento de Microbiología
Facultad de Biología
(E.I.T. Agrícolas)
ctr. Circunvalacion, s/n.
León, Spain

José M. Castro
Universidad de León
Departamento de Microbiología
Facultad de Biología
(E.I.T. Agrícolas)
ctr. Circunvalacion, s/n.
León, Spain

Ching-jer Chang
The Ohio State University
Department of Chemistry
140 West 18th Avenue
Columbus, Ohio 43210, U.S.A.

Keith F. Chater
John Innes Institute
Department of Genetics
Colney Lane
Norwich NR4 7UH, England

Sheri P. Cole
The Ohio State University
Department of Chemistry
140 West 18th Avenue
Columbus, Ohio 43210, U.S.A.

Jesús Cortés
Universidad de León
Departamento de Microbiología
Facultad de Biología
(E.I.T. Agrícolas)
ctr. Circunvalacion, s/n.
León, Spain

Arnold L. Demain
Massachusetts Institute of Technology
Fermentation Microbiology Laboratory
Department of Nutrition and Food Science
Cambridge, Massachusetts 02139, U.S.A.

Hans von Döhren
Technical University of Berlin
Institute of Biochemistry and Molecular
  Biology
Franklinstr. 29
D-1000 Berlin 10 (West)

Horst Dornauer
HOECHST AG
Department of Microbiology
D-6230 Frankfurt/Main 80, FRG

Modesta G. Domínguez
Universidad de León
Departamento de Microbiología
Facultad de Biología
(E.I.T. Agrícolas)
ctr. Circunvalacion, s/n.
León, Spain

Janice Doull
Dalhousie University
Department of Microbiology
Halifax, Nova Scotia
Canada B3H 4J1

Janice Duncan
The Ohio State University
Department of Chemistry
140 West 18th Avenue
Columbus, Ohio 43210, U.S.A.

Inge Eritt
GDR Academy of Sciences
Central Institute of Microbiology and
Experimental Therapy
DDR-6900 Jena, GDR

Karl Esser
Ruhr-Universität
Lehrstuhl für Allgemeine Botanik
Postfach 10 21 48
D-4630 Bochum 1, FRG

Heinz G. Floss
The Ohio State University
Department of Chemistry
140 West 18th Avenue
Columbus, Ohio 43210, U.S.A.

Walter Friedrich
GDR Academy of Sciences
Central Institute of Microbiology and
Experimental Therapy
DDR-6900 Jena, GDR

Isao Fujii
The Ohio State University
Department of Chemistry
140 West 18th Avenue
Columbus, Ohio 43210, U.S.A.

Udo Gräfe
GDR Academy of Sciences
Central Institute of Microbiology and
Experimental Therapy
DDR-6900 Jena, GDR

Hans Grisebach
Albert-Ludwigs-Universität
Institut für Biologie II/
Biochemie der Pflanzen
Schänzlestr. 1
D-7800 Freiburg, FRG

J. Guijarro
Harvard University
Department of Cellular and
Developmental Biology
The Biological Laboratories
16 Divinity Avenue
Cambridge, Massachusetts 02138, U.S.A.

Frank Hänel
GDR Academy of Sciences
Central Institute of Microbiology and
Experimental Therapy
DDR-6900 Jena, GDR

Xian-Guo He
The Ohio State University
Department of Chemistry
140 West 18th Avenue
Columbus, Ohio 43210, U.S.A.

Geoffrey Holt
The Polytechnic of Central London
School of Biotechnology
Faculty of Engineering and Science
115 New Cavendish Street
London W1M 8JS, England

David A. Hopwood
John Innes Institute
Department of Genetics
Colney Lane
Norwich NR4 7UH, England

Paul J. Keller
The Ohio State University
Department of Chemistry
140 West 18th Avenue
Columbus, Ohio 43210, U.S.A.

Ullrich Keller
Technical University of Berlin
Institute of Biochemistry and
Molecular Biology
Franklinstr. 29
D-1000 Berlin 10 (West)

Horst Kleinkauf
Technical University of Berlin
Institute of Biochemistry and
Molecular Biology
Franklinstr. 29
D-1000 Berlin 10 (West)

Werner Lerbs
Academy of Sciences of GDR
Institute of Plant Biochemistry
Weinbergweg 3
DDR-4020 Halle, GDR

Paloma Liras
Universidad de León
Departamento de Microbiología
Facultad de Biología
(E.I.T. Agrícolas)
ctr. Circunvalación, s/n.
León, Spain

Manuel J. López-Nieto
Universidad de León
Departamento de Microbiología
Facultad de Biología
(E.I.T. Agrícolas)
ctr. Circunvalación, s/n.
León, Spain

Richard Losick
Harvard University
Department of Cellular and
Developmental Biology
The Biological Laboratories
16 Divinity Avenue
Cambridge, Massachusetts 02138, U.S.A.

Martin Luckner
Martin-Luther-University
Halle-Wittenberg
Section of Pharmacy
Weinbergweg 15
DDR-4020 Halle, GDR

Nurit A. Magal
Tel-Aviv University
The George S. Wise Faculty of Life
* Sciences*
Department of Microbiology
Ramat-Aviv
69978 Tel-Aviv, Israel

Francisco Malpartida
John Innes Institute
Department of Genetics
Colney Lane
Norwich NR4 7UH, England

Juan F. Martín
Universidad de León
Departamento de Microbiología
Facultad de Biología
(E.I.T. Agrícolas)
ctr. Circunvalacíon, s/n.
León, Spain

Simona Mendelovitz
Tel-Aviv University
The George S. Wise Faculty of Life
    Sciences
Department of Microbiology
Ramat-Aviv
69978 Tel-Aviv, Israel

Georg Nesemann
HOECHST AG
Department of Microbiology
D-6230 Frankfurt/Main 80, FRG

Yoshiro Okami
Microbial Chemistry Research
Foundation
Institute of Microbial Chemistry
3-14-23, Kamiosaki 3-chome
Shinagawa-ku
Tokyo, Japan

Satoshi Ōmura
Kitasato University
The Kitasato Institute and School of
    Pharmaceutical Sciences
5-9-1 Shirokane, Minato-Ku
Tokyo 108, Japan

Filomena R. Ramos
Universidad de León
Departamento de Microbiología
Facultad de Biología
(E.I.T. Agrícolas)
ctr. Circunvalacíon, s/n.
León, Spain

Monica Ranes
Harvard University
Department of Cellular and
Developmental Biology
The Biological Laboratories
16 Divinity Avenue
Cambridge, Massachusetts 02138, U.S.A.

Bernd Röder
GDR Academy of Sciences
Central Institute of Microbiology
and Experimental Therapy
DDR-6900 Jena, GDR

Mark E. Rogers
The Polytechnic of Central London
School of Biotechnology
Faculty of Engineering and Science
115 New Cavendish Street
London W1M 8JS, England

Jorge Romero
Universidad de León
Departamento de Microbiología
Facultad de Biología
(E.I.T. Agrícolas)
ctr. Circunvalación, s/n.
León, Spain

Werner Roos
Academy of Sciences of GDR
Institute of Plant Biochemistry
Weinbergweg 3
DDR-4020 Halle, GDR

Martin Roth
GDR Academy of Sciences
Central Institute of Microbiology
and Experimental Therapy
DDR-6900 Jena, GDR

Brian A. M. Rudd
The Ohio State University
Department of Chemistry
140 West 18th Avenue
Columbus, Ohio 43210, U.S.A.

Gunter Saunders
The Polytechnic of Central London
School of Biotechnology
Faculty of Engineering and Science
115 New Cavendish Street
London W1M 8JS, England

Stuart Shapiro
Dalhousie University
Department of Biology
Halifax, Nova Scotia
Canada B3H 4J1

Colin Stuttard
Dalhousie University
Department of Microbiology
Halifax, Nova Scotia
Canada B3H 4J1

Yoshitake Tanaka
Kitasato University
The Kitasato Institute and School of
Pharmaceutical Sciences
5-9-1 Shirokane, Minato-Ku
Tokyo 108, Japan

Sushma Vats
Dalhousie University
Department of Biology
Halifax, Nova Scotia
Canada B3H 4J1

Leo C. Vining
Dalhousie University
Department of Biology
Halifax, Nova Scotia
Canada B3H 4J1

Janet Westpheling
Harvard University
Department of Cellular and
Developmental Biology
The Biological Laboratories
16 Divinity Avenue
Cambridge, Massachusetts 02138, U.S.A.

Genetic Aspects of Mycotoxin Formation

John D. Bu'Lock

Victoria University of Manchester, Weizmann Microbial Chemistry Laboratory, Department of Chemistry, Manchester M13 9PL, England

1. Abstract

Genetic aspects of mycotoxin production are discussed in general terms and with particular reference to two instances; in both A. parasiticus (aflatoxin) and F. graminearum (zearalenone) there is evidence of a pleiotropic activating system that is relatively labile and independent of the structural genes for the biosynthetic process.

2. Introduction

Despite the fairly continuous attention being given to mycotoxins, there has been relatively little work on their genetics. However this is not surprising. The mycotoxins are produced by fungi, not bacteria; the genetics of fungi is based on systems which are much more versatile than those in prokaryotes, and although our knowledge of fungal genetics is considerable, very little of their more complex behaviour can yet be interpreted in the fashionable terms used in modern molecular genetics, which is still largely restricted to dealing with relatively simple events on single chromosomes.

Moreover like all secondary metabolites the mycotoxins are produced by pathways which involve multiple genes, whose expression is not at all essential for the organism in culture and whose operation is actuated and co-ordinated by mechanisms which are largely unknown. As with other secondary metabolites, their extreme diversity makes it very difficult to select particular systems for the kind of detailed study that is really needed. Their toxicity makes them relatively unpopular for laboratory studies, while the commercial incentive that helps to motivate fundamental research on antibiotic production is less immediately apparent.

This account, therefore, is necessarily a very limited one. It is based on three main sources: firstly, some general considerations drawn from the field of mycotoxin studies as a whole; second, an analysis of particular data for the aflatoxins which is very directly based on the work done by J. W. Bennett and her associates at Tulane University [1]; third, some much more tentative conclusions from work on zearalenone in my own laboratory, initiated with Janice S. Duncan[2] and being continued by J. P. Mooney and C. E. Wright.

3. General considerations

There are some general problems, and some tentative conclusions drawn from limited evidence, that emerge from an examination of the mycotoxins as a whole. These include:

- their status as secondary metabolites,
- their structural and biosynthetic diversity,
- their production in response to environmental parameters,
- their occurrence (non-occurence) in related (un-related) species/strains,
- the problem of their selection value, if any, in evolution of the genotype.

My view of these topics has been set out fully elsewhere [3] and they need not be discussed at any great length here. However it will be helpful for the subsequent more specific accounts to summarise these considerations, because they do underly the matters dealt with in later sections.

3.1   The mycotoxins are fully representative of fungal secondary metabolites as a whole, and their only specific categorisation is for extrinsic reasons. Why these secondary metabolites display such a wide range of physiological activities in other organisms is as unknown as their function,if any, in the producing species.

3.2   The biosynthetic pathways leading to mycotoxins show general features which partly explain the diversity of products: first there are a variety of rather specific synthetic processes which assemble unique molecular structures; second there are an equally varied range of further metabolic steps, often of rather lower specificity, whose interaction leads to a considerably greater variety of end-products. It is apparent that pathways thus structured offer a comparable scope for diversity in the occurrence of particular products in different fungal isolates.

3.3   Present systems of classifying fungi bear only an approximate relationship to the phylogenetic relationships that appear to exist between isolates producing similar or identical mycotoxins, implying that the production of a particular mycotoxin may not be very closely integrated into the total complex of genetic traits that defines a species, and perhaps also that some interspecies transfer of genes has occurred.

3.4   Mycotoxin production is a very variable characteristic in otherwise defined species [4][5]. Where the genetic capability to produce a particular mycotoxin exists in a strain, the actual level of production by that strain varies over a wide range, including virtual non-production, according to the culture history and with environmental/nutritional parameters.

3.5   Where the regulation of mycotoxin biosynthesis has been studied, it has been found to include both specific mechanisms of repression or derepression, and a generalised type of regulatory mechanism, common indeed to all secondary metabolism, which is somehow related to growth-restricting nutrient conditions. This is often referred to as "generalised catabolite repression". Since this type of regulation also governs important aspects of morphological differentiation in many fungi, correlations between specific metabolite production and particular differentiation phenomena are to be expected, and indeed are being defined with increased precision [6][7].

3.6   The complexity of the regulation mechanisms, coupled with the relatively lower specificity of some of the "diversifying" steps in mycotoxin synthesis, must be borne in mind in interpreting the results of mutational studies, for which the non-essential status of the mycotoxins already presents operational difficulties.

4. Aflatoxins in Aspergillus

4.1 Aflatoxins.

The aflatoxins present the most extensively studied of the mycotoxins, reflecting their particular economic importance as well as their comparatively early discovery. Biosynthetically, they are a group of highly-modified polyketides and the sequence of reactions by which they are formed is now relatively well understood [8][9]. A number of intermediates have been characterised and shown to accumulate in specific blocked mutants (see below, 4.3); from our overall understanding of the biosynthesis we can suppose that the whole pathway includes up to twenty or so distinct enzymes or multienzyme complexes, which implies a corresponding number of structural genes together with a full (and unknown) complement of regulatory genes. At least part of the regulation falls within the pleiotropic "general catabolite repression" mechanisms already referred to.

The genetic basis of aflatoxin production in <u>Aspergillus</u> has been examined in three aspects:-

(a) the comparative incidence of toxin production and non-production in natural isolates and laboratory strains of <u>A. flavus</u> and <u>A. parasiticus</u>;

(b) mutant blocks affecting successive steps in aflatoxin biosynthesis;

(c) the genetic basis of certain classes of non-producing variants obtained from producing strains.

These are considered in sections 4.2 and 4.3, below.

4.2 Incidence of Aflatoxin Production.

Aflatoxin production is "characteristic" of <u>A. flavus</u> and <u>A. parasiticus</u>. The taxonomic relationship between the toxigenic <u>A. flavus</u>, the conflated species <u>A. flavus-oryzae</u>, and the commercially-significant <u>A. oryzae</u> (which virtually all authorities agree does not produce aflatoxins) is not entirely convincing (see above, <u>3.2</u>, <u>3.3</u>). Among isolates of <u>A. flavus</u>, Hesseltine found high, low, and non-producing strains, and Diener and Davis found an essentially similar range within <u>A. parasiticus</u> [4]. The problem has recently been re-examined by Wicklow [5], who has concluded that <u>A. oryzae</u> has originated as a "domesticated" strain of <u>A. flavus</u>, with a similar relationship between <u>A. sojae</u> and <u>A. parasiticus</u>; the phenotypic aspects of such domestication were rather fully analysed but with no real clues as to the genetic basis of such changes. In both of the "non-toxigenic" species, the implication is not that the correct conditions for phenotypic toxin production were not applied, but rather that the non-producing strains are genetically incapable of aflatoxin production. <u>A fortiori</u> this should also be the case for strains derived in the laboratory by mutation or other manipulation of toxin-producing strains (see 4.3 and 4.4, below), but for the "wild" non-toxigenic strains we have no easy way of determining how much of the total genetic complement needed for aflatoxin synthesis is present, absent, or in some way suppressed.

In addition (see above, <u>3.2</u>, <u>3.3</u>) key (early) parts of the aflatoxin pathway are found independently in several other species of <u>Aspergillus</u> [8][9]. This situation is not uncommon and is due to the branching nature of the basic biosynthetic pathways (above, <u>3.2</u>).

Finally, it should be noted that both <u>A. flavus</u> and <u>A. parasiticus</u> are imperfect species for which conventional genetic crossing and analysis is not possible. However the parasexual cycle can be employed.

4.3 Mutants blocked in toxin production.

As already indicated, the biosynthetic pathway leading to the aflatoxins is now known in some detail, and a high proportion of the intermediates have been fully characterised. Some of these intermediates have been found to accumulate in mutants which are blocked in the following steps, or as a consequence of external inhibition of particular steps; others have been inferred, and in some cases subsequently demonstrated, on chemical grounds. There is no need to re-present the details of this work since it has been very fully reviewed by the Pretoria group [9].

I propose to concentrate here on some implications of the work[1][10] of Bennett and co-workers on certain types of blocked mutants, and for this discussion it will be sufficient to use a very simplified version of the overall pathway in terms of some specific intermediates, that is:

[acetate/malonate] $\longrightarrow$ norsolorinic acid $\longrightarrow$ versicolorin $\longrightarrow$ aflatoxin

abbreviated as:

$$A/M \longrightarrow NSA \longrightarrow VSA \longrightarrow AFL$$

In this simplification, the step A/M $\longrightarrow$ NSA comprises the assembly and cyclization of the basic polyketide assembly,and there are no known free intermediates. The step NSA $\longrightarrow$ VSA includes a redox conversion of norsolorinic acid to averantin, oxygenation of averantin to averufin, an oxygenase-type cleavage and rearrangement of the latter to versicolorin acetate, and hydrolysis to versicolorin. The step VSA $\longrightarrow$ AFL involves successive oxygenase-type (Bayer-Villiger) ring cleavages and re-cyclisations, first to the sterigmatocystin system and thence to the aflatoxins themselves.

Bennett's group used strains carrying nutritional and spore-colour markers which had this pathway in various forms:

- "complete" : high aflatoxin levels;
- "limited" : low aflatoxin levels due to limited activity in the early steps A/M to VSA;
- "blocked" : blocked either before or after VSA and accumulating either NSA or VSA correspondingly.

An important additional feature of their work was the observation that repeated sub-culturing of A. parasiticus by serial transfer of mycelial inocula between submerged cultures on nutritionally rich media, in which sporulation is suppressed, generates a high proportion of a distinctive type of morphological mutants, with reduced sporulation and distinctive mycelial colony appearance. Such "strain degeneration" had of course been observed previously with these as with other fungi, but specific metabolic aspects of the phenomenon had received relatively little serious attention. Bennett and co-workers studied two such variants (their <u>fan</u> and <u>fluff</u> strains) and showed (by the heterokaryon test) that the characteristic is not extrachromosomal; they also showed that it is accompanied by a failure to accumulate any of the aflatoxin intermediates and also by either a leaky (<u>fluff</u>) or complete (<u>fan</u>) block in the ability to transform exogenous aflatoxin precursors. Here we shall refer to both these variants as "lazy" or <u>lz</u>. Bennett and co-workers obtained <u>lz</u> variants from marked strains with both "blocked" and "complete" versions of the aflatoxin pathway by the serial transfer technique.

In heterozygous diploids from marked strains blocked or limited in the aflatoxin pathway, complementation is observed and aflatoxins can be synthesized. This is also true when one of the components is a <u>lazy</u> variant; the <u>lz</u> characteristic is recessive, at least insofar as it afects the aflatoxin pathway.

Thus, for example, Bennett's diploid SM-2 derived from;
 (a) a limited strain, in which the steps A/M $\rightarrow$ NSA $\rightarrow$ VSA are limiting and which is therefore a low AFL-producer
& (b) a <u>lz</u> variant derived from a VSA-accumulating blocked strain.
The diploid, although still containing the <u>lz</u> character, showed complementation and produced a high level of aflatoxins. Similarly diploid SM-5, derived from the same limited strain and a <u>lz</u> variant of a NSA-accumulating strain (originally blocked between NSA and VSA) only produced low AFL levels (since the block between NSA and VSA was only partly complemented); again, however, the <u>lz</u> character was recessive in the diploid.

In segregants from such diploids there were both <u>lz</u> and <u>lz</u>[+] (morphologically wild-type) haploids. Where the <u>lz</u> character was present it was again dominant and neither aflatoxins nor intermediates accumulated. However in a proportion of the <u>lz</u>[+] segregants the <u>lz</u> character had been dissociated from the aflatoxin pathway as present in the original strain from which the <u>lz</u> component derived; thus from SM-5 some <u>lz</u>[+] haploids displayed the NSA accumulation characteristic of the aflatoxin pathway in the blocked strain from which the <u>lz</u> component of the diploid had been prepared.

For the full details of this analysis, which incidentally showed that neither the <u>lz</u>/<u>lz</u>[+] character nor the individual steps of the aflatoxin pathway are in detectable linkage groups, the original papers should be consulted. Here, for the purpose of comparison with our own evidence about zearalenone in <u>Fusarium</u> (below, 5) just one interpretative suggestion will be added to Bennett's analysis.

From the recessive nature of the <u>lz</u> character in diploids, and from the pleiotropic nature of its effect in haploids, it can be suggested that the "lazy" strains have lost – whether by deletion or, perhaps more plausibly, by some kind of transposition – some genetic determinant which in $\underline{lz}^+$ activates the whole secondary biosynthetic sequence as well as some morphological programmes. In the diploids described above, the necessary activation is adequately conferred by the $\underline{lz}^+$ component. The existence of such activators, either as genes or as gene products, has often been suspected, but only in a few cases has it been proven; the most similar situation seems to be that involving the "A-factors" in some actinomycetes [11].

The mechanism by which the $\underline{lz}$ mutants are generated in the serial transfer procedure is not clear; however the change is not easily reversed, either by futher serial transfers or by UV irradiation. This aspect is considered further below, 5.3.

5. Zearalenone in Fusarium

5.1 Zearalenone as a mycotoxin

Zearalenone is a resorcylic acid derivative with a 14-membered lactone ring. Biosynthetically it is a simple polyketide formed by only a few transformations subsequent to the condensation of one acetate and eight malonyl units. Thus it differs from the aflatoxins which result, as already noted, from a long sequence of subsequent changes. Physiologically it shows oestrogenic and anabolic activity and figures both as a mycotoxin and as an approved animal feed additive ! [12]. It is formed by most but not all strains of <u>Fusarium graminearum</u>, but a non-toxigenic strain of <u>F. graminearum</u> is an approved source of food-grade "mycoprotein" [13].

5.2. Mutants of F. graminearum.

Most of our work on this metabolite has been done with the NRRL strain 3198. This is classed as a high producer, and under standardized assay conditions [2] produces around 700 µg of zearalenone per plate culture. Following mutagen or UV treatment (to $\underline{ca}$ 1% survival), zearalenone levels in the survivors with wild-type morphology range from low (0–100 µg/plate) to very high (1400 µg), with a normal distribution about the "wild-type mean". However the same treatments also generate a surprisingly large proportion of morphologically distinctive mutants which we designated "RUP" (red under-pigment), which we found always produced very low levels of zearalenone. One set of experimental data is summarized in Fig. 1.

Similar RUP strains are generated with almost total efficiency by repeated serial transfers of mycelial inocula grown for 24-48 hours in well-aerated shake cultures on a rich medium. If the transfers are continued, the RUP strains similarly generate a further variant we designated PR (pale RUP). Typical data for one such experiment are presented in Fig. 2.

FIGURE 1 : CLASSIFICATION OF SURVIVORS FROM UV IRRADIATION OF NRRL-3198 BY
COLONY MORPHOLOGY AND ZEARALENONE LEVEL

[The spore suspension was irradiated to 1% survival; 76 survivors were screened
unstable isolates (4) and aberrant morphologies (3) were excluded from the final
analysis]

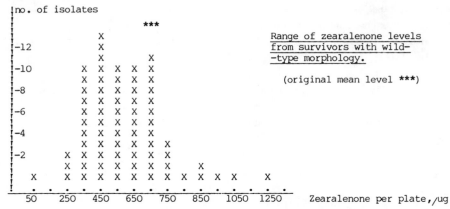

| | Range of zearalenone levels from survivors with wild--type morphology. |
| | (original mean level ***) |

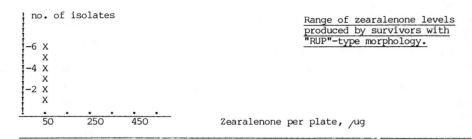

| | Range of zearalenone levels produced by survivors with "RUP"-type morphology. |

FIGURE 2   GENERATION OF "LAZY" VARIANTS (RUP) AND (PR)
FROM NRRL 3198 BY REPEATED SERIAL TRANSFERS

[The cultures were run in malt extract broth, 30 ml per 300 ml shake flask,
inoculated with 3 ml of briefly-macerated mycelium from the previous culture;
at each transfer an aliquot of the culture was macerated and plated out on
ground rice / corn-steep agar and the colonies scored for morphology]

Transfer no.	%wild-type	%RUP	%PR
inoculum	100	0	0
1	100	0	0
2	99	1	0
3	72	28	0
4	7	93	0
5	4	96	0
6	0	98	2
7	0	86	13
8	0	20	80
9	0	28	71
10	0	28	71

Both the RUP and the PR strains show all the features of "degenerated" strains, including reduced sporulation in PR and (in submerged culture) lower maximum specific growth rates in both RUP and PR.   The RUP strains produce only very low levels of zearalenone and the PR strains produce no detectable zearalenone at all.   In heterokaryon tests the RUP character was shown to arise from chromosomal rather than extrachromosomal changes [2].

At one stage we considered that the successive changes in serial transfer cultures might be due to changes in ploidy, starting from an original diploid. However, measurements of the amount of nuclear DNA in RUP spores show no marked difference from the wild-type NRRL 3198; the test is a crude one but sufficient to suggest there is no difference in ploidy.   Measurements on other F. graminearum strains similarly suggest that NRRL 3198 is a haploid, at least one apparent diploid having been found amongst the other isolates measured (Figure 3).

FIGURE 3

MEASUREMENTS OF SPORE DNA IN DIFFERENT F. GRAMINEARUM STRAINS

The DNA content of suspensions of macroconidia was determined; the number of macroconidia per unit volume of the suspension and the average number of spore compartments per macroconodium were also determined. The results are expressed as grams DNA per nucleus, $\pm$ standard deviation, x 10^{12}.

Strain	NRRL 3198 wild type	NRRL 3198 "RUP"	NRRL 5883	A3/5
mean compartments per macroconidium	4.6	4.3	4.1	3.9
DNA/Nucleus	5.95 $\pm$ 0.3	5.37 $\pm$ 0.8	10.8 $\pm$ 1.9	5.96 $\pm$ 0.6

Thus far, the RUP and PR strains of F. graminearum appear to be quite analogous to the "fan" and "fluff" variants of A. parasiticus already discussed, and we shall again use the term lazy for both.   Again, we suggest that what is lost in generating these strains is a pleiotropic activator, rather than any of the genes directly concerned with zearalenone synthesis.   However, our evidence for this, as yet, falls short of the comparable data for the lz strains of A. parasiticus investigated by Bennett.

One piece of our present evidence does point in the same direction.   For the heterokaryon test we prepared auxotrophically-marked wild-type and RUP strains; in minimal medium (appropriately supplemented for the auxotrophs) the wild-type auxotroph produced 30-50 µg zearalenone per plate and the RUP auxotroph none. (These figures are of course considerably less than those given earlier, which are for zearalenone production on an optimized assay medium that would be inappropriate for the forced heterokaryons). Again on minimal medium, the forced heterokaryon, which morphologically clearly showed the effects of the lz character of its RUP component, nevertheless produced 90 µg of zearalenone. This suggests that the lz character is recessive in the heterokaryon, just as it appears to be in the A. parasiticus diploids.

A more definitive test would be to combine in a heterokaryon one of the low-producing strains with wild-type morphology that can also be generated from NRRL 3198 by UV treatment (cf. figure 1), and which apparently carry lesions in genes directly responsible for zearalenone synthesis, with a RUP strain which — on the above argument — has all the structural genes for zearalenone synthesis but lacks the activator. Such a heterokaryon should produce zearalenone even though neither component haploid can do so. Generation of the necessary strain for this experiment is under way.

5.3 The nature of "lazy" mutations.

As already noted, the lz mutations that have been discussed — that is, the fan and fluff mutations in A. parasiticus and the RUP and RP mutations in F. graminearum — have significant common features:
- all are apparently spontaneous, positively selected for under conditions that favour rapid vegetative growth, and do not readily revert;
- all are located chromosomally but (in A. parasiticus) demonstrably not linked to any structural genes for mycotoxin synthesis;
- all are accompanied by losses of other non-vegetative functions; thus fan, fluff, and PR all show reduced sporulation (though sporulation is not affected in RUP);
- biosynthesis of secondary metabolites shows general impairment (fan and fluff neither form nor interconvert aflatoxin precursors; RUP and PR form little or no zearalenone and at the same time their synthesis of other (unidentified but chromatoghraphically distinct) metabolites is also reduced);
- in diploids, fan and fluff are recessive; in heterokaryons, the morphological effect of RUP is still apparent but its effect on zearalenone synthesis seems to be recessive;
- in A. parasiticus (at least) the loss of non-vegetative functions in the lz mutants is not due to loss of genes coding for those functions, which are recoverable from lz$^+$ segregants that have lost the lz character.

The frequency of the lz type of mutation under suitable conditions is high. In F. graminearum, up to 10% of isolates after UV or mutagen treatment to 1% survival show the RUP character either stably or in unstable colonies that soon segregate. For comparison, the yield of auxotrophs is less than 0.1% under these conditions. After six serial transfers under optimal conditions the yield of RUP and PR variants is 100% (Figure 2); similarly in A. parasiticus, up to 100% of the lz variants is obtained after a few serial transfers.

This frequency, especially in the serial transfer experiments, at first suggested that some extrachromosomal element was involved, and indeed in other systems this may still be the case; however in both the A. parasiticus and F. graminearum systems such elements are excluded by the evidence. A second possible explanation is that some kind of chromosomal transposition is involved. The high efficiency of serial transfer must then be due to the irreversibility of the changes rather than to selection. Measurements of specific growth rate under optimum conditions show that this increases in the order PR < RUP < Wild Type (Figure 4), so that the spontaneous variants should be outgrown in simple competition; only the constant and irreversible generation of the variants will explain their eventual predominance under these conditions.

FIGURE 4

MAXIMUM SPECIFIC GROWTH RATES OF F. GRAMINEARUM WILD TYPE AND "LAZY" VARIANTS

Growth rates were measured from the steepest portion of plots of (log dry wt) against time for shake flask cultures; the plots were lionear for up to 20 hr.

Strain (NRRL 3198)	wild type	RUP	PR
$/u_{max}$ (hour)$^{-1}$	0.35	0.31	0.29

Thus with the "lazy" mutation we are dealing with a relatively high-frequency chromosomal event, which results in apparently irreversible inactivation (or loss) of a gene, or group of genes. This loss results in failure to activate a multiplicity of other genes, concerned with secondary biosynthesis, and apparently with some other non-vegetative functions. The loss could occur through some kind of transposition, but there is no direct evidence of this. In both diploids and heterokaryons, lz$^+$ is apparently dominant; i.e. lz$^+$ in one component can activate mycotoxin genes in the other.

The genes thus regulated are not demonstrably linked to the lz character or to each other (i.e. in the wild type, lz$^+$ regulates batteries of unlinked genes). One aspect that is not clear is the relationship between the different lz mutants; in F. graminearum the change to RUP can be followed by the generation of PR; in A. parasiticus the relation between fan and fluff may be different.

6. References

(1) J. W. Bennett in V. Krumphanzl, B. Sikyta and Z. Vanek (Eds) Overproduction of Microbial Products, Academic Press, London New York etc., 1982, pp 549-561.

(2) J. D. Bu'Lock, J. S. Duncan, Experimental Mycology 9, in press (1985).

(3) J. D. Bu'Lock in P. S. Steyn (Ed.) The Biosynthesis of Mycotoxins, Academic Press, New York London etc., 1980, pp 1-17.

(4) cited in J.W. Bennett, J. Gen. Microbiol. 113 (1979) 127-136.

(5) D. T. Wicklow, in H. Kurata and Y. Ueno (Eds) Toxigenic Fungi: Their Toxins and Health Hazards (Proc. 3rd International Mycological Congress) Tokyo 1983; II-2, pp 78-86.

(6) I. M. Campbell, D. L. Doerfler, B. A. Bird, A. T. Remaley, L. M. Rosato and B. N. Davis in V. Krumphanzl, B. Sikyta and Z. Vanek (Eds) Overproduction of Microbial Products, Academic Press, London New York etc., 1982, pp 141-152.

(7) M. Luckner, present volume.

(8) M. O. Moss in J. E. Smith and J. A. Pateman (Eds) Genetics and Physiology of Aspergillus, Academic Press London etc., 1977, 499-525.

(9) P. S. Steyn, R. Vleggaar and P. S.Wessels, in P. S. Steyn (Ed.) The Biosynthesis of Mycotoxins, Academic Press, New York London etc., 1980, pp 105-156.

(10) J. W. Bennett, D. G. Wheeler, J. J. Dunn in M. Moo-Young, C. Vezina,K.Singh, Advances in Biotechnology Vol.3, Pergamon Press, Toronto, pp 417-422.

(11) e.g. A. S. Khokhlov in V. Krumphanzl, B. Sikyta and Z. Vanek (Eds) Overproduction of Microbial Products, Academic Press, London New York etc., 1982, pp 97-109; M. Yanagimoto, Y. Yamada, G. Terui, Hakkokokau 57 (1979), 6-14; U. Grafe et al. Biotech. Lett. 5 (1983) 591-596; U. Grafe, this volume.

(12) J. D. Bu'Lock, in M. O. Moss and J. E. Smith (Eds) The Applied Mycology of Fusarium (Cambridge University Press, 1984) pp 215-230; M. O. Moss, ibid, 195-214.

(13) C. Anderson and G. L. Solomons, in M. O. Moss and J. E. Smith (Eds) The Applied Mycology of Fusarium (Cambridge University Press, 1984) pp.231-250.

Acknowledgement   The author's work with J.S.Duncan was assisted by the Science & Enginering Research Council in association with RHM Research Ltd, and the current work with J.P.Mooney and C.E.Wright is supported by the European Community under the Biomolecular Engineering programme.

Streptomyces have Multiple Forms of RNA Polymerase Which Differ in Their Transcription Specificities and Their Sigma Subunits

Janet Westpheling, Monica Ranes, J. Guijarro and Richard Losick

Harvard University, Department of Cellular and Developmental Biology,
The Biological Laboratories, 16 Divinity Avenue, Cambridge, Massachusetts 02138, U.S.A.

SUMMARY

   Two forms of RNA polymerase holoenzyme have been identified in the filamentous, differentiating bacterium Streptomyces coelicolor. These forms contain different species of sigma factor and are distinguishable by their ability to recognize different promoter classes from Bacillus subtilis and Streptomyces plicatus. These and other holoenzyme forms may in part determine the selective expression of different gene sets in this mophologically complex bacterium.

This article is reprinted with the permission of the American Society for Microbiology from Microbiology 1985.

INTRODUCTION

Streptomyces are interesting from a biological point of view in that they have
an unusually complex cycle of morphological differentiation and they are important
from an industrial point of view in that they produce as secondary metabolites more
than half of the known antibiotic compounds, including most of the medically and
agriculturally important ones produced commercially. The production of antibiotics
and other secondary metabolites often occurs coincidently with the onset of
morphological development in Streptomyces and it is possible that these two
parallel pathways of biochemical and morphological differentiation might be
regulated by the same mechanisms.

Another group of Gram-positive bacteria that exhibit an elaborate cycle of
differentiation (endospore formation) are members of the genus Bacillus. One
important feature of the transcriptional machinery of these bacteria which is
relevant to the expression of developmental genes is the existence of multiple
forms of RNA polymerase holoenzyme, each with the capacity to utilize a
characteristic class of promoters (4, 8). Each of these holoenzyme forms is made
up of a core moiety (β, β' and α) which is associated with one of several species
of sigma factor. Sigma is the subunit of RNA polymerase which confers on core the
ability to recognize and respond to transcription initiation signals. We wondered
whether, as in Bacillus, transcription from different gene sets in Streptomyces is
determined, in part, by multiple forms of RNA polymerase, and if so, whether some
of these holoenzymes forms might be homologous in their promoter recognition
specificity to forms of RNA polymerase from B. subtilis.

RESULTS

We chose Streptomyces coelicolor for this study because of its well defined
genetic map (2) and because of the tools developed for its easy manipulation (2)
which are invaluable for the long term study of developmental processes. To
examine promoter recogntion specificity of RNA polymerase from S. coelicolor, we
used as templates for in vitro transcription plasmid DNAs containing either of two
promoters from B. subtilis known as veg and ctc. These promoters and their
interactions with RNA polymerases from B. subtilis have been well characterized.

The veg promoter is utilized by the predominant form of RNA polymerase in vegetatively growing B. subtilis cells, which has a sigma subunit of 55,000 daltons ($E\sigma^{55}$). This form of RNA polymerase is known to recognize B. subtilis promoters that, like veg, strongly conform to the consensus E. coli promoter sequence regarded as prototypical for eubacteria (10). The ctc promoter, on the other hand, is not recognized by σ^{55}. Instead it is utilized by minor forms of RNA polymerase in B. subtilis, including in particular a form which has a sigma subunit of 37,000 daltons ($E\sigma^{37}$) whose interaction with the ctc promoter has been studied in (6, 13). To detect transcription initiation from the veg and ctc promoters, S. coelicolor RNA polymerase was partially purified from a cleared cell lysate by stepwise elution from a heparin agarose column and used to generate RNA transcripts in "run off" transcription assays. In these assays, preparations of RNA polymerase are incubated with linearized plasmid DNA templates containing the veg or ctc promoters. DNAs containing these promoters were cut at known endonuclease restriction sites downstream from the B. subtilis $E\sigma^{55}$ and $E\sigma^{37}$ transcription startsites and incubated with S. coelicolor RNA polymerase under conditions which allowed RNA synthesis (9). For both veg and ctc templates, run-off RNAs were generated by the S. coelicolor extracts that were indistinguishable in size from the corresponding RNAs produced by B. subtilis $E\sigma^{55}$ and $E\sigma^{37}$. Thus, a relatively crude preparation of RNA polymerase from S. coelicolor was shown to accurately utilize both these heterologous promoters, initiating at sites close to or identical with those from which the corresponding B. subtilis enzymes initiate transcription.

These results allowed two possible interpretations: either RNA polymerase from S. coelicolor existed as a single form of enzyme which was incapable of distinguishing between these two promoters or there were two forms of RNA polymerase in S. coelicolor, one which transcribed veg and another which transcribed ctc. It was possible to resolve this issue by further purification of the enzyme. When RNA polymerase from S. coelicolor was purified by phase partitioning, ammonium sulphate precipitation, gel filtration, and heparin-agarose and DNA-cellulose column chromotography (14) and polymerase in the fractions from the DNA cellulose column were used to generate run-off transcripts from a mixture

of the veg- and ctc-containing templates, gradient elution partially resolved
veg-transcribing activity (eluting at lower salt concentrations) from ctc
transcribing activity (eluting at higher salt concentrations). This finding
indicates that the veg and ctc promoters are separately utilized by different forms
of S. coelicolor RNA polymerase.

   The form of the enzyme responsible for ctc transcription was purified further
by a protocol in which the peak fractions of ctc-transcribing enzyme were
repeatedly pooled and re-chromatographed on heparin-agarose and DNA-cellulose. The
figure shows RNAs generated by highly purified ctc-transcribing enzyme which had
been eluted in a gradient of KCl from DNA-cellulose. To visualize the polypeptide
composition of the DNA-cellulose-purified transcribing activity in these fractions,
protein in samples from the gradient elution was subjected to SDS polyacrylamide
gel electrophoresis as shown in the figure. Gradient-purified polymerase
contained, in addition to several unidentified polypeptides, core RNA polymerase
subunits $\beta, \beta' \alpha$ and   as previously observed for RNA polymerase from S. antibioticus
(7) and S. coelicolor (3), and two polypeptide species of approximately 49,000 and
37,000 daltons whose elution profile coincided closely with that of the
ctc-transcribing activity.

   To determine whether the 49,000 or the 37,000 dalton polypeptides were
responsible for the ctc-transcribing activity, we performed reconstitution
experiments in which RNA polymerase-associated polypeptides from S. coelicolor were
tested with core RNA polymerase from S. coelicolor for their ability to stimulate
transcription from the ctc promoter and heterologous complementation experiments in
which RNA polymerase-associated proteins form S. coelicolor were tested for their
ability to stimulate transcription from the ctc pormoter. As a source of RNA
polymerase-associated polypeptides we used a relatively impure preparation of
enzyme which contained both veg- and ctc-transcribing activity. Protein in slices
from a gel in which RNA polymerase had been separated was eluted and renatured by
the method of Hager and Burgess (5). These gel purified polypeptides were then
added to core and tested for their effect on run-off transcription in reaction
mixtures containing veg or ctc templates. We found that proteins eluted in the
size range of 49,000 daltons as well 37,000 daltons conferred upon both S.

coelicolor and B. subtilis core enzymes the ability to recognize and transcribe
from the ctc promoter. It is not clear whether the 37,000 dalton protein is a
proteolytic fragment of the 49,000 dalton protein or a distinct species of sigma
factor. In any event, both these proteins dictate recognition of the ctc promoter
and we have designated them σ^{49} and σ^{37} in accordance with their apparent molecular
weight. In addition, we were able to identify a polypeptide in the size range of
35,000 daltons (clearly smaller that the 37,000 dalton ctc stimulatory factor)
which strongly enhanced veg RNA synthesis. We have designated this protein σ^{35}.

We have identified a promoter from Streptomyces plicatus, which is transcribed
by the ctc-transcribing RNA polymerase but not by the veg-transcribing enzyme. The
gene product from this promoter, known as endoH, is a secreted endo- -N-
acetylglucosaminidase that hydrolyzes bonds between the N-acetylglucosamine
residues of high mannose oligosaccharides (11, 12). We used the cloned endoH gene
as a hybridization probe to identify the transcription start site in vivo and as a
template for reconstructing its transcription in vitro. S1 nuclease mapping
experiments (1) with RNA isolated from S. plicatus cells revealed an apparent
transcription start site approxamately 70 base pairs upstream from a Hinf
endonuclease restriction site and 115 base pairs upstream from a NarI site.
Specific transcription of the endoH promoter in vitro was demonstrated in run-off
transcription experiments. Using highly purified preparations of the
ctc-transcribing enzyme RNAs were generated which originated close to or identical
with sites used for initiation of RNA synthesis in vivo. In contrast, the veg
transcribing enzyme was inactive with the endoH promoter template. We believe that
the endoH promoter is transcribed by either σ^{49} or σ^{37} from Streptomyces since
highly purified preparations of these enzymes utilize endoH efficiently and since
the elution of endoH- and ctc-transcribing activities were indistinguishable during
gradient elution of RNA polymerase from DNA cellulose.

There are several interesting similarities between the endoH and ctc promoters
in positions relative to the transcription start site that are known to be
important in the utilization of ctc by $E\sigma^{37}$ from B. subtilis. While the overall
sequence homology is somewhat limited, bases thought to signal recognition by
polymerase as judged by homology to other $E\sigma^{37}$ promoters (9), methylation

protection experiments (9) and by base substitution mutations (13) for <u>ctc</u>

utilization are conserved in the <u>endoH</u> sequence.

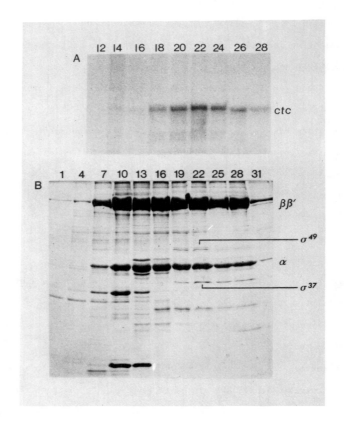

Fig. 1. <u>Subunit composition of the ctc-transcribing form of S. coelicolor</u>
<u>RNA polymerase.</u> <u>S. coelicolor</u> A3(2) cells (350 g) which had been grown in YEME
medium to early stationary phase were disrupted in a French press and RNA
polymerase was partially purified by phase partitioning and gel filtration as
described in ref. 14. Fractions containing the peak of RNA polymerase activity as
determined by incorporation of ^{3}H-UTP into RNA with poly(dA-dT) as template were
pooled and purified by gradient elution from heparin-agarose and then from a
DNA-cellulose column. The heparin agarose column was eluted with a 0.15 to 0.8 M

linear gradient of KCl. The DNA-cellulose column was eluted with a 0.2 to 0.8 M
linear gradient of KCl. 3 ml fractions were collected (fraction 1 was from the low
end of the salt gradient) and 10 µl samples were assayed by run-off transcription
using ctc containing template. The ^{32}P-labelled products of RNA synthesis were
displayed by electrophoresis in a 6% polyacrylamide gel containing 7 M urea and
visualized by autoradiography.

A, run-off RNAs were generated from the ctc promoter by RNA polymerase in
fractions from a DNA-cellulose gradient elution. The position of authentic ctc
run-off RNA generated by Eσ^{37} from B. subtilis is indicated at the right. B,
proteins contained in fractions from the gradient elution were subjected to
electrophoresis in a 10% SDS polyacrylamide gel and then stained with Coomassie
brilliant blue. Molecular weights were determined from BRL molecular weight
markers (not shown) in the range of 13,000 to 200,000 daltons.

CONCLUSION

We conclude that there are at least two distinct forms of RNA polymerase in
Streptomyces which differ in their promoter recognition specificities and their
sigma subunits. Evidence of the significance of these holoenzyme forms to the
transcription of Streptomyces genes is the utilization by one of them of the endoH
gene of S. plicatus. We propose that endoH which has a non-E. coli like promoter
sequence, is an example of a ctc-like promoter in Streptomyces. The demonstration
of RNA polymerase heterogeneity in Streptomyces raises the possibility that the
activity of different sets of genes, including those involved in differentiation
and secondary metabolism, may be determined in part by a variety of holoenzyme
forms which have the capacity to utilize selectively, characteristic classes of
promoters.

REFERENCES

1.   **Berk, A.J. and Sharp, P.A.** 1977. Sizing and mapping of early adenovirus mRNAs
     by gel electrophoresis of S1 endonuclease-digested dhybrids. Cell 12:721-732.

2.   **Chater, K. and Hopwood, D.A.** 1984. Streptomyces Genetics, p. 229-286. In

Goodfellow, M., Mordarski, M. & Williams, S.T. (eds), The Biology of the Actinomycetes, Academic Press, London.

3.   Chater, K.F. and Cooper, C.S. 1975. Purified DNA-dependent RNA polymerase from Streptomyces coelicolor A3(2). Annual Report of the John Innes Institute 66:83-84.

4.   Doi, R.H. 1982. Multiple RNA polymerase holoenzymes exert transcriptional specificity in Bacillus subtilis. Archives of Biochemistry and Biophysics 214:772-782.

5.   Hager, D. and Burgess, R. 1980. Elution of proteins from SDS polyacrylamide gels, removal of SAS, and renaturation of enzymatic activity: results with subunit of E. coli RNA polymerase, wheat germ DNA topoisomerase and other enzymes. Analyt. Biochem. 109:76-86.

6.   Haldenwang, W.G. and Losick, R. 1980. Novel RNA polymerase of   factor from Bacillus subtilis. Proc. natl. Acad. Sci. USA 77:7000-7004.

7.   Jones, G. 1979. Purification of RNA Polymerase from Actinomycin Producing and Nonproducing Cells of Streptomyces antibioticus. Archives of Biochem. Biophys. 198:195-204.

8.   Losick, R. and Pero, J. 1981. Cascades of sigma factors. Cell 25:582-584.

9.   Moran, C.P., Jr., Johnson, W.C. and Losick, R. 1982. Close contacts between [37]-RNA polymerase and a Bacillus subtilis chromosomal promoter. J. molec. Biol. 162:709-713.

10. Moran, C.P.,Jr., Lang, N., LeGrice, S.F.J., Lee, G., Stephens, M., Sonenshein,A.L., Pero, J. and Losick, R. 1982. Nucleotide sequences that

signal the initiation of transcription and translation in <u>Bacillus</u> <u>subtilis</u>.
Mol. gen. Genet. <u>186</u>:339-346.

11. **Robbins, P.W., Trimble, R.B., Wirth, D.F., Hering, C. and Maley, F., Maley,
    G.F., Das, R., Gibson, B.W., Royal N. and Bieman K.** 1984. Primary structure of
    the <u>Streptomyces</u> Enzyme Endo- -N-Acetylglucosaminidase H (Endo H). J. biol.
    Chem. <u>259</u>:7577-7583.

12. **Robbins, P.W., Wirth, D.F. and Hering, C.** 1981. Expression of the <u>Streptomyces</u>
    Enzyme Endoglycosidase H in <u>Escherichia</u> <u>coli</u>. J. biol. Chem. <u>256</u>:10640-10644.

13. **Tatti, K.M. and Moran, C.P., Jr.** 1984. Utilization of one promoter by two
    forms of RNA polymerase from <u>Bacillus</u> <u>subtilis</u>. J. molec. Biol. <u>175</u>:285-297.

14. Westpheling, J., Ranes M. and Losick, R. 1984. RNA Polymerase Heterogeneity in
    <u>Streptomyces</u>. Nature <u>313</u>:22-27.

Gene Cloning to Analyse the Organization and Expression of Antibiotic Biosynthesis Genes in Streptomyces

David A. Hopwood, Francisco Malpartida and Keith F. Chater

John Innes Institute, Department of Genetics, Colney Lane, Norwich NR4 7UH, England

SUMMARY

   Techniques for cloning genes for the biosynthesis of antibiotics
in Streptomyces are now well advanced. Their use has resulted in the
isolation of segments of DNA that control the production of several
antibiotics, notably actinorhodin and methylenomycin in Streptomyces
coelicolor. For each antibiotic, a contiguous stretch of DNA carries
structural biosynthetic genes as well as regulatory and resistance
determinants. The manipulation of such cloned genes can lead to
rational procedures for increasing antibiotic titre, as well as to
the generation of hybrid antibiotics.

1 INTRODUCTION

   Vectors and techniques for gene cloning in Streptomyces are now
developed to the point where the isolation and subsequent analysis of
Streptomyces genes has become relatively straightforward (1). Over
the last two years, this methodology has been applied to cloning DNA
concerned with the biosynthesis of several streptomycete antibiotics:
candicidin in S. griseus (2); undecylprodigiosin, methylenomycin and
actinorhodin in S. coelicolor A3(2) (3-5); oxytetracycline in S.
rimosus (6); clavulanic acid in S. clavuligerus (7); actinomycin in
S. antibioticus (8); and bialaphos in S. hygroscopicus (9,10). This
work has been reviewed elsewhere (11,12). Here we summarise recent
advances in understanding the organization of antibiotic biosynthetic

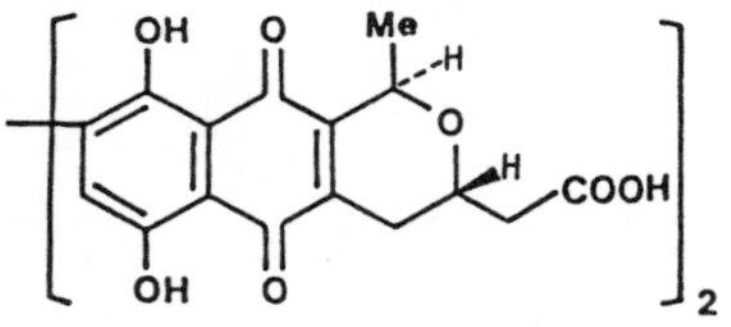

Fig. 1. Actinorhodin.

genes, using actinorhodin and methylenomycin as examples. We then
discuss some implications and potential applications of the cloned
genes for increasing antibiotic "yield" and for generating novel
antibiotics.

2 THE ACTINORHODIN GENE CLUSTER

    Actinorhodin (Fig. 1) is an isochromanequinone antibiotic made
in S. coelicolor via a typical polyketide biosynthetic pathway (13).
Although the pathway is not known in detail, reasonable assumptions
based on limited knowledge of the chemistry of the pathway
intermediates suggest 10-12 steps to convert acetate to the final
product, counting the assembly of eight acetate units to form each
primary polyketide chain as a single step. Seventy-six act blocked
mutants were classified into seven classes (I-VII) on the basis of
the varied colours of the intermediates or shunt products that they
accumulated, and on co-synthetic reactions between mutants (15). The
order of the biosynthetic blocks in six mutant classes appeared to
be: $\xrightarrow{\text{I,III}} \xrightarrow{\text{VII}} \xrightarrow{\text{IV}} \xrightarrow{\text{VI}} \xrightarrow{\text{V}}$ actinorhodin. Class II mutants, which
did not co-synthesise actinorhodin with any other mutants, had the
properties expected of defects in a regulatory gene whose product is
required for expression of the other genes. Mutations in each of the
seven act classes were mapped to a short segment of the chromosomal
linkage map, suggesting that all structural genes for the pathway
were closely linked (but this was a provisional conclusion since the
seven classes of mutants probably did not represent a complete set of
the genes). The act genes were cloned by inserting MboI fragments of
wild-type DNA into the BamHI site of a stable, single copy number
plasmid vector, pIJ922 (16), and recognising blue colonies after
transformation of a class V act mutant. Plasmids from two of the
colonies restored the blue colour, not only to the act mutant used to
isolate them, but also to various other classes of mutants. Indeed,
all seven act classes were complemented by one or both of the clones.
Subsequent in vitro manipulation of the two initial clones led to the
construction of a plasmid, pIJ2303, carrying a 32.5kb insert of

S. coelicolor DNA that complemented all seven classes of act mutants
and also gave rise to actinorhodin when introduced into S. parvulus,
a strain not known to produce any polyketide antibiotic (5).
Subsequently, pIJ2303 was found to generate actinorhodin in at least
five other streptomycetes, providing even stronger evidence that this
clone carries all of the essential genetic information for the
conversion of acetate into actinorhodin.

Success in these experiments may well have depended on the use
of a low copy number vector, rather than a high copy number plasmid.
Earlier extensive attempts to isolate act clones using pIJ702, a
vector derived from the high copy number pIJ101 (17), were unsuccessful (18). Moreover, attempts to sub-clone parts of the act cluster
from pIJ2303 on to pIJ702 yielded clones with significant rearrangements of the DNA and a loss of its biological activity. While the
causes of these problems have not been investigated, it seems likely
that they stem from the deleterious effect, on either the plasmid or
its host, of multiple copies of the act DNA.

Recently, the organization and expression of the act genes
cloned in pIJ2303 have been studied by complementation tests to
locate the various classes of act genes, and by gene disruption
studies (mutational cloning) and S_1 nuclease mapping to define the
pattern of transcription of the DNA (18). In parallel with these
direct studies of the DNA and its transcripts, information on the
functions of the various segments of the act region is coming from:
identification of the compounds accumulated by the act mutants (14);
analysis of the ability of various parts of the cloned DNA to be
expressed in producers of other isochromanequinone antibiotics to
generate novel compounds or to complement blocked mutants (19); and
studies of the effects of extra copies of parts of the cloned DNA on
the level of actinorhodin production by S. coelicolor (20).

Fig. 2 shows the current picture of the organization of the act
region. Complementation tests of the ability of a set of sub-clones
of the region to restore actinorhodin production to at least two act
mutants of each class indicated that genes controlling early steps in
the pathway (mutant classes III, I, VII and IV) lie to the right of
the region, those for some late steps (VI and V) to the left, with
the putative regulatory class II in the centre of the cluster. When
segments of the DNA were sub-cloned into att⁻ phage øC31 vectors
KC515 or KC516 (21) and the recombinant phages were used to generate
lysogens of the act⁺ strain, act mutants were generated in some cases

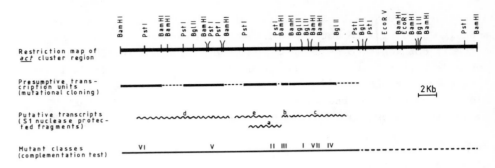

Fig. 2 Organization of the actinorhodin gene cluster (18).

(those in which the cloned fragment was internal to a transcription
unit: ref. 4) but not in others. The pattern of mutagenic and non-
mutagenic fragments identified five apparent transcription units.
Subsequent low resolution S_1 nuclease protection experiments have
confirmed the transcription pattern deduced from the results of gene
disruption, for the right-hand side of the act region. A large
polycistronic transcript (6.2kb) corresponds to classes I, VII and IV
and a small transcript (1kb) corresponds to class III. In the
central and left-hand segments of the region the picture appears to
be more complex, with indications of alternative transcripts from the
same region of the DNA.

There are other pieces of information which bear out the correct-
ness of the above interpretations and provide further pointers to the
functions of the various regions of the DNA. A clone (pIJ2315) which
carries the putative class V region functions in Streptomyces sp.
AM-7161 to hydroxylate medermycin to mederrhodin A (see below),
suggesting that it carries a transcription unit, since the
chromosomal DNAs of S. coelicolor A3(2) and Streptomyces sp. AM-7161
lack sufficient homology for recombination to reconstitute a
transcript; similarly, pIJ2308, which carries the putative class I,
VII, IV transcript, complements a blocked mutant of S. violaceoruber
Tü22 to restore its granaticin production (19). Experiments on the
effect of introducing extra copies of the cloned DNA into the act[+] S.
coelicolor corroborate the idea that the class II DNA region is
involved in activating the act biosynthetic genes (see below).
Finally, actinorhodin resistance must be determined by some part of
the cloned act DNA, since pIJ2303 converts the normally actinorhodin-
sensitive S. parvulus to actinorhodin-resistance. It is tempting to
speculate that resistance might result from expression of the class

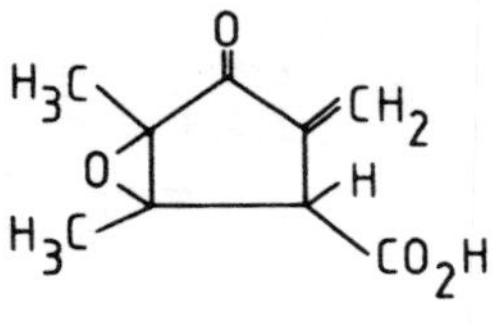

Fig. 3 Methylenomycin A.

II transcript(s): a mechanism in which a resistance determinant, alone or in conjunction with an activator, was required for expression of the biosynthetic genes could ensure that antibiotic was never present in a culture before it had developed resistance (S. parvulus carrying pIJ2303 is sensitive to actinorhodin at an early stage of growth and later becomes resistant).

3 THE METHYLENOMYCIN GENE CLUSTER

A special interest of the antibiotic methylenomycin A (Fig. 3) is its biosynthesis by the products of structural genes borne on the SCP1 plasmid of S. coelicolor A3(2) (22), and on pSV1 of S. violaceus-ruber SANK 95570 (23). Although pSV1 could be visualised on agarose gels after particularly careful lysis of the host (23), it could not be isolated in amounts required for cloning; SCP1 is even harder to detect physically (24). Thus shotgun cloning from total genomic DNA was required in order to isolate the mmy genes. The approach was mutational cloning: the insertion of DNA fragments into the att⁻ φC31 vector KC400, use of the clones to generate lysogens of an SCP1-containing S. coelicolor strain, and the isolation of mmy mutants amongst these lysogens (4). The experiments were aided by the use of donor DNA from SCP1⁺ S. parvulus so that the only complete homology between the DNA of donor and recipient (an SCP1-containing S. coelicolor strain) was provided by SCP1 sequences (which were, moreover, present in multiple copies in the donor). Thus, a very high proportion of the S. coelicolor lysogens isolated in the experiment carried SCP1 fragments, and nine out of 278 of them were mmy mutants. (There is no reason to believe that this approach to the cloning of antibiotic biosynthetic genes would not work in the commoner situation when donor and recipient DNA are totally homologous, and indeed the frequency of blocked mutants generated by mutational cloning should be no lower than that of similar mutants induced by conventional mutagenesis: (25).)

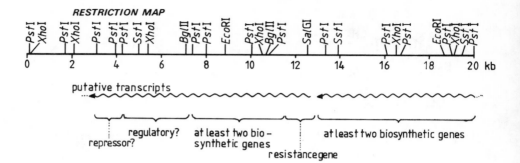

Fig. 4 Organization of the methylenomycin gene cluster (29).

The cloning of <u>mmy</u> DNA was done with <u>Pst</u>I and yielded several
non-overlapping <u>Pst</u>I fragments of SCP1. All of them, by definition,
must be internal to transcription units. Their relationships to each
other were next determined by Southern hybridisation to the DNA of
SCP1-containing <u>S. coelicolor</u> cut with several restriction enzymes,
and the results were confirmed and extended by re-cloning, in plasmid
vectors, the DNA of KC400 lysogens carrying certain of the original
cloned <u>mmy</u> segments with selection for the antibiotic resistance
marker of the phage vector (25). In this way, a continuous 20kb
segment of SCP1 DNA was mapped (Fig. 4). Interestingly, it carries
several <u>mmy</u> structural genes on either side of the gene for
methylenomycin resistance (<u>mmr</u>) that was originally cloned by direct
selection (26). Gene disruption studies have revealed two long
transcripts in this segment of DNA, one of 9.5kb to the left of (and
probably including) <u>mmr</u> and one of at least 6.5kb extending to the
right of <u>mmr</u>. Co-synthesis studies with <u>mmy</u> mutants generated by
gene disruption indicate at least two biosynthetic genes in each
transcription unit (the biosynthetic pathway of methylenomycin,
except for the final step, is unknown: (27)). In addition, it is
clear that the left-hand transcript is also involved in regulation of
the <u>mmy</u> structural genes since DNA segments at its left-hand end,
cloned into KC515, disrupted the transcript to over-produce
methylenomycin rather than abolishing its production. Thus, the <u>mmy</u>
region is an organized segment of DNA that includes resistance and
regulatory functions as well as some (perhaps all) of the structural
genes required for biosynthesis of the antibiotic. As we saw above,
the same appeared to be true of the <u>act</u> cluster. However,
interesting differences between the two systems probably exist.
Thus, regulation of <u>mmy</u> expression apparently involves a negatively-
acting function (since mutants generated by gene disruption over-

produce methylenomycin), while the control function so far recognised for the act region is positively-acting.

4 APPROACHES TO ANTIBIOTIC "YIELD" IMPROVEMENT VIA THE CLONING OF ANTIBIOTIC PRODUCTION GENES

The titre ("yield") of antibiotic produced by a microorganism depends on a large number of genes (perhaps hundreds), including many that are not directly involved in the biosynthetic pathway itself. Thus, simple approaches to yield improvement by overcoming metabolic bottlenecks through increased gene dosage using cloned DNA may not be very fruitful (28). More tangible benefits of gene cloning in the context of yield improvement are likely to accrue through the increased understanding of the normal genetic regulation of antibiotic biosynthesis that will follow analysis of the cloned bio-synthetic genes. Studies of the cloned act and mmy genes already provide grounds for optimism.

Fig. 5 shows the effect on actinorhodin titre of introducing an extra copy of the whole set of act genes on pIJ2303 into the wild-type act$^+$ strain. We see a dramatic enhancement of actinorhodin production, with a titre increase of 30-40 fold under these particular culture conditions. The increase in titre is out of proportion to the increased copy number of the genes (which is probably little over 2-fold); and some of it is probably attributable to effects of the vector. However, when the effect on yield of introducing plasmids carrying each transcript in turn into the wild-type strain was investigated, a specific stimulus was attributable to the class II region (20). This result reinforces the idea that the class II region codes for an activator of the biosynthetic genes: increasing its concentration above a sensitive threshold would have a disproportionate effect on antibiotic yield.

As was mentioned above, marked methylenomycin titre increases have also resulted from manipulation of the cloned mmy DNA, in this case by disrupting one end of a transcript that also carries two or more of the biosynthetic genes. An increase of methylenomycin production of about tenfold was observed.

These two observations are little more than anecdotal at present, and indeed they did not arise from a deliberate effort to increase antibiotic titre. Nevertheless, they indicate that a

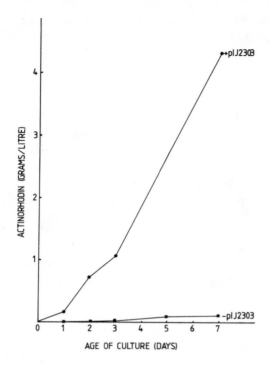

Fig. 5 Production of actinorhodin by a "wild-type" culture of
Streptomyces coelicolor containing (+pIJ2303) or not containing
(-pIJ2303) an extra cloned set of actinorhodin biosynthetic genes
(20).

systematic study of the mechanisms of regulation of antibiotic biosynthetic pathways will be well worthwhile as part of a strategy of
titre improvement.

5 GENERATION OF "HYBRID" ANTIBIOTICS

The availability of the various act clones and sub-clones
offered an opportunity to test the idea that novel antibiotics might
result when biosynthetic genes for one antibiotic are transferred to
strains making other members of the same chemical class of compounds:
the so-called "hybrid antibiotic" concept (19). When pIJ2303 was
transferred to S. violaceoruber Tü22, which produces granaticin and
dihydrogranaticin (Fig. 6), a novel compound, "dihydrogranatirhodin",
was produced. This compound has the stereochemistry of actinorhodin

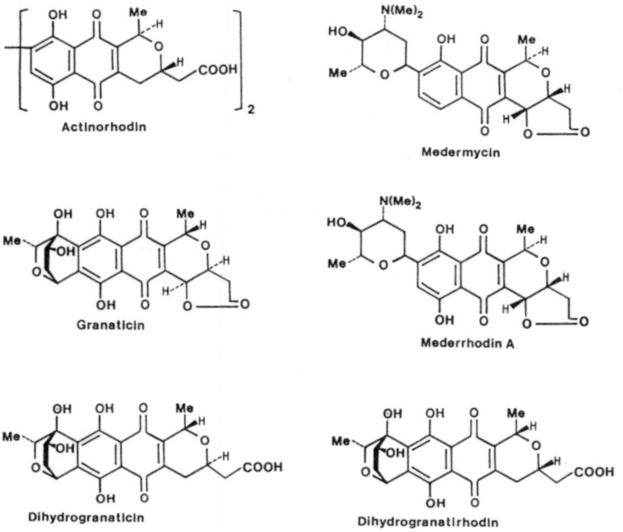

Fig. 6 Structures of actinorhodin and of some related antibotics. Mederrhodin A and dihydrogranatirhodin are "hybrid" molecules produced by transferring biosynthetic genes for actinorhodin into the producers of medermycin and of granaticin and dihydrogranaticin respectively (19).

at one of its two asymmetric carbon atoms and that of dihydro-granaticin at the other (Fig. 6). Some actinorhodin was found in the hybrid strain, but very little of the normal antibiotics of the recipient (granaticin and dihydrogranaticin). When pIJ2303 was introduced into Streptomyces sp AM-7161, which produces medermycin (Fig. 6), a mixture of medermycin and actinorhodin was found, but no novel metabolites. However, when a set of act sub-clones was used, one of them (pIJ2315), which carries a class V transcript (see above), led to the production of two novel compounds, one of which was identified as 6-hydroxymedermycin, or "mederrhodin A" (Fig. 6). The fact that the class V clone produced this result was consistent with the finding (14) that class V act mutants of S. coelicolor fail to attach the -OH at C-6 of actinorhodin: presumably pIJ2315 codes for a hydroxylase capable of introducing oxygen at C-6 of the actinorhodin precursor or of medermycin.

It is interesting that pIJ2303, carrying the complete set of act genes, gave different results in Tü22 and in AM-7161: in the former, gene products of the cloned DNA co-operated with those of the recipient to generate a novel metabolite, but not in the latter case. Only when one or more "late" enzymes of the actinorhodin pathway lacked the normal substrate did they accept intermediates (or more probably the end product) of the medermycin pathway. This varied behaviour presumably reflects such factors as differences in the relative affinities and specificities of the enzymes for their substrates, possible interactions between regulatory molecules for the two sets of pathway enzymes, possible intracellular channelling of intermediates, and others. Such factors must be understood if future attempts to generate hybrid antibiotics by gene cloning are to be made more rational.

6 REFERENCES

(1)   M.J. Bibb, K.F. Chater, D.A. Hopwood, In M. Inoue (Ed.), Experimental Manipulation of Gene Expression, Academic Press, New York (1983), pp. 53-82.

(2)   J.A. Gil, D.A. Hopwood. Gene 25 (1983) 119-132.

(3)   J.S. Feitelson, D.A. Hopwood. Molec. Gen. Genet. 190 (1983) 394-398.

(4)   K.F. Chater, C.J. Bruton. Gene 26 (1983) 67-78.

(5)   F. Malpartida, D.A. Hopwood. Nature 309 (1984) 462-464.

(6)   P.M. Rhodes, I.S. Hunter, E.J. Friend, M. Warren. Biochem. Soc. Trans. 12 (1984) 586-587.

(7)   C.R. Bailey, M.J. Butler, I.D. Normansell, R.T. Rowlands, D.J. Winstanley. Bio/Technology 2 (1984) 808-811.

(8)   G.H. Jones, D.A. Hopwood. J. Biol. Chem. 259 (1984) 14151-14157.

(9)   T. Murakami, H. Anzai, S. Imai, T. Kazahaya, R. Ito, M. Matsunaga, M. Sato, K. Nagaoka, C.J. Thompson. Abstr. Ann. Meeting Soc. Fermentation Technol., Japan (1984).

(10) C.J. Thompson, personal communication.

(11) D.A. Hopwood, M.J. Bibb, C.J. Bruton, J.S. Feitelson, J.A. Gil. Trends in Biotechnol. 1 (1983) 42-48.

(12) D.A. Hopwood, F. Malpartida, H.M. Kieser, H. Ikeda, S. Ōmura. In S. Silver (Ed.) Microbiology - 1985, American Soc. for Microbiol., Washington D.C. (1985) (In press).

(13) C.P. Gorst-Allman, B.A.M. Rudd, C-J. Chang, H.G. Floss. J. Org. Chem. 46 (1981) 455-456.

(14) S.P. Cole, Ph.D. Thesis, University of Ohio, Columbus (1985).

(15) B.A.M. Rudd, D.A. Hopwood. J. Gen. Microbiol 114 (1979) 35-43.

(16) D.J. Lydiate, F. Malpartida, D.A. Hopwood. Gene (1985) (In press).

(17) E. Katz, C.J. Thompson, D.A. Hopwood. J. Gen. Microbiol. <u>129</u>
      (1982) 2703-2714.
(18) F. Malpartida, unpublished results.
(19) D.A. Hopwood, F. Malpartida, H.M. Kieser, H. Ikeda, J. Duncan,
      I. Fujii, B.A.M. Rudd, H.G. Floss, S. Ōmura. Nature <u>314</u> (1985)
      642-644.
(20) D.A. Hopwood, F. Malpartida, H.M. Kieser, unpublished results.
(21) M.R. Rodicio, C.J. Bruton, K.F. Chater. Gene (1985) (In press).
(22) R. Kirby, D.A. Hopwood. J. Gen. Microbiol. <u>98</u> (1977) 239-252.
(23) A. Aguilar, D.A. Hopwood. J. Gen. Microbiol. <u>128</u> (1981) 1893-
      1901.
(24) D.A. Hopwood, M.J. Bibb, J.M. Ward, J. Westpheling, In Plasmids
      of Medical, Environmental and Commercial Importance (Ed. K.N.
      Timmis and A. Pühler) Elsevier/North Holland, Amsterdam (1979).
      pp. 245-258.
(25) K.F. Chater, A.A. King, M.R. Rodicio, C.J. Bruton, S.H. Fisher,
      J.M. Piret, C.P. Smith, S.G. Foster, In S. Silver (Ed.)
      Microbiology - 85. American Soc. for Microbiol., Washington
      D.C. (1985) (In press).
(26) M.J Bibb, J.L. Schottel, S.N. Cohen. Nature <u>284</u> (1980) 526-531.
(27) U. Hornemann, D.A. Hopwood, In J.W. Corcoran (Ed.) Antibiotics
      IV Biosynthesis. Springer-Verlag, Berlin (1981) pp. 123-131.
(28) D.A. Hopwood, K.F. Chater. Phil. Trans. Royal Soc. B <u>290</u> (1980)
      313-328.
(29) K.F. Chater, C.J. Bruton. EMBO J. (submitted).

Vectors for Eucaryotic Cloning Based on Organellar DNA

Karl Esser

Ruhr-Universität, Lehrstuhl für Allgemeine Botanik, Postfach 102148, D-4630 Bochum 1, FRG

SUMMARY
Based on the homology of mitochondria and chloroplasts to bacteria and due to the fact that both organelles may contain in addition to circular ds DNA also plasmids, a concept is presented to use their DNA to construct vectors for eukaryotic cloning.

According to the endosymbiotic theory for the origin of the eukaryotic cell, mitochondria and chloroplasts are thought to have bacterial ancestry (for literature review see 1 and 2). One argument in favour of this theory is based mainly on the fact that genetic information in these organelles consists of circular ds DNA (3). The theory finds further support in the recent detection of plasmids in mitochondria, both replicative and integrative plasmids, which may be homologous to the plasmids found in bacteria. From this discovery it was logical to propose the use of mitochondrial plasmids and also mt DNA integrated plasmid sequences for construction of eukaryotic vectors (4). As such, gene sequences from mitochondria (mt) and probably also from chloroplasts (cl) , whether represented in the organellar DNA or identified as extrachromosomal elements, may be expected to function as integrative vectors and/or as replicons in the development of eukaryotic cloning vectors (fig. 1).

---

*This paper is based on some chapters of a book: Esser K, Kück U, Lang-Hinrichs C, Lemke P, Osiewacz H D, Stahl U, Tudzynski P (1985) Plasmids of Eukaryotes, Fundamentals and Applications. Springer-Verlag, Berlin, Heidelberg, New York 1985.

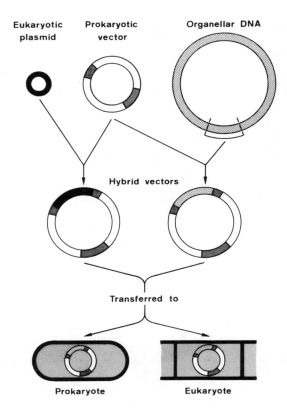

Fig. 1: Generalized scheme for the construction of an autonomous replicating eukaryotic/prokaryotic hybrid vector. The eukaryotic part may be derived from eukaryotic plasmid (left) or from either nuclear of organellar DNA (right). The prokaryotic part, usually obtained from a common E.coli vector, encodes for convenient maintenance (replication and selection) in the bacterial host.

Vectors constructed from organellar DNA would not be expected to differ basically from vectors made on the basis of naturally-occurring plasmids. Requirements for a selective marker and for a prokaryotic part of the vector would have to be fulfilled in the same way (fig.2). However, the source of a eukaryotic origin of replication would differ. An ori might be derived from any of the eukaryotic DNA components, that is, either from nuclear (n) DNA, or organellar (mt or cl) DNA. Examples are available for such types of vector construction (5,6,7).

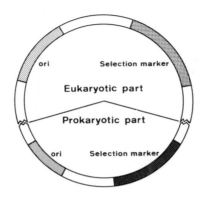

Fig. 2: Generalized scheme of a vector for eukaryotic cloning. It consists of
eukaryotic   and   prokaryotic   parts   represented   by different hatching. The
latter part is optional but enables the vector to be efficiently propagated
and selected in a host such as E.coli. By analogy to the prokaryotic part
the eukaryotic part is composed of three functional domains:

(1)   a selection marker   (genes for an appropriate antibiotic resistance or
for complementation in an essential biosynthetic pathway)

(2)   a sequence inducing autonomous replication   which serves as a start
signal for the DNA polymerase of the host and

(3)   a region for the   insertion of genes   to be transferred. It is
advantageous if host-specific transcriptional and translational signals are
present in this third region.

The isolation of ori regions can be achieved principally by two strategies.

The first is based on the identification and localization of sequences used

in vivo   for replication (8,9,10).The second approach is a more general way

which relies on the yeast Saccharomyces cerevisiae as a tester strain for

the isolation of sequences functional as ori in this host (5,11,12). This

strategy is only applicable for an ori that replicates autonomously in

S.cerevisiae. Its authenticity as an actual ori in the donor cell has to be

confirmed in each case. Both strategies have been used successfully.

In the above mentioned book on Eukaryotic Plasmids both types of vectors,

those based on confirmed replication origins and those based on random DNA

segments as autonomously replicating sequences are described in detail. The

results   obtained   with these vectors are compiled in lists and their application is discussed.

In practise special attention has to be given to a maintenance of vector transferred genes. Vectors that replicate stably are desirable for gene cloning, whether homologous or heterologous in origin. Two requirements have to be fulfilled to make the expression of vector-encoded genes effective: mitotic instability of the vector must be kept to a minimum and expression of the cloned gene must be rendered as efficient as possible.

Stabilization of vectors in host cells may be obtained by various strategies, such as stabilizing genes, centromeres, efficiency of the ori region, integration into nuclear DNA.

The expression of foreign genes in cells is dependent on a variety of factors, the most important of which are related to transcriptional and translational efficiencies and post translational events, such as product activation. Since there are striking differences between prokaryotic and eukaryotic gene organization no predictions can be made at present for efficiency of any vector albeit that there are many examples obtained with eukaryotic vectors on transcription, translation and post translational level. (For detailed references see footnote on p.1.) In each case empirical experience is needed to obtain a cloning system which is not only successful on test tube level but also applicable for industrial production.

REFERENCES

(1) Gray MW (1981) Mitochondrial genome diversity and the evolution of mitochondrial DNA. Can J Biochem 60: 157-171

(2) Wallace DC (1982) Structure and evolution of organelle genomes. Microbiol Rev 46: 208-240

(3) Gray MW, Doolittle WE (1982) Has the endosymbiont hypothesis been proven? Microbiol Rev 46: 1-42

(4) Esser K, Kück U, Stahl U, Tudzynski P (1983) Cloning vectors of mitochondrial origin for eukaryotes: a new concept in genetic engineering. Curr Genet 7: 239-243

(5) Stinchcomb DT, Thomas M, Kelly J, Selker E, Davis RW (1980) Eukaryotic DNA segments capable of autonomous replication in yeast. Proc Natl Acad Sci 77: 4559-4563

(6) Hyman BC, Harris Cramer J, Rownd H (1982) Properties of a Saccharomyces cerevisiae mt DNA segment conferring high-frequency yeast transformation. Proc Natl Acad Sci 79: 1578-1582

(7) Stahl U, Tudzynski P, Kück U, Esser K (1982) Replication and expression of a bacterial mitochondrial hybrid plasmid in the fungus Podospora anserina. Proc Natl Acad Sci 79: 3641-3645

(8) Zakian VA (1981) Origin of replication from Xenopus laevis mitochondrial DNA promotes high-frequency transformation in yeast. Proc Natl Acad Sci 78: 3128-3132

(9) Kojo H, Greenberg BD, Sugina A (1981) Yeast 2μm plasmid DNA replication in vitro:origin and direction. Proc Natl Acad Sci 78: 7261-7265

(10) Skryabin KG, Eldarov MA, Larionov VL, Bayer AA, Klootwijk J, de Regt VCHF, Veldman GM, Planta RJ, Georgiev OI, Hadjiolov AA (1984) Structure and function of the nontranscribed spacer regions of yeast rDNA Nucl Acids Res 12: 2955-2968

(11) Chan CSM and Tye BK (1980) Autonomously replicating sequences in Saccharomyces cerevisiae. Proc Natl Acad Sci 77: 6329-6333

(12) Beach D, Piper M, Shall S (1980) Isolation of chromosomal origins of replaction in yeast. Nature 284: 185-187

Enzymes Involved in ß-Lactam Biosynthesis Controlled by Carbon and Nitrogen Regulation

Juan F. Martín, Manuel J. López-Nieto, José M. Castro, Jesús Cortés, Jorge Romero, Filomena R. Ramos, Jesús M. Cantoral, Emilio Alvarez, Modesta G. Domínguez, José L. Barredo and Paloma Liras

Universidad de León, Departamento de Microbiología, Facultad de Biología, (E.I.T. Agrícolas), ctr. Circunvalacíon, s/n., León, Spain

Abstract

Carbon catabolite regulation of penicillin biosynthesis is exerted by glucose and other sugars, except lactose. It involves repression, but not inhibition, of the formation of α-aminoadipyl-cysteinyl-valine (ACV) and isopenicillin N synthetase but not of penicillin acyltransferase. On the hand, carbon catabolite regulation of cephalosporin and cephamycin biosynthesis is exerted mainly by repression and inhibition of the deacetoxycephalosporin C synthetase (expandase). In addition, the formation of ACV is strongly repressed by glucose in *Streptomyces lactamdurans*. Nitrogen sources that are easily assimilated (e.g. ammonium) produce a strong negative regulation on penicillin, cephalosporin and cephamycin biosynthesis. Ammonium produces a strong repression, but not inhibition, of ACV formation, isopenicillin N synthetase, isopenicillin N isomerase and deacetoxycephalosporin C synthetase (expandase) in *Streptomyces lactamdurans* and probably also in *Acremonium chrysogenum*. The penicillin biosynthetic enzymes regulated by nitrogen sources in *Penicillium chrysogenum* are not known. The nature of the intracellular effectors that mediate carbon catabolite regulation, or nitrogen source control, of the biosynthesis of ß-lactam antibiotics, remains obscure.

1. Introduction

1.1. Regulatory mechanism and antibiotic production

The genes coding for antibiotic biosynthesis are usually chromosomal although in some cases they may be extrachromosomal (1,2). These genes are expressed only under certain nutritional conditions. Most genes coding for antibiotic biosynthesis are not expressed when the producer microorganism is growing at high specific growth rates (see below). This phenomenon suggest that during rapid growth either antibiotic synthetases are not formed or, if formed, their activity is inhibited (3).

There are several general regulatory mechanisms that control antibiotic biosynthesis: carbon catabolite regulation, nitrogen source control and phosphate regulation. These are usually exerted on the biosynthetic pathways of many different antibiotics belonging to unrelated biosynthetic groups. In addition, there are many specific mechanisms that control the biosynthesis of one particular antibiotic, or a group of chemically related antibiotics (e.g. lysine feedback regulation of penicillin biosynthesis in *Penicillium chrysogenum* (4), methionine induction of cephalosporin production in *Acremonium chrysogenum* (5) or feedback inhibition of candicidin biosynthesis by aromatic amino acids at the PABA synthetase level (6) among others).

The control of the biosynthesis of antibiotics may be exerted at least at four different levels during expression of genes coding for antibiotic biosynthesis. Intracellular effectors formed in response to the nutrient composition may repress enzyme synthesis by blocking the formation of specific mRNA for antibiotic synthesis. A second level involving processing (splicing) of mRNAs is likely to occur in β-lactam-producing filamentous fungi. Thirdly, control of antibiotic synthesis, may be exerted in some cases at the translational and post-translational levels. Finally, inhibition of enzyme activities of antibiotic synthetases, is in some cases a well documented mechanism of control of antibiotic biosynthesis (see below).

1.2. Removal of regulatory mechanisms lead to antibiotic overproduction

Overproducing mutants are routinely used in most antibiotic fermentations. However, it is really surprising how little it is known about the genetics and physiology of these overproducing strains. In a few cases, evidence has been obtained indicating that high producing mutants are deregulated either in the pathways that provide the primary metabolites that are precursors of antibiotics (7), or in the specific enzymes involved in the formation of the antibiotic structure.

Goulden and Chattaway (8) reported many years ago, that a high penicillin yielding mutant was less sensitive to valine inhibition of acetohydroxyacid synthetase (the first enzyme of the valine biosynthetic pathway) than its ancestral strain. More recently we found that a high penicillin-producing strain of *P. chrysogenum* was slightly less sensitive to lysine regulation than low producing strains (9). Similarly, aspartokinase mutants of *Streptomyces clavuligerus* resistant to the lysine analog S-(2-aminoethyl)-L-cysteine produced up to five times more cephamycin C, as a result of the removal of feedback regulation by lysine (10). Many other examples of improved β-lactam-producing strains are known, although the mutations involved have not been characterized (11).

In addition to these examples of increasing yields by removal of control mechanisms that limit the supply of antibiotic precursors, high penicillin-producing mutants are known that contain greatly increased levels of one or more of the biosynthetic enzymes (Table 1) (12). *P. chrysogenum* Wis 54-1255 a strain that originated from *P. chrysogenum* Wis 49-2166 by about eight nitrosoguanidine and UV mutagenesis and clone screening steps (11) contains more than 10-fold higher specific activity of isopenicillin N synthetase (cyclase), that correlates with an increase in penicillin titers from less than 100 µg/ml to ca. 800 µg/ml. The high-producing strain *P. chrysogenum* AS-P-78 (producing ca 4,500 µg/ml under the same conditions) contains a sixfold-higher isopenicillin N synthetase activity than strain Wis 54-1255, thus correlating well with the five to sixfold increase in penicillin production observed.

Table 1. Isopenicillin N synthetase activity of strains with different
       penicillin producing ability

Strains	Penicillin (μg/ml)	Isopenicillin N synthetase* Specific activity (nkat/g protein)	% activity
P. chrysogenum AS-P-78	4,500	121.7	100
P. chrysogenum Wis 54-1255	810	18.3	16.2
P. chrysogenum Wis 49-2105A (Leu$^-$ PABA$^-$)	70	Traces	1.0
P. chrysogenum Wis 49-2105B (Leu$^-$ Met$^-$)	90	Traces	1.0

*In the 50-80% fraction of ammonium sulfate saturation;from Ramos et al
(12)

       Industrial strains of *P. chrysogenum* have been reported
that accumulate 6-APA a shunt metabolite that is formed when penicillin-producing strains lack enough transacylase activity or when
the side-chain precursor (e.g. phenylacetic acid) is limiting (13,14).
Similarly, strains of *P. chrysogenum* have been reported to excrete
large amounts of modified di- or tri-peptides which can not be converted into penicillin, apparently because of late enzyme bottlenecks (15).

       In summary, the removal of bottlenecks that limit the
supply of precursor amino acids for α-aminoadipyl-cysteinyl-
valine biosynthesis, methionine (a precursor of the methoxy group
at C-7 of cephamycins), acetyl or carbamoyl groups (precursors of
the side chain at C-3 of cephalosporins or cephamycin C, respectively), seem to be of upmost interest. In addition, increasing the
specific activity of enzymes involved in the formation of the
β-lactams, may improve further antibiotic production. Removal of
these bottlenecks may be achieved by empirical mutation and selection, but the availability of cloning vectors suitable for β-lactam
producing actinomycetes (16) and *A. chrysogenum* (17,18), will make
it possible in the near future to approach the removal of enzyme
bottlenecks in a rational way (19).

2. Enzymes involved in β-lactam biosynthesis

2.1. Penicillin-synthesizing enzymes

Penicillins, cephalosporins and cephamycins are formed in Penicillium, Acremonium and Streptomyces respectively, by a series of reactions that include two common steps in all cases: 1) formation of the tripeptide δ(L-α-aminoadipyl-cysteinyl-valine (ACV) by the so-called ACV synthetase complex and 2) cyclization of the tripeptide ACV to isopenicillin N by isopenicillin N synthetase (cyclase) (Fig 1). In the penicillin biosynthetic pathway, the α-aminoadipyl side chain of isopenicillin N is later exchanged by phenylacetic acid. This reaction is carried out by an acyltransferase found in crude extracts of *P. chrysogenum* (20) but not in extracts of *A. chrysogenum*.

2.1.1. α-Aminoadipyl-cysteinyl-valine synthesis

The peptide ACV, an intermediate in penicillin biosynthesis (21) has been found both in cell extracts and the culture broth of the high and low penicillin-producing strains of *P. chrysogenum* (22). The presence of ACV in the culture broth filtrates, observed also by Adriaens et al (23), is intriguing, since such peptide is not available for the cyclization enzyme and therefore is lost for penicillin production. Formation of the ACV tripeptide in *P. chrysogenum* has been studied in our laboratory by following the incorporation of (^{14}C)valine and α-(^{14}C)aminoadipic acid into ACV. The low ACV-forming activity found in a low-producing strain correlates well with the small isopenicillin N synthetase activity found in this strain. (^{14}C)Valine, α-(^{14}C)aminoadipic acid and (^{14}C)cysteine are efficiently incorporated into ACV. The excellent incorporation of L-valine supports previous suggestions that this amino acid is incorporated at the L-form and isomerized to D-valine during ACV biosynthesis (23).

ACV formation is stimulated by phenylacetic acid when added during growth of the culture (22). This stimulatory effect is higher in the high producing strain, what lends support to the empirical method of isolating penicillin overproducing mutants by resistance to toxic levels of phenylacetic acid (24). ACV formation is clearly stimulated when protein synthesis was inhibited with cycloheximide or anisomicin, indicating that this peptide is formed by a non-ribosomal condensation of the three component amino acids as suggested by Fawcett and Abraham (25). Blocking protein synthesis may

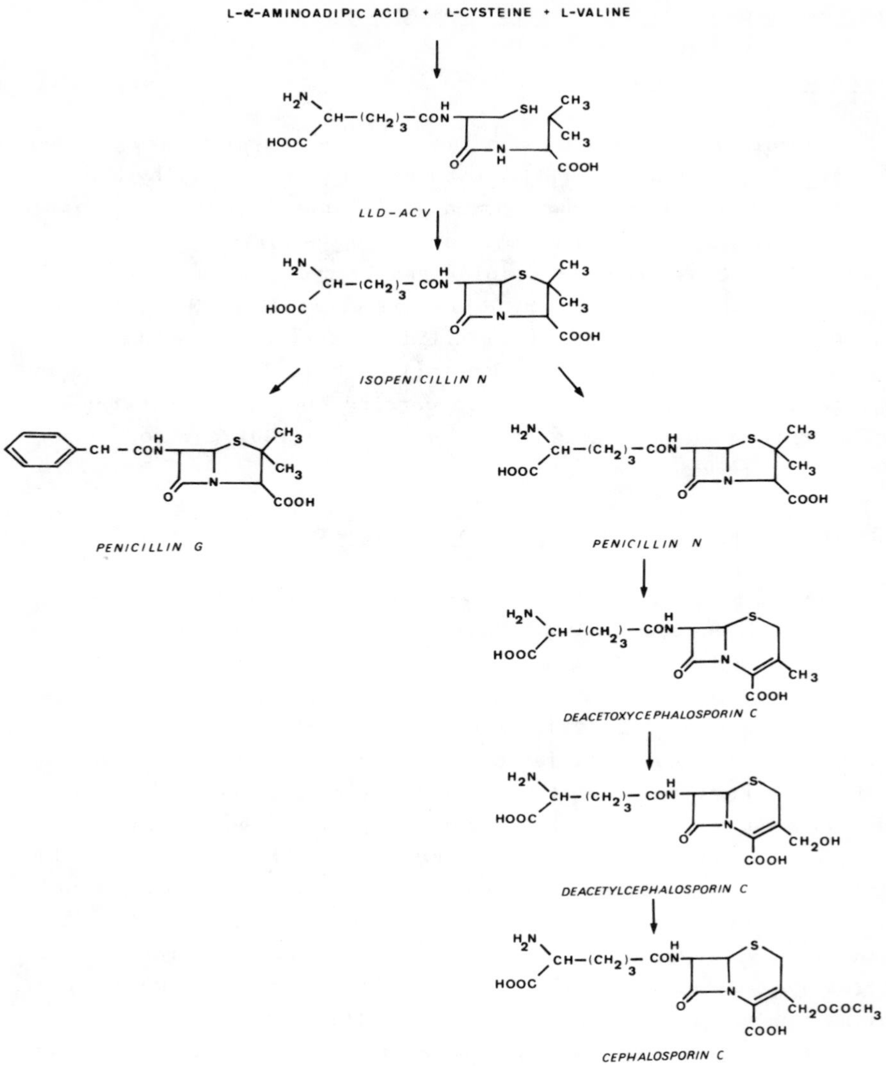

Fig 1. Biosynthetic pathways of penicillin G and cephalosporin C.

channel amino acids towards non-ribosomal ACV formation, as suggested by Katz and Weissbach (26) in the actinomycin producing actinomycete. ACV formation is also stimulated by α-aminoadipic acid,
and inhibited by leucine, isoleucine and D-valine (27).

The ACV-synthesizing activity of the culture increases
between 24 and 48 h of incubation preceding penicillin biosynthesis
and remains constant thereafter. A decay of ACV-forming activity
with an apparent half life of 25 h is observed when *de novo* protein
synthesis is inhibited with cycloheximide. Glutathione (γ-glutamyl-
cysteinyl-glycine) exerts an inhibitory effect on ACV formation in
P. chrysogenum . Penicillin G (end product of the pathway) inhibits
the conversion of ACV into penicillin G, producing an accumulation
of tripeptide (28). ACV-forming enzymes are very unstable *in vitro*
and there are difficulties to purify them.

2.1.2. Isopenicillin N synthetase

The second enzyme of the pathway isopenicillin N synthetase has been purified from extracts of the high producing strain
P. chrysogenum AS-P-78. The cyclase requires dithiothreitol and is
stimulated by ferrous ions and ascorbate, all of which are cofactors
of oxygenases. Co^{2+} and Mn^{2+} completely inhibit the enzyme activity
apparently due to competition with Fe^{2+}. The optimal temperature
is 25ºC, similar to best temperature for penicillin production, and
the optimal pH 7.8. The reaction requires O_2 (Table 2) and is stimulated by increasing the dissolved oxygen concentration of the reaction mixture (12). Cyclization, therefore, appears to proceed by
oxygen-mediated removal of hydrogen atoms during formation of the
B-lactam and thiazolidine rings. These requirements are similar to
those of the cyclases of *A. chrysogenum* , *S. clavuligerus* and *S. lactamdurans* (see below) (29).

The role of DTT in the cyclization reaction is dual: it
protects the enzyme against inactivation by oxygen (itself required
in the reaction) and it keeps the substrates in the adequate monomer
form. The dimer ACV substrate is reduced to the monomer by DTT (30).
The monomer form of ACV appears to be the true substrate of the
reaction. Moreover, DTT estabilizes the enzyme against inactivation
during storage, indicating that the thiol groups of the enzyme are
essential for the reaction.

The cyclase of *P. chrysogenum* has been purified 15-fold by
a combination of protamine sulfate precipitation and ammonium sulfate fractionation, followed by dialysis, ion -exchange chromatography on DEAE-Sephacel and gel filtration on Sephacryl S-200. The

estimated molecular weight obtained by gel filtration and polyacrylamide gel electrophoresis is 39,000 $\pm$ 1,000, similar to the reported
molecular weight of the isopenicillin N synthetase of   *Acremonium
chrysogenum* (see below) (12).

        The purified enzyme shows an apparent Km for ACV of 0.13mM
that is slightly lower than the reported value of the Km for the enzyme
from *A. chrysogenum* (see below). The cyclase activity of *P. chrysogenum* was inhibited competitively by glutathione (γ-glutamyl-cysteinyl-
glycine).

        Isopenicillin N synthetase was formed after the initial
rapid growth phase of the culture (about 18 h) (Fig 2) preceding
onset of penicillin biosynthesis (24 to 36 h). A high level of cyclase activity was present throughout the penicillin fermentation
(12) in contrast to the rapid dissapearance of the cyclase in
A. chrysogenum and *S. clavuligerus* (see below). This may account
for the continued synthesis of penicillin during at least 120 h by
the high penicillin producing strain AS-P-78. The time-course of
isopenicillin N synthetase is parallel to the pattern of ACV-forming
activity (22) and to the overall penicillin "synthetase" activity (31).

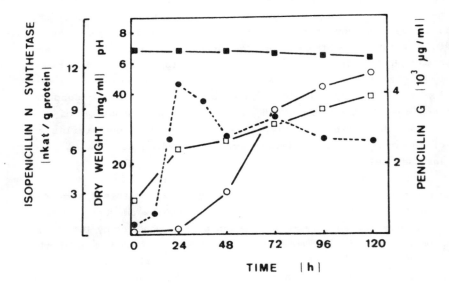

Fig 2. Time-course of growth (cell dry weight ($\square$), isopenicillin N
synthetase activity ($\bullet$), and penicillin G formation ($\circ$) during a
long-term culture of *P. chrysogenum* in complex production medium for
penicillin production $\blacksquare$, pH.

2.1.3. Penicillin acyltransferase

In the last reaction of the penicillin biosynthetic path-way, the α-aminoadipyl side chain is exchanged for phenylacetic acid, previously activated in the form of phenylacetyl-CoA. This reaction is carried out by an acyltransferase found in crude extracts of *P. chrysogenum* (20,32,33). This enzyme also acylates 6-aminopenicillanic acid to penicillin G using phenylacetyl-CoA (33).

The time-course of acyltransferase formation correlates well with that of penicillin production (20,33). Specific activity of the acyltransferase is higher in cells grown in media supporting high penicillin production; this enzyme is absent from fungi that do not produce penicillin and is present at higher levels in superior penicillin-producing mutants than in their predecessors (34).

2.2. Enzymes involved in cephalosporin and cephamycin biosynthesis

2.2.1. Synthesis of ACV

The biosynthetic pathways of cephalosporins and cephamycins resemble that of penicillin (Fig 1). The tripeptide ACV and isopenicillin N, in fact, are intermediates in the biosynthesis of both penicillins and cephalosporins. LLD-α-aminoadipyl-cysteinyl-valine has been found in the cephalosporin producing fungi *A. chrysogenum* (25) and *Paecilomyces persicinus* (36), and also in extracts of the cephamycin producers *S. lactamdurans* (37) and *S. clavuligerus* (38). The tripeptide synthetase of cephalosporin or cephamycin producers is poorly known. Loder and Abraham (39) reported that an extract of *A. chrysogenum* was able to incorporate DL-(^{14}C)valine into ACV when incubated with δ(L-α-aminoadipyl)-L-cysteine, but the enzyme(s) involved have not been fully characterized (25).

2.2.2. Isopenicillin N synthetase (cyclase)

Isopenicillin N is formed by cyclization of the ACV tri-peptide as in penicillin biosynthesis (see above). The isopenicillin N synthetase (cyclase) of *A. chrysogenum* has been extensively studied (40,41,42,43). The cyclization reaction in extracts of *A. chrysogenum* is stimulated by Fe^{2+}, ascorbate and dithiothreitol (44), as occurred in *P. chrysogenum*, but not by ATP or α-ketogluta-rate. The cyclase of *A. chrysogenum* has been highly purified (45,46) and the molecular weight established as 40,000 to 42,000, similar to that reported for the cyclase of *Penicillium* (Table 2).

Table 2. Characteristics of some enzymes involved in biosynthesis of β-lactam antibiotics

Microorganisms	Cofactor Requirement	Stimulators	Inhibitors	M_r
Isopenicillin N synthetase (cyclase)				
P. chrysogenum	O_2, DTT	Fe^{2+}, Ascorbic acid	Co^{2+}, Mn^{2+}, Glutathione	39,000
A. chrysogenum	DTT	Fe^{2+}, Ascorbic acid	Aminoadipyl-cysteinyl-dihidrovaline	41,000
S. clavuligerus	O_2, DTT	Fe^{2+}, Ascorbic acid		36,500
S. lactamdurans	DTT	Fe^{2+}, Ascorbic acid	Glucose-6-phosphate	—
Isopenicillin N epimerase				
A. chrysogenum	ND	ND	ND	ND
S. clavuligerus	None	Pyridoxal-phosphate*	Hydroxylamine, D-Cyclo-Serine, Isoniazid, Iso-proniazid	60,000
S. lactamdurans	None	Pyridoxal-phosphate	ND	ND
Deacetoxycephalosporin C synthetase				
A. chrysogenum	Fe^{2+}, ascorbate	α-ketoglutarate, ATP	ATP (high levels), Cu^{2+}, Zn^{2+}	31,000
S. clavuligerus	α-ketoglutarate, Fe^{2+}, ascorbate	Mg^{2+}	ATP	29,500
S. lactamdurans	Fe^{2+}, α-ketoglutarate	—	Glucose-6-P, Fructose 1,6-diphosphate	—

*Pyridoxal-phosphate is required in the buffer to stabilize the enzyme.

The enzyme accepts in addition to the LLD-tripeptide, analogue tripeptides in which D-valine has been replaced by D-isoleucine (43), and a peptide-like molecule phenylacetyl-cysteinyl-valine containing a phenylacetil residue instead of α-aminoadipic acid (47).

The cyclase of *S. clavuligerus* has been purified a 100-fold and shown to have a molecular weight of 36,500 (48). A similar Mr has been estimated for the cyclase of *S. lactamdurans* (49). All the cyclases appear to have similar DTT and O_2 requirements, although the requirement for O_2 of the enzymes from *A. chrysogenum* and *S. lactamdurans* have not been clearly established. They are all stimulated by Fe^{2+} and ascorbic acid, and do not appear to require ATP, FAD or NAD (Table 2).

The cyclases of *A. chrysogenum* and *S. clavuligerus* exhibit similar specificity toward several unnatural substrates in which the α-aminoadipyl moiety has been changed. The L-glutamyl-, L-aspartyl-, N-acetyl-L-α-aminoadipyl-, and glycyl-α-aminoadipyl-containing peptides are inactive substrates, but adipyl-L-cysteinyl-D-valine is cyclized to its corresponding penicillin, carboxybutylpenicillin (45,50).

2.2.3. Isopenicillin N isomerase (epimerase)

In cephalosporin and cephamycin-producing microorganisms isopenicillin N is converted to penicillin N by isopenicillin N isomerase, an enzyme that converts the L-aminoadipic acid side chain to the D-configuration. This activity that appears to be lacking in *Penicillium*, was initially discovered in *A. chrysogenum* (40) but it is, however, extremely labile (51,52) in extracts obtained from this microorganisms.

On the other hand, *S. clavuligerus* (53) and *S. lactamdurans* (37) have more stable epimerases. The epimerase of *S. clavuligerus* has been purified 35-fold. It is not affected by EDTA or anaerobic incubation, suggesting that it does not require Fe^{2+} or other metal ions, at difference of the cyclase and expandase. Pyridoxal phosphate does not stimulate epimerase activity but partially reverses the inhibitory effect of hydroxylamine (53). The requirement for pyridoxal phosphate of the epimerase of *S. clavuligerus* and *S. lactamdurans* is difficult to prove since this cofactor is required for the stability of the enzyme and must be added to the buffers during purification. The Mr of the epimerase of *S. clavuligerus* has been estimated to be 60,000.

2.2.4. Deacetoxycephalosporin C synthetase

Penicillin N is converted to deacetoxycephalosporin C (DAOC) by the deacetoxycephalosporin C synthetase, the so-called ring-expanding enzyme or expandase (54). The expandase of *A. chrysogenum* is markedly stimulated by Fe^{2+} and ascorbic acid, well known stimulators of dioxygenases (55,56), and also by α-ketoglutarate (57,50). The enzyme from *A. chrysogenum* has a molecular weight of 31,000 and appears to be soluble (50). It expands the thiazolidine ring of the nucleus of penicillin N but it does not accept the isomer isopenicillin N, penicillin G or 6-APA as substrates, i.e. the enzyme shows a high specificity for the side-chain attached to the penicillin nucleus.

The expandase of *S. clavuligerus*, on the other hand, has a strong requirement for Fe^{2+}, α-ketoglutarate, and ascorbate as co-factors while Mg^{2+} and K^+ had a lesser effect (58). Similar requirements have been found for the expandase of *S. lactamdurans* (59), but ferrous ion requirement is very high (60). The molecular weight of the expandase of *S. clavuligerus* has been estimated as 29,500 (61).

2.2.5. Deacetoxycephalosporin C hydroxylase

The following reaction of the cephalosporin and cephamycin biosynthetic pathway is the hydroxylation of deacetoxycephalosporin C to deacetylcephalosporin C (DAC) by an α-ketoglutarate-requiring dioxygenase. This reaction is carried out by cell extracts of *A. chrysogenum* (62) or *S. clavuligerus* (63). The enzyme that catalyzes incorporation of oxygen from O_2 into DAC (64), requires α-ketoglutarate, ascorbate, dithiothreitol and Fe^{2+}. DAOC hydroxylase and DAOC synthetase are both intermolecular dioxygenases that have similar requirements. Scheidegger and coworkers (65) were unable to separate the two enzyme activities in extracts of an industrial strain of *A. chrysogenum* by several steps of purification and proposed, on this basis, that DAOC synthetase and DAOC hydroxylase are located on a single protein of Mr 33,000. The bifunctional role of this protein is supported by the well known result that *A. chrysogenum* accumulates only low concentrations of free deacetoxycephalosporin C. However, the bifunctional role may be due to two linked but different enzyme activities since mutants blocked in the conversion of DAOC to DAC have been isolated that accumulate increased levels of DAOC (66). The two activities, DAOC synthetase and DAOC hydroxylase, are easily separated in extracts of *S. clavuligerus* by anion exchange chromatography (61). A molecular weight of 26,200 has been estimated for the

DAOC hydroxylase as compared to 29,500 for the DAOC synthetase.

2.2.6. Deacetylcephalosporin C acetyltransferase

Acetylation of DAC to cephalosporin C by the enzyme acetyl-CoA:deacetylcephalosporin C acetyltransferase is the terminal reaction in cephalosporin-producing fungi (Fig 1) (67). Mutants blocked in this reaction have been isolated that accumulate DAC (67).

2.3. Late reactions in cephamycin biosynthesis

Cephalosporin C is the end product of the biosynthetic pathway in *A. chrysogenum*. However, further reactions are involved in the introduction of the C-7 methoxy group and the attachment of the carbamoyl group of C-3' during cephamycin biosynthesis in the actinomycetes (Fig 3). Several side chains may be attached to the C-3' hydroxymethyl group of DAC. These include a carbamoyl residue in cephamycin C, an acetyl group in 7-α-methoxycephalosporin C, and aromatic acyl derivates in cephamycins A, B and C-2801X. An enzyme, O-carbamoyl transferase, has been found in extracts of *S. clavuligerus* that transfers a carbamoyl group from carbamoyl phosphate to deacetyl-7-α-methoxycephalosporin C to form cephamycin C (68). The enzyme synthesizes a wide variety of 3-carbamoyloxymethylcephems due to lack of specificity in the substituents of the 7-amino group of cephalosporin. This enzyme requires ATP and is stimulated by Mg^{2+}, Mn^{2+}, and other nucleoside triphosphates.

The methoxy group at C-7 of cephamycins is introduced by an enzyme system containing a dioxygenase and a methyltransferase. The methoxy group derives from molecular oxygen and methionine (69, 70). These enzymes convert cephalosporin C and O-carbamoyl-deacetylcephalosporin C (but not deacetylcephalosporin C) into 7-α-methoxy-derivatives in the presence of Fe^{2+}, α-ketoglutarate, S-adenosylmethionine (SAM) ad ascorbate, suggesting that methoxylation is a late reaction after the side chain at C-3' has been introduced.

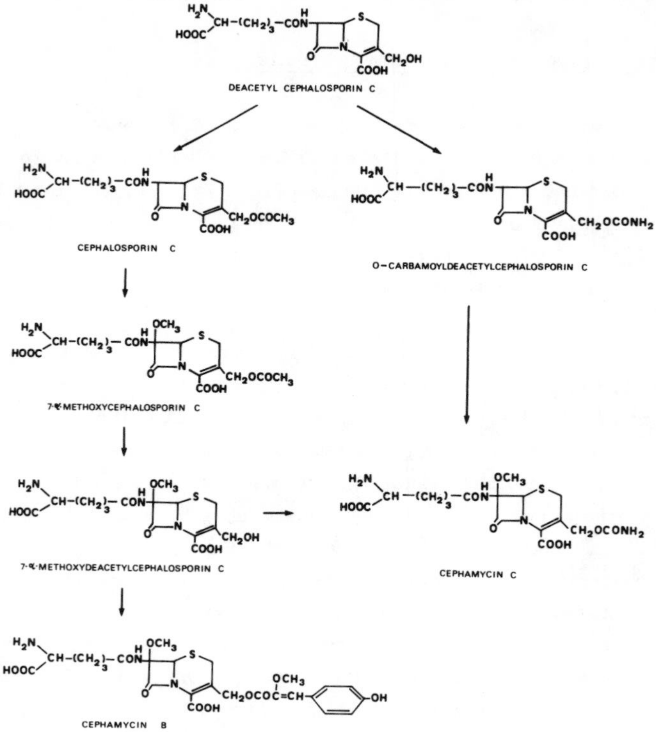

Fig 3. Late reactions of the cephamycin biosynthetic pathway converting deacetylcephalosporin C into cephamycin B or cephamycin C.

3. Mechanisms of control of β-lactam antibiotic production

The biosynthesis of β-lactams and other antibiotics occurs best at low growth rates produced by nutrient inbalance (3). Low specific growth rates can be brought about by limitation of carbon, nitrogen or phosphorus sources. In effect, the biosynthesis of penicillins and cephalosporins is subject to negative regulation by glucose, nitrogen, and to a lesser extent, phosphorus sources (71,72, 19).

Understanding the molecular basis of these regulatory mechanisms will be extremely useful to increase antibiotic yields since one of the direct ways to get high producing strains is the selective removal of bottlenecks in the antibiotic biosynthetic pathways (19).

Two models have been proposed to explain the delay on the onset of antibiotic synthesis until the carbon, nitrogen or phosphorus source is depleted below an ineffective threshold level: 1) A small molecular weight effector acts as a co-repressor or inhibitor, repressing formation or inhibiting action of antibiotic synthetases. Therefore, the corepressor or inhibitor must be depleted before antibiotic synthesis can occur. This model fits some of the experimental data on carbon catabolite regulation, nitrogen metabolite regulation, and phosphate control. 2) In a second regulatory model, an inducer or activator must by synthesized by the producing culture or added to it in order to initiate biosynthesis (3).

3.1. Carbon catabolite regulation

Glucose is usually an excellent carbon source for growth of antibiotic-producing microorganisms but it interferes with the biosynthesis of many antibiotics. An exception is the cephamycin producer *S. clavuligerus*, that does not grow on glucose (73), apparently due to the lack of an efficient glucose transport system (74). This interference with antibiotic production which was initially named the "glucose effect", due to the fact that it was initially observed when glucose was used as carbon source, is exerted by many other carbon sources (31,75) and should named carbon catabolite regulation.

In a medium containing glucose plus a second carbon source, glucose is generally used first thereby suppressing antibiotic biosynthesis. When glucose is depleted,the enzymes required for catabolism of the second carbon source and for antibiotic production are derepressed. This phenomenon is similar to the sequential utiliza-

tion of two different carbon sources by enterobacteria which results
in a diauxic groth pattern. The molecular mechanisms governing sugar
utilization and antibiotic production in *P. chrysogenum* appear to be
similar (76).

3.1.1. Glucose effect on penicillin biosynthesis

Several B-lactam antibiotics are known to be regulated
by glucose or other carbon sources. It is known since the early studies on media development for penicillin production that some di-,
oligo- and polysaccharides are better carbon sources than glucose
for penicillin biosynthesis (77). The rapid use of glucose interferes
with penicillin production by *P. chrysogenum*, in contrast to slowly used
lactose. The degree of reduction of penicillin biosynthesis by glucose is similar in several low and high-producing strains tested,
suggesting that this regulatory mechanism has not been removed during
the mutation procedures for selecting high penicillin producing mutants (78). Industrial production of penicillin has been carried
out for years using lactose, which is slowly metabolized. Carbon
catabolite regulation of penicillin biosynthesis by glucose is by-
passed when glucose is slowly fed to the culture (79).

The mechanism of carbon catabolite regulation of B-lactam
biosynthesis is being elucidated. In batch cultures, glucose addition
(140 mM) drastically reduces penicilin biosynthesis. No significant
levels of penicillin are formed in the first 72 h of fermentation
in glucose-supplemented (140 mM) cultures. However, penicillin biosynthesis starts after penicillin is depleted from the broth. The
negative effect of glucose on penicillin biosynthesis is concentration-dependent in the range of 28-140 mM.

Short-term *in vivo* studies in which we measure the incorporation of (^{14}C)valine into penicillin by nitrogen-limited resting
cells of *P. chrysogenum*, indicate that carbon catabolite regulation of
penicillin biosynthesis is due to repression of enzymes involved in
penicillin biosynthesis. Incorporation of L-(U-^{14}C)valine into penicillin was reduced by 70% when cells were grown on 140 mM glucose as
compared with cells grown in lactose (31).

Cultures of *P. chrysogenum* AS-P-78 show maximal "penicillin
synthetase" activity in complex medium from 24 to 48 h of fermentation, coinciding with the phase of rapid penicillin production. Addition of glucose to the resting cell suspension after the cells have
been grown in absence of glucose have only a small effect on "penicillin synthetase" activity. However, when the cells are grown in
presence of glucose there is a strong repression of the penicillin
synthetase activity (31).

Recently, the three enzyme activities involved in penicillin biosy..thesis that we may consider components of the "penicillin synthetase" complex have been determined. Our results indicate that no δ(α-aminoadipyl)-cysteinyl-valine (ACV) is formed under conditions of total repression of penicillin by glucose; derepression of tripeptide biosynthesis occurs when the level of glucose is reduced (80). No ACV is found in the first 24 h of fermentation in glucose-supplemented cultures whereas a significant amount of tripeptide is formed in control cultures (22). After 48 h, when the level of glucose is depleted, formation of both ACV tripeptide and benzylpenicillin occurs.

Glucose also represses the second enzyme of the pathway, isopenicillin N synthetase. The level of this enzyme is greatly reduced until 72 h in glucose-supplemented cultures as compared with the enzyme levels in control cultures grown in lactose (80). The third enzyme of the pathway penicillin acyltransferase does not seem to be repressed by glucose (80) (Fig 4).

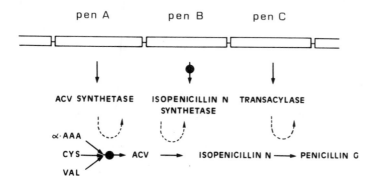

Fig 4. Model of carbon catabolite regulation of the expression of genes involved in penicillin biosynthesis (pen A, pen B, pen C). Formation of ACV and the activity of isopenicillin N synthetase are repressed by glucose (black circles). It is not known whether ACV synthetase activity is also repressed by glucose.

Glucose repression of ACV formation and penicillin biosynthesis is not reversed *in vivo* by addition of the precursor amino
acids. However, the pool of α-aminoadipic acid (α-AAA) in glucose-
supplemented cultures is smaller throughout the fermentation than
in control cultures. To establish whether the glucose effect on penicillin biosynthesis might be explained by a deprivation of α-AAA
we measured the activity of two key enzymes in the formation and
catabolism of α-AAA, homocitrate synthase and saccharopine dehydrogenase (81). Homocitrate synthase is greatly stimulated in glucose-
supplemented cells as compared to control cultures, specially at
24 and 48 h of incubation, coinciding with the phase of rapid growth.
After 72 h, glucose is depleted and homocitrate synthase activity
decreases to normal levels. Saccharopine dehydrogenase activity is
also higher in glucose-supplemented than in control cultures at 12 h
of incubation but returns to normal levels at 24 h. The higher requirement of lysine for growth in glucose-supplemented cells is met
by the increased levels of homocitrate synthase and saccharopine
dehydrogenase activities. A higher flux of intermediates through
the lysine pathway could partially explain the lower pool of α-AAA
(81) (Fig 5). The cellular uptake of α-AAA, that seems to play an
important role of the re-utilization of the α-AAA released in the
last reaction by the acyltransferase (82), is reduced by 50% in glucose-supplemented cultures.

These results suggest that glucose control of penicillin
biosynthesis affects both the activity of the tripeptide synthetase
and also the level of the α-AAA precursor (80).

3.1.2. Regulation by carbon sources other than glucose

Carbon sources other than glucose exert different degrees
of repression on the incorporation of (^{14}C)valine into penicillin
as well as on total antibiotic production (31). Lactose does not
repress penicillin biosynthesis whereas the repressive effect
produced by sucrose, fructose or galactose is similar to the effect
exerted by glucose. Polysaccharides (starch and dextrins) have a
smaller repressive effect than glucose probably reflecting their
slow rate of hydrolysis into glucose.

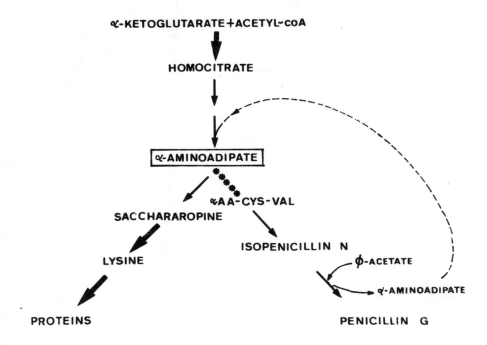

Fig 5. Carbon catabolite regulation of the biosynthesis of ⍺-amino-adipic acid and ACV. Homocitrate synthase (a) saccharopine dehydroge-nase (b) and protein synthesis (c) are stimulated by glucose (thick arrows). Formation of ACV is severely decreased by glucose (stars).

3.1.3. Possible effectors involved in carbon catabolite regulation

        Carbon catabolite regulation of penicillin biosynthesis requires transport of the sugar or at least the interaction of glucose with the permease systems that transport the sugar into the cells. The regulatory mechanism does not seem to be exerted by rham-nose, a sugar that is not easily metabolized by fungi, or by β-methylglucoside and 3-0-methylglucoside used at the same concen-tration as glucose (80).
        2-Deoxyglucose, a glucose analogue that is taken up by cells and phosphorylated although its metabolism does not proceed further, does exert carbon catabolite regulation of penicillin bio-synthesis. 2-Deoxyglucose is taken up by cells of *P. chrysogenum* and converted in 2-deoxyglucose-6-phosphate which accumulate *in vivo* (80). In yeast, accumulation of 2-deoxyglucose-6-phosphate results in

inhibition of the conversion of glucose-6-phosphate to fructose-6-phosphate by phosphoglucose isomerase and a reduction of sugar transport into the cells (83,84).

However, formation of glucose-6-phosphate from glucose (or 2-deoxyglucose-6-phosphate from 2-deoxyglucose) does not appear to be required for carbon catabolite regulation.

The pattern of cyclic-AMP changes during the penicillin fermentation and the response of cyclic-AMP levels to glucose supplementation, does not support a possible involvement of cyclic-AMP on the control of penicillin biosynthesis by glucose (80).

3.1.4. Stimulation of the glucose effect on penicillin biosynthesis by phosphate

Glucose (140 mM) had little effect when added to phosphate-limited medium, even when added at the beginning of the·fermentation. In cultures supplemented with both glucose (140 mM) and inorganic phosphate (100 mM) there was a drastic reduction of penicillin biosynthesis. Almost identical results were obtained when the sugar was added at 36 h, just prior to onset of penicillin biosynthesis (85). This stimulation of the glucose effect by phosphate suggest that a phosphate-activated transport system and/or catabolism of glucose, may be involved in triggering the carbon catabolite regulatory mechanism.

3.1.5. Carbon catabolite regulation of cephalosporin C biosynthesis

Similar carbon effects occur in the cephalosporin C fermentation using *A. chrysogenum*. Glucose, maltose and glycerol reduce cephalosporin biosynthesis, whereas sucrose and galactose favour antibiotic production (86,87). There is an inverse relationship between the ability of a carbon source to support growth and the production of cephalosporin by cells grown on that particular carbon source. Similar results have been obtained by Matsumura et al (88) in continuous fermentations. The highest cephalosporin yields are obtained in continuous culture at low dilution rates, using glucose-limited cultures.

In cephalosporin fermentations the biosynthetic intermediate penicillin N is formed about 24 h earlier than cephalosporin C, when a synchronized culture, obtained by inoculating with conidia, is used (89). The sequential formation of penicillin N and cephalosporin C appears to be the result of a differential derepression of enzyme formation at different threshold levels of glucose.

Cephalosporin C biosynthesis is strongly depressed by glucose whereas penicillin N accumulates in cultures supplemented with glucose (Fig 6). These results have been explained by the *in vivo* lability of the enzyme deacetoxycephalosporin C synthetase (expandase) (90,91). Carbon catabolite regulation by rapidly used carbon sources is enhanced by the *in vivo* instability of the expandase as compared to the cyclase (92), since the repressive effect of glucose prevents the expandase level from being replenished.

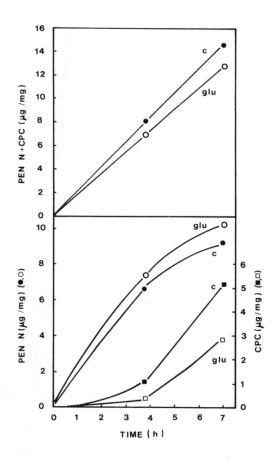

Fig 6. Accumulation of penicillin N and repression of conversion of penicillin N into cephalosporin C by glucose in resting cell cultures of *A. chrysogenum*.

3.1.6. <u>Cumulative effect</u> of glucose and phosphate on cephalosporin biosynthesis

Formation of penicillin N and cephalosporin C in *A. chryso-genum* is clearly affected by phosphate, at difference of penicillin biosynthesis in *P. chrysogenum*, where inorganic phosphate by itself does not exert a significant effect. Inorganic phosphate at low concentrations (1 to 30 mM) does not affect the early steps of the cephalosporin biosynthetic pathway leading to penicillin N, but higher concentrations (30 to 300 mM) are clearly inhibitory. Conversion of pen N to cephalosporin C is strictly dependent on phosphate concentration. Low phosphate concentrations are limiting for conversion of pen N to cephalosporin C whereas concentrations above 100 mM are extremely inhibitory (85).

In addition to the phosphate effect, glucose exerts an independent repression on the expandase. Glucose and phosphate combined exert a synergistic effect on the regulation of expandase. In conclusion, our results and those of Demain and coworkers, suggest that phosphate decreases the overall flux of precursors through the cephalosporin biosynthetic pathway, whereas glucose specifically affects the ring expansion system (85). Kuenzi (93) has suggested that phosphate exerts its negative effect on cephalosporin biosynthesis, in an industrial strain of *A. chrysogenum*, by stimulating the rate of glucose consumption. However, although the glucose effect on expandase might be enhanced by increasing the glucose uptake, the effect of phosphate seems to be more complex since it affects early and late steps of the biosynthetic pathway, at difference of glucose that specifically represses the expandase.

Glucose also controls the undesirable degradation of cephalosporin C to deacetylcephalosporin C by acetylhydrolase (94).

3.1.7. <u>Carbon catabolite regulation of the biosynthesis of cepha-mycins</u>

Actinomycetes produce a large number of antibiotics containing the β-lactam nucleus, including cephamycins, clavulanic acid, carbapenems and monobactams. In addition, monobactams are produced by strains of *Chromobacterium violaceum*, *Acetobacter sp.* and *Agrobacterium radiobacter*. The cephamycins are synthesized by a pathway similar to that of cephalosporin with some differences in the last steps of the pathway (Fig 3). The other β-lactams from actinomycetes or Gram-negative bacteria are synthesized by peptide-like condensation mechanisms also similar to those of penicillins and cephalosporins (96,97,98).

S. *clavuligerus* is capable of utilizing starch, maltose, glycerol, α-ketoglutarate or succinate as sole carbon sources for growth, but it is incapable of using glucose. Carbohydrates support better growth than organic acids. The specific production of cephamycin decreases as the concentration of glycerol or maltose increase above the growth-limiting concentration (73). The differential effect exerted by glycerol on cephamycin and clavulanic formation by S. *clavuligerus* has been used to dissociate cephamycin C formation from clavulanic acid biosynthesis, two of the antibiotics produced by this strain (99). Glycerol, a direct precursor of clavulanic acid, is indispensable for production of this B-lactamase inhibitor. In absence of glycerol no clavulanic acid is formed but cephamycin production occurs. At concentrations above 110 mM glycerol exerts a small inhibitory effect on cephamycin biosynthesis (99) in agreement with the results of Aharonowitz and Demain (73).

Unfortunately, S. *clavuligerus* does not grow on glucose and therefore, a standard regulation of cephamycin biosynthesis by glucose can not be studied in this microorganism. It is unclear whether the effect exerted by glycerol at high concentration on cephamycin biosynthesis resembles the well-established carbon catabolite regulation of penicillin and cephalosporin biosynthesis; probably the mechanims of control of β-lactam biosynthesis by glucose and glycerol are different since glycerol is taken up by a distint transport system. To solve this problem we have isolated glucose-utilizing mutants of S. *clavuligerus* that indeed provide an insight into the mechanism of glucose control of cephamycin biosynthesis (74).

We have also studied the mechanism of glucose control of cephamycin biosynthesis in S. *lactamdurans,* a strain that grows perfectly on glucose (59,60,100). Glucose exerts a strong negative regulation on cephamycin biosynthesis by S. *lactamdurans*, similar to the effect produced by glucose on penicillin formation by P. *chrysogenum* (100). Glucose strongly represses both ACV formation and the ring expansion in S. *lactamdurans*, but had little effect on the cyclase and epimerase (60) (Fig 7). Repression of ACV formation by glucose is entirely similar to the effect observed in P. *chrysogenum* during penicillin biosynthesis. It is interesting that glutathione formation is not affected by glucose in the same experiments, in contrast to the strong effect-exerted on ACV biosynthesis, although both tripeptides appear to be formed by similar non-ribosomal enzyme systems (25,22). The strong repression of the expandase is similar to the effect observed in A. *chrysogenum* during cephalosporin biosynthesis (89,90,91).

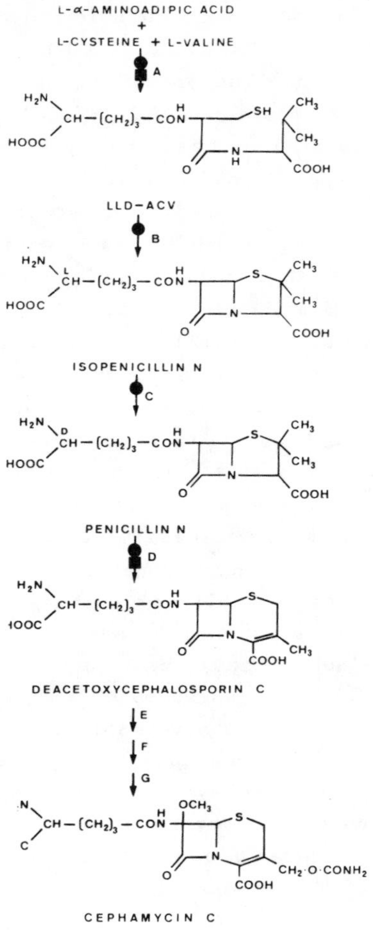

Fig 7. Enzymes of the biosynthetic pathway of cephamycin C known to be repressed by carbon catabolite (●) and nitrogen source regula- tion (■).

The control exerted by glucose on ACV formation and on the expandase, appears to be due mainly to a repression of enzyme synthesis. However glucose derivatives had also an inhibitory effect on the activity of preformed enzymes. The expandase activity of *S. lactamdurans* is strongly inhibited *in vitro* by glucose-6-phosphate, fructose-1,6-diphosphate and inorganic phosphate, and the cyclase is inhibited by glucose-6-phosphate (60) (Fig 7). Fructose 2,6-diphosphate, that has been described as a regulatory effector of glycolysis in higher cells had a significant inhibition effect on expandase but showed no effect on the other two enzymes. The inhibitory effect of phosphate on the expandase of *S. lactamdurans* is not reversed by Fe^{2+} ions (60) at difference of what has been reported by Lubbe et al (102) in *S. clavuligerus*.

The time-course of intracellular cyclic-AMP during the culture, that decreases sharply in parallel to glucose depletion, (contrarily to what occurs in enterobacteria), indicates that carbon catabolite regulation of cephamycin biosynthesis is probably not mediated by c-AMP. These results agree with similar observations made by Vining and coworkers who also found that c-AMP was not involved in the onset of streptomycin biosynthesis in *S. griseus* (103). Cyclic-AMP in *Streptomyces* follows the same pattern as intracellular ATP and other nucleotides involved in the control of phosphate-sensitive antibiotic biosynthesis (104,105) but does not appear to be involved in carbon catabolite regulation of antibiotic production.

3.2. Nitrogen source regulation of β-lactam biosynthesis

Regulation of the biosynthesis of β-lactam antibiotics by rapidly assimilable nitrogen sources, mainly ammonium ions and certain amino acids, has been attracting a great deal of interest (106). Ammonium regulation of the expression of genes coding for enzymes required for the catabolism of other nitrogen sources in bacteria is well-established (107) and the mechanisms of nitrogen source regulation of gene expression in yeast and fungi are beginning to be understood (108,109).

3.2.1. Control by ammonium of penicillin and cephalosporin biosynthesis

Inhibition of penicillin biosynthesis in *P. chrysogenum* by high levels of NH_4^+ has been reported in *P. chrysogenum*. The ammonium effect was correlated with low levels of glutamine synthetase (110).

Unfortunately, the penicillin biosynthetic enzymes affected by NH_4^+ are not known.

Production of cephalosporin by *A. chrysogenum* is also depressed by nitrogen sources at concentrations above 100 mM (111). The nitrogen effect was reversed by addition of tribasic magnesium phosphate to the ammonium-containing medium. Nitrogen control of cephalosporin biosynthesis was exerted mainly by repression of the expandase. A decrease of the ammonium nitrogen level in the broth leads to derepression of expandase (111). Other early enzymes of the pathway (tripeptide synthetase and/or cyclase) are probably also repressed by ammonium since depletion of this nitrogen source leads not only to increases in cephalosporin C but, to a lesser extent, of penicillin N also.

3.2.2. Nitrogen source control of cephamycin production

The biosynthesis of cephamycin by *S. clavuligerus*, *S. lactamdurans* and *S. cattleya*, is regulated by the concentration of some nitrogen sources in the medium.

S. clavuligerus uses a variety of nitrogen sources for growth including ammonium salts, amino acids and urea. The production of cephamycin by *S. clavuligerus* is strongly reduced when ammonium sulfate serves as the sole nitrogen source or when added to an amino acid based medium (99, 112). Glutamic acid at high concentrations also exerts a negative effect on cephamycin biosynthesis (99).

Ammonium salts and asparagine produce a concentration-dependent reduction of cephamycin C biosynthesis by *S. lactamdurans*. Addition of ammonium salts at 1 mM concentration reduce cephamycin biosynthesis in this microorganism by 50% whereas concentrations of asparagine above 10 mM are required to get the same effect (37). A similar nitrogen source control operates on the production of cephamycin C by *S. cattleya* (113,114). In ammonium-limited chemostat cultures of *S. cattleya* high cephamycin titers are achieved at low-specific growth rates at which ammonium utilization rates are greatly reduced.

The enzymes of cephamycin biosynthesis affected by nitrogen source regulation have been studied in *S. clavuligerus* and *S. lactamdurans*. In a preliminary report, repression of isopenicillin N synthetase by ammonium was suggested (114a). In *S. lactamdurans* the pool of ACV was drastically reduced by ammonium (Fig 8) due probably to a depressive effect on the tripeptide synthetase . It is unclear to what extent ammonium may affect the availability of amino acids for tripeptide formation since the direct precursor amino acids (cysteine, valine and ⍺-aminoadipic acid) were barely detectable in cultures with or without ammonium supplementation (37). Isopenicillin N synthetase (cyclase), isopenicillin N isomerase and deacetoxycephalosporin C synthetase were also drastically reduced in ammonium-supplemented cultures (Fig 8). However the activities of these enzymes were not inhibited *in vitro* by 40 mM ammonium, suggesting that the enzymes were repressed but not inhibited by ammonium *in vivo*. The main mechanism of control of enzymes involved in biosynthesis of β-lactam antibiotics appear, therefore, to be repression of enzyme formation that was observed also in carbon catabolite regulation of penicillin and cephalosporin formation, and in nitrogen source regulation of cephalosporins in *C. acremonium* (see above).

Since formation of ACV and the activities of cyclase, epimerase, and expandase were depressed to about the same extent by ammonium, we proposed that most, and probably all the enzymes, of the cephamycin biosynthetic pathway in *S. lactamdurans* are probably coordinately regulated. However, it would be convenient to establish if this coordinate regulation holds true for the very late enzymes of the pathway that convert deacetoxycephalosporin C into cephamycin C (37). Coordinate regulation of biosynthetic enzymes of secondary metabolites has not been reported so far, but it is an attractive mechanism to modulate synchronously the expression of genes leading to a product that is formed only under certain circumstances (e.g. low specific growth rate), as occurs with the induction and repression mechanisms that control the pathways for biosynthesis of primary metabolites.

The model of coordinated regulation of β-lactam biosynthetic enzymes by ammonium may not however be true in all β-lactam producing microorganisms, since in *A. chrysogenum* the expandase appears to be more sensitive than other enzymes to nitrogen regulation (111). However, this enzyme seems to be very unstable *in vivo* in *A. chrysogenum* (90) and mechanisms such as enzyme inactivation, in addition to repression by nitrogen sources, may explain the apparently higher sensibility of this enzyme to nitrogen regulation.

3.2.3. Nitrogen source regulation of clavulanic acid biosynthesis

Production of clavulanic acid by *S. clavuligerus* is also regulated by glutamic acid and ammonium. Both produce a concentration-dependent reduction of clavulanic acid at concentrations above 10 mM. Glutamic acid at concentrations above 40 mM completely suppress clavulanic acid biosynthesis. Onset of clavulanic acid only occurs

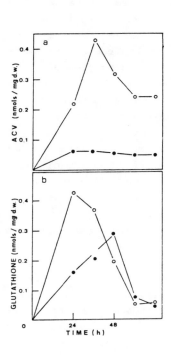

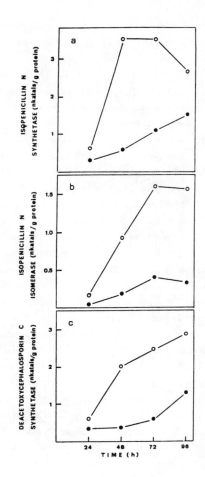

Fig 8. Left: Intracellular levels of ACV (a) and glutathione (b) in control (O) and NH_4Cl (40 mM)-supplemented cells (●). Right: Isopenicillin N synthetase (a), isopenicillin N isomerase (b) and deacetoxycephalosporin C synthetase (c) in control (O) and NH_4Cl (40 mM)-supplemented cells (●).

after glutamic acid is depleted (99). The enzymes involved in clavulanic acid biosynthesis have not been characterized so far.

3.2.4. Glutamine   synthetase and nitrogen regulation

The possible involvement in the control of antibiotic biosynthesis of glutamine synthetase (GS), a key enzyme in the control
of general nitrogen metabolism, has attracted considerable attention
(115,116,106). However, the role of GS proposed by Magasanik a decade
ago on the control of nitrogen metabolism in bacteria, is now being
reconsidered (107).

High specific cephamycin production is always obtained
under growth conditions that lead to high GS activity. Studies in
S. clavuligerus (112), *S. cattleya* (113,117) and *S. lactamdurans* (37)
showed that GS activity peaked during the late stages of growth, when
ammonia was depleted in the medium, coinciding with the phase of
rapid antibiotic synthesis. Inactivation of glutamine synthetase by
adenylation, as occurs in enteric bacteria, has been reported in
Streptomyces (117,118). However, there is no evidence for or against
the involvement of glutamine synthetase as a regulatory protein in
the control of gene expression during antibiotic biosynthesis.

GS activity decreases in cells grown in media containing
excess ammonium as also did antibiotic production. Glutamic acid is,
by far, the most abundant amino acid in the pool of *S. lactamdurans*
(60-70% of the total pool) and also in *S. clavuligerus* (10). The relative concentration of glutamic acid and glutamine in the amino acid
pool decreases in ammonium-supplemented cultures of *S. lactamdurans*,
while alanine and phosphoserine increases (37).

3.2.5. Coordinate regulation of proteases and cephamycin biosynthesis

Extracellular proteases in *S. clavuligerus* (116) and *S. lactamdurans* (119,37) are decreased by ammonium in parallel to repression of cephamycin biosynthesis. In *S. lactamdurans* the formation of
aerial mycelium and sporulation is also repressed by ammonium, in
addition to serine proteases and cephamycin (119). Spontaneous *amy*⁻
mutants arise that have lost the ability to form proteases, aerial
mycelium and cephamycin (119,120).

It appears that a pleiotropic intracellular effector that
transmits signals from nitrogen metabolism, affects the expression of
genes involved in antibiotic biosynthesis, proteases formation and
differentiation. Mutations affecting the formation of this pleiotropic effector result, therefore, in a variety of phenotypes including
lack of proteases, antibiotic and aerial mycelium formation (120).

4. Removal of carbon and nitrogen regulatory bottlenecks

The advances in the knowledge of the mechanisms of carbon and nitrogen catabolite regulation suggest that mutants insensitive to carbon or nitrogen source regulation may be easily selected. Some of these mutants may be higher producers. For example a deacetoxycephalosporin C synthetase glucose-derepressed mutant having a more stable enzyme with a longer half-life probably would have an increased cephalosporin production. Mutants of *P. chrysogenum* insensitive to carbon catabolite regulation have been obtained; they show   an increased penicillin production in glucose rich medium (76).

5. Future outlook

Cloning vectors and transformation systems in β-lactam producing *Streptomyces* are being improved (2). The genes of *S. clavuligerus* for clavulanic acid biosynthesis have been cloned recently (16). Cloning vectors in β-lactam-producing fungi have been constructed using either mitochondrial DNA or autonomous replicating sequences *(ars)* of *A. chrysogenum* (17,18). A *leu* gene of *A. chrysogenum* has been cloned that it will be useful as a marker for bifunctional vectors, since it is expressed in *E. coli* (121).

Using molecular genetic techniques it should be possible, in a few years, to characterize the molecular mechanisms of carbon and nitrogen control of β-lactam biosynthesis, and to remove the bottlenecks in the pathways by obtaining deregulated mutants by *in vitro* mutagenesis.

Acknowledgements

The work on penicillin and cephamycin has been supported by two grants of the CAICYT, Madrid, and by Antibióticos, S.A. León, Spain. We thank L. Vara for typing the manuscript and B. Martín, and M.P. Puertas for technical assistance.

References

(1) D. Hopwood, K.F. Chater, In: Genetics and Breeding of Industrial Microorganisms (Ball, ed.). CRC Press. Boca Raton (1984) 7.

(2) J.F. Martín, J.A. Gil, Biotechnology 2 (1984) 63.

(3) J.F. Martín, A.L. Demain, Microbiol. Rev. 44 (1980) 230.

(4) J.M. Luengo, G. Revilla, M.J. López-Nieto, J.R. Villanueva, J.F. Martín, J. Bacteriol. 144 (1980) 869.

(5) S.W. Drew, A.L. Demain, J. Antibiot. 28 (1975) 889.

(6) J.A. Gil, G. Naharro, J.R. Villanueva, J.F. Martín, J. Gen. Microbiol. 131 (1985) 1279.

(7) S.W. Drew, A.L. Demain, Ann. Rev. Microbiol. 31 (1977) 343.

(8) S.A. Goulden, F.W. Chattaway, J. Gen. Microbiol. 59 (1969) 111.

(9) J.M. Luengo, G. Revilla, J.R. Villanueva, J.F. Martín, J. Gen. Microbiol. 115 (1979) 207.

(10) Y. Aharonowitz, S. Mendelowitz, F. Kirenberg, V. Kuper, J. Bacteriol. 157 (1984) 337.

(11) R.P. Elander, In: Antibiotics containing the β-lactam structure I. (A.L. Demain, N.A. Solomon, eds.) Springer-Verlag, Berlin (1983) 97.

(12) F.R. Ramos, M.J. López-Nieto, J.F. Martín, Antimicrob. Agents Chemother. 27 (1985) 380.

(13) R.C. Erickson, R.E. Bennet, Appl. Microbiol. 13 (1965) 738.

(14) K. Kitano, K. Kintaka, K. Katamato, K. Nara, Y. Nakao. J. Ferm. Technol. 53 (1975) 339.

(15) F. Avanzini, P. Valenti, Abstr. 6th Intern. Ferm. Symp. London, Ontario (1980) 18.

(16) C.R. Balley, M.J. Butler, I.D. Normansell, R.T. Rowlands, D.I. Winstanley, Biotechnology 2 (1984) 808.

(17) P. Tudzynski, K. Esser, Curr. Genet. 6 (1982) 153.

(18) P.L. Skatrud, S.W. Queener, Curr. Genet. 8 (1984) 155.

(19) J.F. Martín, P. Liras, Trends Biotechnol. 3 (1985) 39.

(20) D.L. Pruess, M.J. Jhonson, J. Bacteriol. 94 (1967) 1502.

(21) P.A. Fawcett, J.J. Usher, J.A. Huddleston, R.C. Bleaney, J.J. Nisbet, E.P. Abraham, Biochem. J. 157 (1976) 651.

(22) M.J. López-Nieto, F.R. Ramos, J.M. Luengo, J.F. Martín, Appl. Microbiol. Biotechnol. 21 (1985), in press.

(23) P. Adriaens, B. Meeschaert, W. Wuyts, H. Vanderhaegue, H. Eyssen. Antimicrob. Agents Chemother. 8 (1975) 638.

(24) M.M. Dhar, A.W. Khan, Nature 233 (1971) 182.

(25) P.A. Fawcett, E.P. Abraham, Methods Enzymol. 43 (1975) 471.

(26) E. Katz, H. Weissbach, J. Biol. Chem. 238 (1963) 666.

(27) M.J. López-Nieto, J.F. Martín, in preparation.

(28) G. Revilla, M.J. López-Nieto, J.F. Martín, in preparation.

(29) C.P. Pang, B. Chakravarti, R.M. Adlington, H.H. Ting, R.L. White, G.S. Jayatilake, J.E. Baldwin, E.P. Abraham, Biochem. J. 222 (1984) 789.

(30) S.E. Jensen, D.W.S. Westlake, S. Wolfe, J. Antibiot. 35 (1982) 1026.

(31) G. Revilla, M.J. López-Nieto, J.M. Luengo, J.F. Martín, J. Antibiot. 37 (1984) 27.

(32) P.B. Loder, Postepy Hig. Med. Dosw. 26 (1972) 493.

(33) E. Alvarez, J.F. Martín, unpublished results.

(34) A.L. Demain, In: Antibiotics containing the B-lactam structure I. (A.L. Demain, N.A. Solomon, eds.), Springer-Verlag, Berlin (1983) 189.

(35) P.B. Loder, E.P. Abraham, Biochem. J. 123 (1971) 471.

(36) L.A. Eriquez, M.A. Pisano, Antimicrob. Agents Chemother. 16 (1979) 392.

(37) J.M. Castro, P. Liras, J. Cortés, J.F. Martín, Appl. Microbiol. Biotechnol. 21 (1985), in press.

(38) J. Romero, P. Liras, J.F. Martín, unpublished results.

(39) P.B. Loder, E.P. Abraham, Biochem. J. 123 (1971) 477.

(40) T. Konomi, S. Herchen, J.E. Baldwin, M. Yoshida, N.A. Hunt, A.L. Demain, Biochem. J. 184 (1979) 427.

(41) J. O'Sullivan, R.C. Bleaney, J.A. Huddleston, E.P. Abraham. Biochem. J. 184 (1979) 421.

(41) J.E. Baldwin, B.L. Johnson, J.J. Usher, E.P. Abraham, J.A. Huddleston, R.L. White. J. Chem. Soc. Chem Commun. (1980) 1271.

(43) G. Bahadur, J.E. Baldwin, L.D. Field, E.M.M. Lehtonen, J.J. Usher, C.A. Vallejo, E.P. Abraham, R.L. White, J. Chem. Soc. Chem. Commun (1981) 917.

(44) Y. Sawada, J.E. Baldwin, P.D. Singh, N.A. Solomon, A.L. Demain, Antimicrob. Agents Chemother. 18 (1980) 485.

(45) J. Kupka, Y.Q. Shen, S. Wolfe, A.L. Demain, Can. J. Microbiol. 29 (1983) 488.

(46) I.J. Hollander, Y.Q. shen, J. Heim, A.L. Demain, S. Wolfe, Science 224 (1984) 610.

(47) J.M. Luengo, M.T. Alemany, F. Salto, F.R. Ramos, M.J. López-Nieto, J.F. Martín, Science (1985), Submitted.

(48) S. Wolfe, A.L. Demain, S.E. Jensen, D.W.S. Westlake. Science 226 (1984) 1386.

(49) J.M. Castro, P. Liras, J.F. Martín, unpublished results.

(50) J. Kupka, Y.Q. Shen, S. Wolfe, A.L. Demain, FEMS Microbiol. Lett. 16 (1983) 1.

(51) J.E. Baldwin, J.W. Keeping, P.D. Singh, C.A. Vallejo, Biochem. J. 194 (1981) 649.

(52) S. Jayatilake, J.A. Huddleston, E.P. Abraham, Biochem. J. 194 (1981) 645.

(53) S.E. Jensen, D.W.S. Westlake, S. Wolfe, Can. J. Microbiol. 29 (1983) 1526.

(54) M. Kohsaka, A.L. Demain, Biochem. Biophys. Res. Commun 70 (1976) 465.

(55) Y. Sawada, N.A. Hunt, A.L. Demain, J. Antibiot. 32 (1979) 1303.

(56) D.J. Hook, L.T. Chang, R.P. Elander, R.B. Morin, Biochem. Biophys. Res. Commun. 87 (1979) 258.

(57) H.R. Felix, H.H. Peter, H.J. Treichler, J. Antibiot. 34 (1981) 567.

(58) S.E. Jensen, D.W.S. Westlake, R.J. Bowers, S. Wolfe, J. Antibiot. 35 (1982) 1351.

(59) J. Cortés, P. Liras, J.M. Castro, J. Romero, J.F. Martín, Biochem. Soc. Trans. 12 (1984) 863.

(60) J. Cortés, P. Liras, J.M. Castro, J.F. Martín, J. Gen. Microbiol. (1985), submitted manuscript.

(61) S.E. Jensen, D.W.S. Westlake, S. Wolfe, J. Antibiot. 38 (1985) 263.

(62) Y. Fujisawa, M. Kikuchi, T. Kanzaki, J. Antibiot. 30 (1977) 775.

(63) M.K. Turner, J.E. Farthing, S.J. Brewer, Biochem. J. 173 (1978) 839.

(64) C.M. Stevens, E.P. Abraham, F.C. Huang, C.J. Sih, Fed. Proc. 34 (1975) 625.

(65) A. Scheidegger, M.T. Kuenzi, J. Nuesch, J. Antibiot. 37 (1984) 522.

(66) Y. Fujisawa, T. Kitano, T. Kanyaki, Agric. Biol. Chem. 39 (1975) 2049.

(67) Y. Fujisawa, T. Kanzaki, Agric. Biol. Chem. 39 (1975) 2043.

(68) S.J. Brewer, P.M. Taylor, M.K. Turner, Biochem. J. 185 (1980) 555.

(69) J. O'Sullivan, R.C. Bleaney, J.A. Huddleston, E.P. Abraham, Biochem. J. 184 (1979) 421.

(70) J. O'Sullivan, E.P. Abraham, Biochem. J. 186 (1980) 613.

(71) A.L. Demain, Proc. of the Fourth. Intern. Symp. on Genetics of Industrial Microorganisms (Y. Ikeda, T. Beppu, eds.) Kodansha Ltd., Tokyo (1982) 79.

(72) J.F. Martín, Y. Aharonowitz, In: Antibiotics containing the B. lactam Structure I. (A.L. Demain, N.A. Solomon, eds.) Springer-Verlag, Berlin (1983) 229.

(73) Y. Aharonowitz, A.L. Demain, Antimicrob. Agents Chemother. $\underline{14}$ (1978) 159.

(74) M.G. Domínguez, P. Liras, J.F. Martín, unpublished results.

(75) L.A. Kominek, Antimicrob. Agents Chemother. $\underline{1}$ (1972) 123.

(76) J.L. Barredo, J.F. Martín, unpublished results.

(77) F.V. Soltero, M.J. Jhonson, Appl. Microbiol. $\underline{1}$ (1953) 52.

(78) J.F. Martín, F. Antequera, J. Antibiot., submitted manuscript.

(79) F.V. Soltero, M.J. Jhonson, Appl. Microbiol. $\underline{2}$ (1954) 41.

(80) G. Revilla, M.J. López-Nieto, F.R. Ramos, E. Alvarez, J.F. Martín, submitted manuscript.

(81) J.F. Martín, G. Revilla, M.J. López-Nieto, F.R. ramos, J.M. Cantoral, Biochem. Soc. Trans. $\underline{12}$ (1984) 866.

(82) C.G. Friedrich, A.L. Demain, Arch. Microbiol. $\underline{119}$ (1978) 43.

(83) S.C. Kuo, J.D. Lampen, J. Bacteriol. $\underline{111}$ (1972) 419.

(84) C.F. Heredia, G. de la Fuente, A. Sols, Biochem. Biophys Acta. $\underline{86}$ (1964) 216.

(85) J.F. Martín, G. Revilla, D.M. Zanca, M.J. López-Nieto, In: Trends in Antibiotic Research (H. Umezawa, A.L. Demain, T. Hata, C.R. Hatchinson, eds.) Japan Antibiotics Research Association, Tokyo (1982) 258.

(86) A.L. Demain, V.M. Kennel, J. Ferm. Technol. $\underline{56}$ (1978) 323.

(87) R.J. Mehta, C.H. Nash, J.L. Speth, Y.K. Oh., Dev. Ind. Microbiol. $\underline{21}$ (1980) 227.

(88) M. Matsumura, T. Imanaka, T. Yoshida, T. Taguchi, J. Ferm. Technol. $\underline{56}$ (1978) 345.

(89) D.M. Zanca, J.F. Martín, J. Antibiot. $\underline{36}$ (1983) 700.

(90) C.J. Behmer, A.L. Demain, Curr. Microbiol. $\underline{8}$ (1983) 107.

(91) J. Heim, Y.Q. Shen, S. Wolfe, A.L. Demain, Appl. Microbiol. Biotechnol. $\underline{19}$ (1984) 232.

(92) Y.M. Kennel, C.J. Behmer, A.L. Demain, Enzyme Microbiol. Technol. $\underline{3}$ (1981) 243.

(93) M.T. Kuenzi, Arch. Microbiol. $\underline{128}$ (1980) 78.

(94) A. Hinnen, J. Nuesch, Antimicrob. Agents Chemother. $\underline{9}$ (1976) 824.

(95) J.O. O'Sullivan, C. Ball, In: Biochemistry and Genetic Regulation of Commercially Important Antibiotics (L.C. Vining, ed.) Addison-Wesley, Reading (1983) 73.

(96) J. O'Sullivan, A.M. Gillum, C.A. Aklonis, M.L. Souser, R.B. Sykes, Antimicrob. Agents Chemother. $\underline{21}$ (1982) 558.

(97) S.W. Elson, R.S. Oliver, J. Antibiot. $\underline{31}$ (1978) 586.

(98) S.W. Elson, R.S. Oliver, B.W. Bycroft, E.A. Faruk, J. Antibiot. $\underline{35}$ (1982) 81.

(99) J. Romero, P. Liras, J.F. Martín, Appl. Microbiol. Biotechnol. 20 (1984) 318.

(100) J. Cortés, J.M. Castro, P. Liras, J.F. Martín, Preprints of the Third European Congress on Biotechnology, Vol I, Verlag-Chemie, Weinheim (1984) 21.

(101) H.G. Hers, L. Hue, E.U. Schaftingen, Trends Biochem. Sci. 7 (1982) 329.

(102) C. Lubbe, S.E. Jensen, A.L. Demain, FEMS Microbiol. Lett. 25 (1984) 75.

(103) C.M. Ragan, L.C. Vining, Can. J. Microbiol. 24 (1978) 1012.

(104) J.F. Martín, A. L. Demain, Can. J. Microbiol. 23 (1977) 1334.

(105) J.F. Martín, P. Liras, A.L. Demain, Biochem. Biophys. Res. Commun. 83 (1978) 822.

(106) Y. Aharonowitz, Ann. Rev. Microbiol. 34 (1980) 209.

(107) B. Magasanik, Ann. Rev. Genet. 16 (1982)1 135.

(108) F. Sánchez, M. Compomanes, C. Quinto, W. Hansberg, J. Mora, R. Palacios, J. Bacteriol. 136 (1978) 880.

(109) T.G. Cooper, R.A. Sumrada, J. Bacteriol. 155 (1983) 623.

(110) S. Sánchez, L. Paniagua, R.C. Mateos, F. Lara, F. Mora, In: Advances in Biotechnol. 3 (L.C. Vining, K. Singh, eds.), Pergamon Press, Toronto (1980) 147.

(111) Y.Q. Shen, J. Heim, N.A. Solomon, S. Wolfe, A.L. Deamin, J. Antibiot. 37 (1984) 503.

(112) Y. Aharonowitz, A.L. Demain, Can. J. Microbiol. 25 (1979) 61.

(113) G. Lilley, A.E. Clark, G.C. Lawrence, J. Chem. Tech. Biotechnol. 31 (1981) 127.

(114) M.E. Bushell, A. Fryday, J. Gen. Microbiol. 129 (1983) 1733.

(114a) A.L. Demain, A. Braña, Abstracts Ann. Meeting Amer. Soc. Microbiol. (1984) 198.

(115) B. Tyler, Ann. Rev. Biochem. 47 (1978) 1127.

(116) Y. Aharonowitz, In: Genetics of Industrial Microorganisms (O.K. Sebek, A.I. Laskin, eds.), American Society for Microbiology, Washington, D.C. (1979) 210.

(117) R. Wax, L. Snyder, L. Kaplan, Appl. Env. Microbiol. 44 (1982) 1004.

(118) S.L. Streicher, B. Tyler, Proc. Natl. Acad. Sci. USA 78 (1981) 229.

(119) C.L. Ginther, Antimicrob. Agents Chemother. 15 (1979) 522.

(120) J.F. Martín, M.T. Alegre, J.M. Castro, P. Liras, In: Biological Biochemical and Biomedical Aspects of Actinomycetes (L. Ortiz-Ortiz, L.F. Bojalil, V. Yakoleff). Academic Press, Orlando (1984) 273.

(121) E. Friedlin, J. Nüesch. Current Genet. 8 (1984) 271

Control of Cephamycin Formation in Streptomyces clavuligerus by Nitrogenous Compounds

Arnold L. Demain and Alfredo F. Braña*

Massachusetts Institute of Technology, Fermentation Microbiology Laboratory, Department of Nutrition and Food Science, Cambridge, Massachusetts 02139, U.S.A.

*Universidad de Oviedo, Departamento Interfacultativo de Microbiologia, Oviedo, Spain

Abstract

Production of cephalosporins by Streptomyces clavuligerus is negatively affected by ammonium salts as nitrogen source. The mechanism involves repression of enzyme synthesis, not inhibition of enzyme action. Of the three pathway enzymes examined, the enzyme most severely repressed is isopenicillin N synthetase (cyclase). Desacetoxycephalosporin C synthetase (expandase) was repressed to a lesser degree whereas penicillin epimerase was unaffected by growth in NH_4^+. It appears that cyclase may be the rate-limiting enzyme in S. clavuligerus NRRL 3585. Mutants lacking glutamine synthetase, glutamate synthase or alanine dehydrogenase still were subject to ammonium repression indicating that these enzymes are not acting as regulatory proteins with respect to antibiotic bio-synthesis.

Streptomyces clavuligerus NRRL 3585 is a producer of several β-lactam anti-biotics, mainly cephamycin C. Antibiotic production in this species has been shown to be deeply influenced by the nitrogen source used in the culture medium (1). Ammonium salts were found to depress cephalosporin production, but no data were available on the mechanism mediating this negative effect.

In our studies, all fermentations were carried out in the buffered defined medium described by Aharonowitz and Demain (1), using different nitrogen sources.

*Present address: Department of Microbiology, University of Oviedo, Spain.

The standard medium, which contained 15 mM L-asparagine as the only nitrogen source, allowed relatively good production. When increasing concentrations of ammonium chloride were added to this medium, a progressive and strong decrease in cephalosporin production was observed. With ammonium chloride as the sole nitrogen source, optimal production was found at about 30 mM ammonium, although the antibiotic titer was much lower than that obtained with asparagine. In all fermentations, the pH was maintained within a narrow range (6.3 - 7.0). These pH values were found not to interfere with production in independent experiments with resting cells buffered between those limits. Thus, the ammonium effect cannot be explained by a drop in pH due to the utilization of ammonium.

HPLC analysis of fermentation broths showed the presence of two cephalosporins, cephamycin C and its precursor o-carbomoyldesacetylcephalosporin C (A16886A), the former in far higher amounts than the latter (Fig. 1). The use of asparagine or

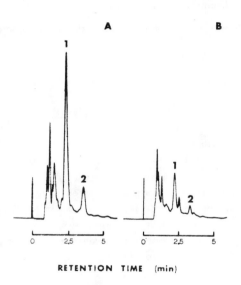

RETENTION TIME (min)

Fig. 1 HPLC analysis of fermentation broths in media with (A) 15mM L-asparagine or (B) 40 mM NH_4Cl. Two peaks corresponding to cephamycin C (1) and A 16886 A (2) were found in both samples.

ammonium chloride as nitrogen sources influenced the total amount of antibiotic, but did not change the relative proportions of the two compounds produced. No penicillin N was detected in any case.

In order to find out whether ammonium inhibited or repressed one or several steps in the biosynthesis of cephalosporins, several fermentations with different ammonium concentrations were conducted. Samples of mycelium from the exponential phase of growth were collected, washed, resuspended in a small volume of MOPS buffer with 100 μg/ml of chloramphenicol, and incubated for 2 hours. The specific production of cephalosporins under these conditions (resting cell activity) reflected the biosynthetic potential of the mycelium at the moment of harvest. At the same time, another part of the culture was used to prepare crude extracts. The activities of three enzymes of the biosynthetic pathway of the cephalosporins present in extracts were measured: isopenicillin N synthetase (cyclase) which catalyzes the cyclization of the tripeptide δ-(L-α-aminoadipyl)-L-cysteinyl-D-valine to isopenicillin N, the first antibiotic in the pathway; isopenicillin N epimerase, which catalyzes the epimerization of isopenicillin N to penicillin N; and desacetoxycephalosporin C synthetase (expandase), which catalyzes the expansion of the penicillin ring to give the first cephalosporin, desacetoxycephalosporin C.

The presence of ammonium in the fermentation medium caused a decrease in the specific production of antibiotic to a degree proportional to its concentration (Table 1). Similarly, the resting cell activity of cells previously grown with ammonium was lowered. Among the three antibiotic synthetases determined, the cyclase was strongly repressed by ammonium, especially at high concentrations. The expandase was also repressed, although to a lower extent. In the case of the epimerase, there was no clear correlation between the amount of ammonium in the cultures and the enzymatic activity. On the other hand, ammonium was found not to be inhibitory when added during short periods to resting cell systems or to the assay mixtures of the three enzymes studied. Experiments with mixed crude extracts from repressed and derepressed cultures ruled out the possibility of an intracellular inhibitor being synthesized in the cultures with ammonium. In conclusion, ammonium represses, but does not inhibit, the synthesis of cephalosporins by S. clavuligerus.

The degree of repression, as measured by resting cell activity, was found to correlate with the cyclase levels (Fig. 2). No such correlation was observed with the epimerase or expandase activities. Since the resting cell activity reflects the overall antibiotic biosynthetic activity, it appears that biosynthesis is dependent on the cyclase level. In other words, the data suggest that the cyclase may be the rate-limiting enzyme in the pathway.

Table 1

Effects of ammonium on production, resting cell activity and enzymatic activity

N source	Cephalosporins (u/mg·h)	Resting cell activity (u/mg·h)	Cyclase	Epimerase	Expandase
				(u/mg prot)	
15 mM asparagine (asn)	35.0	1.50	28.0	28.3	24.3
asn + 10mM NH_4Cl	26.7	1.00	19.0	22.5	18.6
asn + 30mM NH_4Cl	11.3	1.07	21.0	19.5	14.8
asn + 80mM NH_4Cl	6.8	0.40	7.0	18.6	17.0
20mM NH_4Cl	10.5	0.64	9.3	15.0	21.9
30mM NH_4Cl	6.5	0.53	10.0	22.0	20.2
50mM NH_4Cl	2.3	0.36	7.0	ND	12.1
80mM NH_4Cl	1.7	0.18	3.7	23.3	13.0

The values of antibiotic production are the maximum achieved throughout the fermentations. Samples for determination of resting cell activity and enzymatic activities were taken in **exponential phase** of growth. ND = not determined.

Several of these findings were confirmed by following different parameters during fermentations with either asparagine or ammonium chloride, at equivalent concentrations, as the only nitrogen source (Fig. 3). Growth was slightly slower with ammonium, although the final cell yield was identical. Production of cephalosporins took place during growth in both cases, but it was 60% reduced in the ammonium medium. Both cyclase and expandase showed maximum activities during late exponential phase, and both, especially the cyclase, were repressed by ammonium. The epimerase activity increased during growth, with similar values in the two cultures.

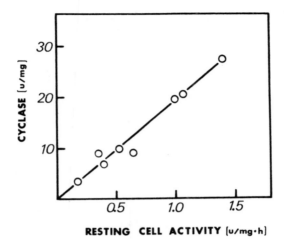

Fig. 2 Correlation between cyclase specific activity and resting cell activity.

When the values of the cyclase activity and the specific rate of production throughout the fermentation were plotted as a function of growth, both parameters were roughly similar (Fig. 4). Maximum values were observed about one doubling time before the end of growth. Similar correlations were found in fermentations with asparagine or ammonium chloride as nitrogen source. These data gave further support to the above mentioned possibility of the cyclase as a limiting step in the biosynthetic pathway of cephalosporins in this organism.

Antibiotic production was strongly influenced by the nature of the nitrogen source when different compounds were tested at equivalent concentrations (30 mM nitrogen) (Table 2). Ammonium and alanine were the poorest, and asparagine and aspartate the best sources for production among those tested that supported good growth. A rough correlation between the cyclase activities in exponential phase and specific cephamycin production was observed. The growth rates were not related to the production or the enzymatic activities.

Next, we began to study the mechanism of the repression produced by ammonium. For that purpose, the activities of enzymes mediating assimilation of ammonium in microorganisms (2) were measured in crude extracts (Table 3). Significant levels of glutamine synthetase (GS), glutamate synthase (GOGAT), and alanine dehydro-genase (ADH) were detected in different media. GS activity varied markedly

82   *Arnold L. Damain and Alfredo F. Braña*

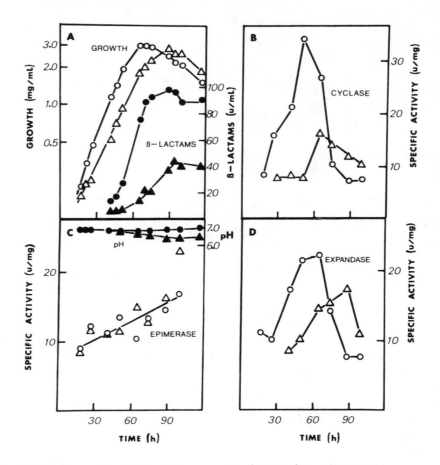

Fig. 3 Effect of growth with 15 mM L-asparagine (circles) or 30mM NH₄Cl
(triangles) as nitrogen sources on formation of antibiotic synthetases.

depending on the nitrogen source, although repressed levels were always found in
the presence of ammonium. Ammonium shock of cultures with high GS activity caused
a rapid inactivation of the enzyme. GOGAT activities were rather constant,
independent of the nitrogen source, whereas ADH was increased by alanine or
ammonium in the culture medium. Glutamate dehydrogenase and alanine-2-ketoglutarate
aminotransferase were not found under any growth conditions.

Table 2

Growth, production and antibiotic synthetases with
different nitrogen sources

N source	Cephalosporins (u/mL)	Cyclase	Epimerase (u/mg protein)	Expandase	Doubling time (h)
L-asparagine	69.0	40.1	52.0	17.4	11.5
L-aspartate	65.0	30.6	50.0	10.1	9.0
L-glutamine	52.5	24.8	66.0	12.7	11.0
urea	38.0	26.1	36.0	6.2	17.0
L-histidine	37.0	26.1	42.0	9.2	10.0
L-glutamate	31.0	11.5	47.0	7.3	6.3
L-alanine	25.0	13.6	27.0	4.2	13.5
NH_4Cl	17.5	15.2	42.0	6.0	13.5

The cephalosporin values are the maximum achieved throughout the fermentation.
Samples for the determination of enzymatic activities were taken in exponential
phase. All nitrogen sources were used at a concentration equivalent to 30 mM
nitrogen.

In order to obtain mutants impaired in assimilation of ammonium, spores of
S. clavuligerus were mutagenized with N-methyl-N'-nitro-N-mitrosoguanidine.
After selection, two types of mutants were found: the first class could not grow in
any medium in the absence of glutamine. They did not have detectable GS activity.
The second class could grow with different amino acids yielding glutamate by
transamination (aspartate, asparagine, lysine) or degradation (glutamine, proline,
arginine, histidine), but not with ammonium or alanine. These mutants lacked
GOGAT activity. Both types of strains had normal activities and regulation of ADH.
In other experiments, the mutagenized spores were selected for inability to utilize
alanine as the only carbon and nitrogen source. With this procedure, one mutant
lacking ADH activity was isolated. The ADH mutant was able to utilize ammonium

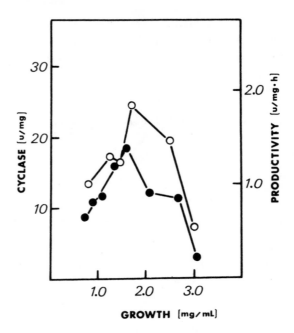

Fig. 4   Profiles of cyclase specific activity (o) and specific productivity (●)
during fermentation in medium with 15 mM L-asparagine as sole nitrogen
source.

at low or high concentration in a way identical to the wild type, but could not
use alanine. All these data indicated that the GS-GOGAT pathway is the only means
of ammonium assimilation in S. clavuligerus. ADH does not seem to play a direct
role in that process, but its induction by ammonium suggests that it might have
some other related function.

The effect of ammonium on cephalosporin production and formation of antibiotic
synthetases in the different classes of mutants was studied. In the case of the
wild type, addition of 40 mM NH_4Cl to the standard medium decreased antibiotic
production and repressed cyclase and expandase (Table 4). It also induced ADH
and did not affect GS and GOGAT. Similar results were found with the mutants
lacking GS or GOGAT (despite the fact that none of them could use ammonium for
growth) or ADH. This behavior contrasts with observations of primary metabolism in
different microorganisms (3,4), where a relief of ammonium repression by mutations
affecting GS are often found. The data also indicate that active GS, GOGAT or ADH
molecules are not functioning as regulatory proteins for antibiotic synthesis since
each mutant still was subject to ammonium regulation.

Table 3

Enzymes of ammonium assimilation in fermentations
with different nitrogen sources

N source	glutamine synthetase	alanine dehydrogenase (u/mg protein)	glutamate synthase
L-asparagine (asn)	2052	51	48
asn + 40mM NH$_4$C1	420	234	65
L-aspartate	495	49	32
L-glutamine	2169	55	62
urea	395	23	51
L-histidine	1410	235	54
L-glutamate	2336	71	31
L-alanine	1848	1060	60
NH$_4$C1	551	817	60

Enzymatic activities were determined in crude extracts from cultures growing in exponential phase.

     Looking for the hypothetical compound responsible for ammonium repression of antibiotic production, we analyzed the intracellular pool of free amino acids in cells grown with a variety of ammonium levels. Among 22 compounds detected by HPLC, only glutamine and alanine showed marked variations in response to the ammonium concentration was raised above 20 mM (Table 5). Therefore, alanine or glutamine could act as an effector of ammonium repression.

     The GS⁻ mutant (gln 2) had reduced intracellular pools of glutamine (Table 5). Repression of antibiotic production in this mutant by addition of ammonium was accompanied by a dramatic increase in the alanine pool but a much weaker effect on the glutamine pool. Conversely, growth of the ADH⁻ mutant (M15) in the presence or absence of ammonium had a strong effect on the glutamine but not in the alanine pool, although ammonium caused a decrease in the levels of cyclase and production

Table 4

Ammonium repression in wild type and mutants
of ammonium assimilation

Strain	N source	Cephalosporins (u/mg)	Cyclase	Expandase	GS	ADH
				(u/mg protein)		
Wild type	L-glutamine	33.0	22.7	7.1	806	67
	gln + NH$_4$C1	9.6	10.2	5.2	446	139
gln 2 (GS⁻)	L-glutamine	11.1	11.5	7.4	< 10	53
	gln + NH$_4$C1	1.5	1.4	3.8	< 10	1850
glu 2 (GOGAT⁻)	L-aspartate	11.4	20.1	9.5	386	306
	asp + NH$_4$C1	4.0	6.3	10.1	448	1346
M15 (ADH⁻)	L-glutamine	18.7	13.8	6.1	3328	6
	gln + NH$_4$C1	3.6	9.9	4.7	663	7

The values of specific production of cephalosporins are the maximum achieved
throughout the fermentation. The enzymatic activities were measured in samples
from cultures growing in exponential phase. Amino acids were used at a concentration providing 30 mM nitrogen. Where indicated, 40 mM NH$_4$C1 was added.

similar to the ones observed in the wild type. Therefore, neither glutamine nor
alanine seemed to play a direct role as effectors of the ammonium control of
cephalosporin biosynthesis. This suggests that either ammonium itself acts as a
corepressor, or that it is incorporated into another compound in a reaction not
affected by these mutations.

Other data indicated that the nitrogen control might be even more complicated.
When poor nitrogen sources such as proline or threonine are used, a very low
production and a strong repression of cyclase, epimerase and expandase was observed
(Table 6). Under these conditions, GS activity was high and ADH low, while the

Table 5

Effect of the addition of ammonium on the intracellular concentrations of free glutamine and alanine

Strain	N source	Pool content	
		glutamine	alanine
		(nmoles/mg protein)	
Wild type	L-asparagine (asn)	36.2	20.5
	asn + 80mM NH$_4$Cl	64.6	56.1
gln 2 (GS-)	L-glutamine (gln)	6.7	18.8
	gln + 40mM NH$_4$Cl	9.7	78.1
M15 (ADH⁻)	L-asparagine	15.6	24.7
	asn + 80mM NH$_4$Cl	70.3	30.0

Asparagine and glutamine were used at 15 mM. The intracellular concentrations of glutamine and alanine were measured in exponentially growing cells.

intracellular pools of glutamine and alanine were low. This type of repression could be partially relieved by addition of small concentrations of ammonium, with simultaneous decrease in the GS activity and increase in the glutamine pool levels. It is unknown whether this effect is related to the ammonium control or it responds to a different regulatory circuit.

From all the data mentioned above, it can be concluded that the production of cephalosporins by S. clavuligerus is regulated by the nitrogen source in a way different from the ones described in enteric bacteria and fungi (3,4). It does not seem to involve the immediate products of ammonium assimilation, glutamine and alanine, or the enzymes mediating that assimilation. Further studies, with isolation of ammonium-derepressed mutants may prove useful in the elucidation of this type of regulation.

Table 6

Effects of supplementation with low ammonium on fermentations with poor nitrogen sources

N source	Cephalosporins (u/mL)	Cyclase (u/mg)	Pool content glutamine (nmoles/mg protein)	Pool content alanine (nmoles/mg protein)	Doubling time (h)
L-proline	<1	<2	6	7	24.0
proline + 10mM NH_4Cl	35	21	40	13	13.5
L-threonine	13	9	15	7	18.5
threonine + 10mM NH_4Cl	27	17	42	5	12.0

Amino acids were used at 30 mM. The antibiotic values are the maximum achieved throughout the fermentation. Cyclase and intracellular pools were measured during exponential phase of growth.

References

(1) Y. Aharonowitz, A.L. Demain, Can. J. Microbiol. 25 (1979) 61.
(2) H. Dalton, Int. Rev. Biochem. 21 (1979) 227.
(3) B. Magasanik, Ann. Rev. Genet. 16 (1982) 135.
(4) G.A. Marzluf, Microbiol. Rev. 45 (1981) 437.

Acknowledgement

Support for this work was provided by National Science Grant PCM82-18029. A.F.B. received a fellowship from the Fundacion Juan March of Spain. We acknowledge the help of Saul Wolfe for preparation of enzyme substrates in the cephalosporin pathway.

Implication of Lysine Metabolism on Regulation of Cephamycin C Biosynthesis in Streptomyces clavuligerus

Yair Aharonowitz, Simona Mendelovitz, Hana Ben-Artzi and Nurit M. Magal

Tel-Aviv University, The George S. Wise Faculty of Life Sciences, Department of Microbiology, Ramat-Aviv, 69978 Tel-Aviv, Israel

SUMMARY

In Streptomyces clavuligerus both L-lysine and diaminopimelic acid stimulated specific production of a β-lactam antibiotic. Since feedback control was found to be exerted on aspartokinase activity by lysine plus threonine and on homoserine dehydrogenase by threonine alone it was assumed that carbon flow from aspartate to lysine and α-aminoadipic acid would be rate-limiting for antibiotic synthesis. It would also be expected that genetic release of aspartokinase from feedback inhibition would result in increased synthesis of the antibiotic. A high percentage of the mutants impaired in feedback regulation of aspartokinase activity produced significantly higher amounts of antibiotics. These lysine analog resistant mutants also contained higher levels of total free amino acid compared to the wild type strain. Diaminopimelic acid accounted for 10 to 20% of the total free amino acid pools of the mutants, as compared to 0.5% in the wild type strain. Our findings that antibiotic synthesis was stimulated by diaminopimelic acid accumulation, either through genetic deregulation

---

Abbreviations: AAA: α-aminoadipate; MOPS: morpholinopropane sulfonic acid; DAP: diaminopimelic acid; DDPS: dihydrodipicolinic acid synthetase; HSD: homoserine dehydrogenase; AEC: S-(2-aminoethyl)-L-cysteine.

or by the addition of the amino acid to the growth medium of a wild
type strain, suggest that individual precursor pool level can control
the biosynthesis of secondary metabolites such as cephamycin C.

1   INTRODUCTION

Many antibiotics are derived from precursors which are themselves
end products or intermediates of primary metabolism (1). This suggests that mechanisms controlling primary metabolic activities, which
supply the required substrates for antibiotic production may affect
the ability of the cell to produce the antibiotics.

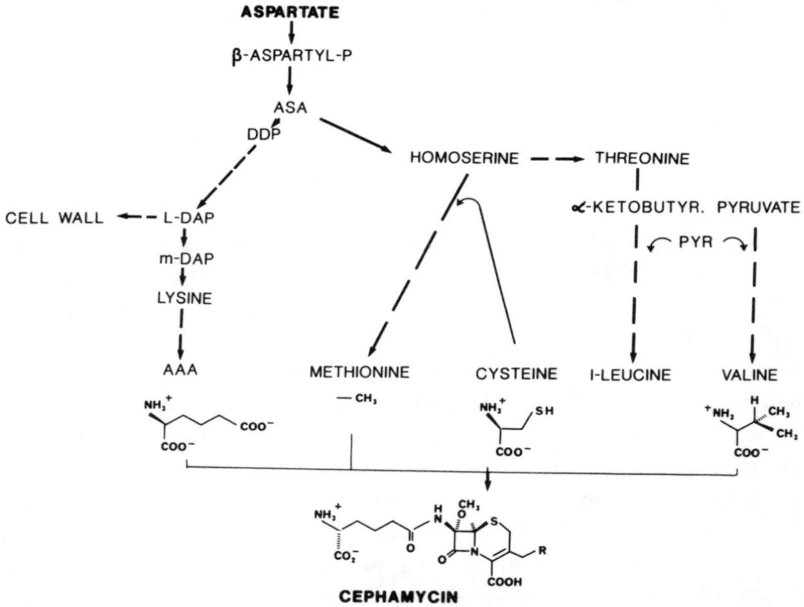

Fig. 1.   The aspartic acid family pathway and its involvement in
          cephamycin biosynthesis.
          Abbreviations not used in text: ASA, aspartic semialdehyde;
          PYR, pyruvate; α-KETOBUTYR, α-ketobutyrate.

In the case of <u>Streptomyces clavuligerus</u>, which produce the β-
lactam antibiotic cephamycin C, (2), the aspartic acid pathway might
serve as target for regulatory mechanisms in controlling antibiotic

biosynthesis. This pathway (Fig. 1), which produces the α-amino-adipate (AAA) side chain of cephamycin C and the methyl group at the C-7 position, involves cysteine as an intermediate and shares common enzymes with the valine biosynthetic pathway. There are both cysteine and valine moieties in the cephamycin molecule.

In the following report, feedback control mechanisms operating at the level of a specific amino acid (lysine) biosynthesis, were shown to be involved in the control of cephamycin C biosynthesis in strepto-mycetes. Mutants insensitive to this control mechanism showed sig-nificant overproduction of ß-lactam antibiotics.

2   PHYSIOLOGICAL AND BIOCHEMICAL STUDIES

2.1 Antibiotic Production Capacity as a Function of Culture Age

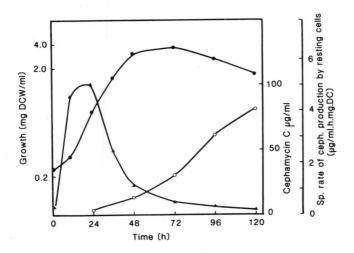

Fig. 2.   Cephamycin C production by growing and resting cells of S. clavuligerus as a function of age of culture. The curves show (●) growth; (▲) specific production by resting cells; (○) cephamycin C, titers in fermentation medium.

Initial experiments were designed to establish at which culture phase cells would possess the highest capacity of antibiotic produc-tion, as assayed in a resting cell system. Fig. 2 shows typical

trophophase-idiophase kinetics of a Streptomyces clavuligerus culture
grown in a chemically defined medium.   It was anticipated that cells
harvested in idiophase when antibiotic production was high would also
possess the highest capacity to produce antibiotics when washed and
resuspended in buffer as a resting cell suspension.   However, as shown
in Fig. 2, the highest potential for antibiotic production was
observed in cells harvested during the early exponential phase of
growth.   Upon cessation of growth, a sharp decrease in the specific
capacity of production was seen.   These results have led us to assume
that the pool level of available primary metabolites, which serve as
direct precursors for antibiotic biosynthesis, may become a key factor
in regulating antibiotic production, especially when the specific antibiotic synthetases are already present in the cell.   This control of
the rate of antibiotic biosynthesis should be greatest when such precursor concentrations are in the range of, or below, the Km value of
the rate limiting steps.   Since availability of precursors of secondary metabolism is clearly affected by mechanisms controlling primary
metabolic pathways it follows that alteration in, or bypassing of
regulatory mechanisms, as well as nutritional deficiencies or excesses
could create conditions that favour secondary metabolism.

2.2   Aspartic Acid Family of Amino Acids and Antibiotic Production

In order to test whether any of the aspartic acid family of amino
acids or their intermediates affect antibiotic synthesis by S. clavuligerus when added to the fermentation media or to a resting cell system, the following experiments were carried out.   S. clavuligerus was
grown in a chemically defined medium which contained glycerol, L-
asparagine, morpholinopropane sulfonic acid buffer (MOPS), mineral
salts and different amino acids.   Cephamycin C production was monitored for 120 h.   None of the direct precursors of cephamycin C
(α-aminoadipate, cysteine, valine or methionine) had any stimulatory
effect on specific production when added at 10 mM final concentration
to the chemically defined medium (3).   L-lysine and also a racemic
mixture of diaminopimelic (DAP) both intermediates in the specific
biosynthetic pathway leading to α-aminoadipic acid, markedly stimulated antibiotic formation.   The stimulatory effect of lysine but not
DAP could be further increased by combining it with threonine and or
with valine (3).   Furthermore, L-lysine was equally effective in stimulating cephamycin C synthesis regardless of the time at which the
addition was made (Table 1).   By contrast the mixture of DAP isomers
stimulated production to the highest extent when added 24 h after the
inoculation of the culture, while, addition of α-aminoadipate

stimulated production of antibiotics only when added at 24 h or later.

Table 1.   Effect of time of addition of precursor amino acids on
           cephamycin C production.

Amino acid added 10 mM	Relative specific production at time of addition (h)[a]		
	0	24	48
No addition	100	100	100
L-Lysine	167	174	199
DAP	166	234	85
AAA	104	133	131

(a)   Specific antibiotic production: 100 = 27 µg/mg DCW

Increased antibiotic biosynthesis as a result of lysine addition could also be observed when lysine was added to a resting cell system depleted from its carbon, nitrogen, and energy source. One possible reason for this stimulatory effect was that the added lysine served as both carbon and nitrogen source, thus permitting reinitiation of growth. However, the data presented in Table 2 show that the lysine effect is specific, since, when lysine, asparagine or maltose was

Table 2.   Cephamycin C production by resting cells[a]

Addition	Cephamycin C µg/ml	Relative Specific Production
No addition	41.6	1.00
Maltose 14 mM	48.0	1.15
Lysine 10 mM	90.2	2.16
Asparagine 10 mM	42.7	1.02

(a)   Cell concentration in production buffer was 8.2 mg DCW/ml in a
      total volume of 10 ml. Production values are the maximum value
      reached after 24 h of incubation at 30°C. All fermentations
      contained chloramphenicol at final concentration of 25 µg/ml.

added to a resting cell system in the presence of chloramphenicol, only lysine stimulated antibiotic production. Since this lysine effect was not dependent on de novo protein synthesis, a possible explanation is that lysine was converted into α-aminoadipate, thus providing a substrate for the specific antibiotic synthetases.

These studies suggested that the carbon flow through the lysine-specific branch of the aspartic acid pathway in S. clavuligerus, might be a rate limiting step in the formation of cephamycins.

2.3 Feedback controls of lysine biosynthesis

The flow of carbon from aspartate through lysine to the α-amino-adipyl side chain of the cephamycin molecule could be subjected to control by regulatory mechanisms operating at the initial and branching steps of the pathway. A study was carried out on the regulation of three key enzyme activities located in such positions: (a) aspartokinase - the first common step of the pathway; (b) dihydrodipicolinic acid synthetase (DDPS) - the first specific step in the lysine branch; and (c) homoserine dehydrogenase (HSD) - the first step of the other branches of the pathway.

Table 3.   Effect of aspartic acid family of amino acids on aspartokinase activity[a]

addition (10 mM)	Relative enzyme activity (%)
None	100
L-threonine	120
L-lysine	150
L-methionine	112
L-isoleucine	96
L-homoserine	105
DL-meso-DAP	84
α-aminoadipate	113
S-(2-aminoethyl)-L-Cysteine (AEC)	118
L-lysine + L-threonine	4
L-lysine + L-methionine	127
L-lysine + L-isoleucine	146
L-threonine + AEC	18

(a) Aspartokinase activity was assayed by the standard hydroxamate assay (3). The protein content in each assay was 0.94 mg. In the reaction with no added amino acid, 21.6 nmol of asparto-hydroxamate per min was formed which was taken as 100% activity.

The results presented in Table 3 show that aspartokinase activity was strongly inhibited by the simultaneous addition of threonine and lysine (3,4). This concerted feedback inhibition effect was very specific; combination of lysine with other amino acids of the aspartic acid family were not inhibitory. The degree by which lysine, threonine and the combination of both affected aspartokinase preparations did not change significantly with culture age (3). Lysine could be substituted by its analogue thiolysine (AEC), and feedback inhibition of aspartokinase by the concerted effect of threonine plus AEC, similar to that obtained by thronine plus lysine could be demonstrated.

Only partial feedback inhibition of the DDPS activity was effected by DAP or AAA. Concentrations of 20 mM DAP or 40 mM AAA were required in order to achieve 50% inhibition of the enzyme. The third enzyme, HSD, was inhibited by threonine or hemoserine, whereas, isoleucine an end product of the homoserine branch had no effect on HSD activity. When the effect of amino acids on enzyme biosynthesis was studied, aspartokinase was shown to be partially repressed by methionine and quite strongly by isoleucine. HSD was repressed partially by isoleucine, while DDPS was not affected significantly by any of the amino acids tested (3).

The data presented thus far indicate that the carbon flow from aspartate to lysine is strictly controlled by a highly sensitive, concerted feedback inhibition mechanism acting on the first enzyme of the biosynthetic pathway, aspartokinase. This enzyme is probably the first rate limiting step in the conversion of aspartate to AAA. The strong feedback inhibition of homoserine dehydrogenase by threonine, and the lack of significant inhibition of DDPS, both support free carbon flow through the initial steps of the lysine branch.

3 MUTANTS IMPAIRED IN REGULATION OF ASPARTOKINASE ACTIVITY

3.1. Antibiotic production by mutant strains

Following the operational approach exploited in the development of lysine overproducing microbial strains (5,6), it was expected that toxic lysine analogs such as S-(2-aminoethyl)-L-cysteine could be used to select for resistant phenotypes, some of which would possess an alterated aspartokinase. Of the several different genotypes that could account for an AEC-resistant phenotype, those possessing a genetic alteration in the aspartokinase regulatory site were of special interest to us. It was expected that in such mutants the concerted

inhibitory effect by threonine plus lysine, or its analogs, on aspartokinase would be absent. Indeed, 44 such mutants were obtained,and
32 were found to have an aspartokinase activity that was not inhibited
by lysine plus threonine (4).

Table 4. Specific antibiotic production by AER-resistant and
          wild-type strains of S. clavuligerus (4).[a]

Mutant no.	Aspartokinase deregulation[b]	Specific production of antibiotic [µg(mg dry cell wt)$^{-1}$]	Relative Specific Production
Wild type	-	47	1.0
aec(R)10	+	94	2.0
aec(R)15	+	323	6.9
aec(R)28	+	313	6.7
aec(R)50	+	270	5.7
aec(R)52	+	237	5.0
aec(R)54	+	209	4.4

(a) Cultures were grown in chemically defined medium without any
     added amino acids except asparagine.
(b) Aspartokinase activity which is not inhibited when assayed in the
     presence of 0.4 mM-L-Lysine plus 0.4 mM L-threonine.

The AEC resistant mutants were grown in the chemically defined
medium for 120 h and samples were assayed for cephamycin C titers.
Among those mutants in which aspartokinase activity was deregulated,
about 70% (23 out of 32) produced antibiotics of higher titers and at
higher specific production values than the wild type (Table 4).
Although the majority of the AEC-resistant aspartokinase-deregulated mutants produced higher antibiotic titers, as well as higher
specific production values, the degree of increase did not correlate
exactly with the degree of impairment in aspartokinase regulation.
The possible involvement of more than a single mutation could not be
ruled out.

3.2. Free amino acid pool studies.

Attempts were made to determine whether these regulatory alterations, which were caused specifically by the aecR mutation, could
affect the composition and relative concentrations of the intracellular free amino acid pool in such a way that might explain antibiotic

overproduction in strains containing this mutation. Thus, cultures of
the wild type and of a few mutant strains were grown for 96 h in the
unsupplemented chemical defined medium and sampled, at different time
intervals, and assayed for biomass, antibiotics and composition of
intracellular amino acid pools (7). A high pool content of free amino
acids always found in cells harvested at early stages of growth. A
sharp decrease in the pool content was observed during the middle and
late log phase of growth. Large differences were observed in concen-

Table 5. Free Intracellular Amino Acid Pool content

| Amino acid | Relative pool content (%) | | | | concentration | |
| | wild type | | aecR28 | | aecR28/WT(a) | |
	24h	72h	24h	72h	24h	72h
ASP	3.0	2.5	3.2	3.0	1.5	1.6
THR	1.8	1.3	2.6	1.7	2.1	1.7
SER	6.2	5.9	5.6	6.7	1.3	1.5
GLU	68.0	63.5	53.7	39.8	1.1	0.85
GLY	1.7	2.2	2.0	8.5	1.7	5.2
ALA	5.3	7.6	3.8	4.6	1.0	0.83
CYS	0.6	0.4	0.8	ND	2.0	ND
VAL	3.2	4.6	1.3	3.9	0.6	1.1
DAP	0.5	0.3	14.9	17.0	44.5	80.0
MET	0.5	0.6	1.3	3.9	3.6	8.8
ILEU	1.0	0.4	0.9	ND	1.2	ND
LEU	ND	1.1	2.1	11.3	ND	1.7
TYR	0.6	0.6	0.6	0.8	1.3	1.8
PHE	0.9	1.4	0.8	1.1	1.2	1.1
HIS	0.5	0.8	0.5	0.6	1.3	1.0
LYS	3.3	3.0	3.1	4.7	1.3	2.1
ARG	3.1	3.6	2.7	2.4	1.2	0.9
100% in nmol/mgDCW						
	103.2	58.4	146.7	79.9	1.4	1.36

(a) The concentration ratio was calculated by dividing the actual
     concentration (in nmol/mgDCW) of each individual amino acid as
     found in extracts of the mutant and wild-type strains.

     ND - could not be detected; DCW - Dry Cell Weight

tration and composition of individual amino acids in the pool between
mutant and wild type strains. Generally, the total pool content of
the AEC resistant mutants tested was higher than that of the wild-type
strain. However, the data presented in Table 5 show that the most
striking individual difference was in the concentration of diaminopimelic acid (DAP).

Elevated DAP pool contents were characteristic of most mutants
which were resistant to AEC and possessed an altered regulation of
their aspartokinase activity. DAP concentration in such mutant
strains could account for about 15% of the total free amino acid pool,
whereas, wild-type extracts contained only 0.5% DAP. The values for
DAP concentrations followed the same pattern throughout the growth
cycle; highest values were always found during the initial growth
phase (7).

The pool content of threonine and lysine was also higher in the
mutant strain as compared to the wild type. In the case of lysine,
the increase occurred mainly during later growth stages. In some of
the mutant strains the lysine content at 72h was two to three times
higher than in the wild-type strain. Glycine, which represented about
2% of the total free amino acid in the pool in the wild-type strain
was usually found at similar concentrations in the mutant cells
extracted at the early growth phase. However, a four-fold increase in
glycine content was observed in samples extracted from mutant cells
late in growth. Small changes in relative concentrations of other
amino acids as a function of growth were observed. However, such
changes showed no consistency with respect to species of amino acid or
to strain of organism.

4   DAP-DECARBOXYLASE ACTIVITY IN S. CLAVULIGERUS EXTRACTS

The large accumulation of DAP indicated the possibility that the
conversion of DAP to lysine by DAP-decarboxylase was also subject to
feedback control. This enzyme was characterized and shown to be susceptible to feedback inhibition by L-lysine. The inhibition was
incomplete, even at lysine concentrations up to 50 mM (Table 6).

The fact that DAP-decarboxylase of S. clavuligerus was feedback
inhibited by lysine could explain the observation that DAP accumulated
in those mutants possessing impaired regulation of aspartokinase. It
is therefore suggested that DAP-decarboxylase can be a rate limiting
step in the carbon flow toward AAA and thus could also affect the rate
of antibiotic production.

Table 6.   Effect of amino acids and lysine analogs on
           DAP-decarboxylase activity[a]

Amino acid added	Concentration mM	Relative Activity
No addition	-	100
Glutamate	10	104
Methionine	10	106
L-Alanine	10	36
D-Alanine	10	107
Valine	10	91
Glycine	10	98
Threonine	10	92
Homoserine	10	104
AEC	10	104
D-Lysine	10	90
Hydroxylysine	10	99
α-AAA	10	101
Cysteine	10	85
Lysine	10	51
Lysine	2	67
Lysine	1	91
Lysine	0.5	104

(a)   DAP-decarboxylase activity was measured by determining the
      release of radioactive CO_2 from mixtures of 14C-labeled DL-meso-
      DAP as substrate; 100% activity is equivalent to the release of
      0.3 μmoles of CO_2 per h per mg protein.

5   CONCLUDING REMARKS

We have attempted to examine the idea whether or not the link
existing between primary and secondary metabolism implies the possibility of obtaining high producer strains, through selection of
mutants that are deregulated in the biosynthesis of a primary metabolite that is directly involved as a precursor in the synthesis of the
antibiotic.   Initially the involvement of the primary metabolite as a
rate-limiting factor in antibiotic biosynthesis must be established.
This was shown to be the case with lysine metabolism in <u>S. clavuli-
gerus</u>.   Physiological experiments have shown the specific effect the

addition of lysine and diaminopimelic acid to the fermentation media
on antibiotic production. Further biochemical analysis of enzyme
activities involved in the aspartic acid pathway revealed the key role
of aspartokinase in controlling the flow of carbon towards the lysine
specific branch in the pathway. Based on this information, mutants
deregulated in their aspartokinase activity were selected. The majority of these AEC-resistant aspartokinase-deregulated mutants produced
higher antibiotic titers as well as higher specific production values.
The free amino acid pool study revealed accumulation of DAP rather
than lysine or AAA. This later observation was found to be a result
of lysine control over the DAP-decarboxylase step similar to that
reported for Streptomyces lipmanii (8).

It should be noted that mutants overproducing lysine (for which
DAP is a biosynthetic intermediate in prokaryotes) have been isolated
from several other microorganisms having a phenotype of lysine analog
resistance. These overproducing mutants were also shown to be
deregulated in their aspartokinase activity (5). Lysine
overproduction was shown primarily to result in an extracellular
accumulation of the amino acid. On the other hand, lysine auxotrophs
of S. lipmanii, blocked in DAP-decarboxylase, accumulated DAP
intracellularly (8).

Comparison of the results obtained from studies on lysine control
of β-lactam antibiotic synthesis in fungi and streptomyces reveals the
difference in production capacity found among the lysine analog-
resistant mutants of these organisms. Lysine analog resistant mutants
of Penicillium chrysogenum were isolated, two of which overproduced
lysine and were inferior to their parent strain in penicillin
production (9). The rationale behind the isolation of lysine
analog-resistant mutants was, in both studies, to obtain a lysine over
producer. However, such mutants gave opposite results with respect to
antibiotic synthesis.

Our finding that antibiotic synthesis in S. clavuligerus was stimulated by DAP accumulation, either through genetic deregulation or by
the addition of DAP to the growth medium of a wild-type strain strongly suggests that individual amino acid pool levels can control the
biosynthesis of secondary metabolites such as cephamycin C. Therefore, we believe that such a study can provide an additional framework
on which to base genetic modification leading to strain improvement.

6 ACKNOWLEDGEMENT

We wish to thank J.N. Campbell for reading the manuscript and for his valuable comments, and Mrs. V. Kervin for the expert typing of the manuscript.

7 REFERENCES

(1) S.W. Drew, A.L. Demain, Ann. Rev. Microbiol. 31 (1977) 343-356.

(2) C.E. Higgens, R.E. Kastner, Int. J. Syst. Bacteriol. 21 (1971) 326-331.

(3) S. Mendelovitz, Y. Aharonowitz, Antimicrob. Agents Chemother. 21 (1982) 74-84.

(4) S. Mendelovitz, Y. Aharonowitz, J. Gen. Microbiol. 123 (1983) 2062-2069.

(5) K. Sano, I. Shiio, J. Gen. Appl. Microbiol. 16 (1970) 373-391.

(6) I. Shiio, R. Miyajima, J. Biochem. (tokyo) 65 (1969) 849-859.

(7) Y. Aharonowitz, S. Mendelovitz, F. Kirenberg, V. Kuper, J. Bacteriol. 157 (1984) 337-340.

(8) J.R. Kirkpatrick, L.E. Doolin, O.W. Godfrey, Antimicrob. Agents Chemother. 4 (1973) 542-550.

(9) P.S. Masurekar, A.L. Demain, Antimicrob. Agents Chemother. 6 (1974) 366-368.

Genetics of Penicillium chrysogenum and Biosynthesis of ß-Lactam Antibiotics

Geoffrey Holt, Mark E. Rogers and Gunter Saunders

The Polytechnic of Central London, School of Biotechnology, Faculty of Engineering and Science, 115 New Cavendish Street, London W1M 8JS, England

Our knowledge of the genetics and biochemistry of the synthesis of penicillin by <u>Penicillium chrysogenum</u> has grown gradually over the last four decades[1,2]. In recent years biochemists have contributed the most significant advances by the purification of several of the enzymes involved and establishing suitable cell free synthetic systems[3,4]. In contrast, genetic investigations other than empirical mutagenesis to increase yield, have not proceeded at the same pace, a consequence no doubt of the fact that genetic analysis via the parasexual cycle is rather long-winded[5]. This situation will be changed when a rational application of recombinant DNA technology is possible.

At the Polytechnic of Central London our studies originally concentrated on the wild type Peoria isolate of <u>P. chrysogenum</u> NRRL 1951[6]. After the isolation of 78 penicillin non-producing (Npe) derivatives from NRRL1951 using a test system involving biological assay, and subsequent complementation analysis, 5 genetic loci were implicated in the secondary metabolic pathway, designated groups V, W, X, Y and Z[7,8]. Biochemical analysis of representatives of each complementation group with respect to intermediates and enzymes involved in the penicillin biosynthetic pathway was also carried out. Briefly, members of complementation groups X, Y and Z appear not to be capable of synthesising tripeptide like material, but do possess an acyl-exchange activity suggesting that they are blocked at an early stage in biosynthesis. Members of groups V and W however, do synthesize

tripeptide and are therefore more likely to be blocked at ring closure
or in the acyl-transferase terminal reactions. Of particular interest
was the observation that in members of complementation groups X and Y
no intermediates were detected and only trace levels of enzymes found.
When coupled with the fact that greater than 50% of Npe isolates are
members of complementation group Y, and that naturally occurring Npe
isolates of P. chrysogenum have been shown to be blocked in synthesis
at this point[9], indicates a possible key role for this particular gene.
Linkage analysis has been carried out for the npe genes and has shown
these genes to be located on 3 separate linkage groups, with three
genes (W, Y, Z) found on linkage group I[10].

Like others we have investigated,in the last few years, a fresh
approach aimed at constructing a usable cloning system for P.
chrysogenum and in addition developing novel analytical techniques for
the detection of intermediates of the biosynthetic pathway.

The advantages of a genetic approach involving recombinant DNA
techniques are manifold and have been discussed elsewhere[11] including
in relation to filamentous fungi producing β-lactams[12]. Cloning vectors
for filamentous fungi are generally rudimentary[11] when compared to
those currently available for prokaryotes including antibiotic-
producing Streptomycetes[13,14]. However, usable systems within the
filamentous fungi have been established most particularly for
Neurospora crassa[15,16,17] and latterly, Aspergillus nidulans[18,19,20,21].
In almost all cases selection of transformants is made on the basis of
complementation of a biochemical deficiency in a specific recipient
strain[22]. In only one published example is selection made on the basis
of resistance to an antibiotic[23]. Usually genes involved in amino acid
metabolism of fungi have been cloned on typical E. coli plasmid vectors,
the clones being detected on the basis of complementation of the
corresponding biosynthetic deficiency in E. coli. The recombinant
plasmid obtained can be used to transform a similar auxotrophic
derivative of the fungus usually by integration of the vector into the
site of homology of the host chromosome(s). Subsequent development of
such vectors has illustrated the potential of fungal satellite DNA in
conferring autonomous replicative ability on integrative vectors or on
elevating transformation frequencies[16].

As a first step an examination has been made of the nucleic acid
content of a range of isolates of P. chrysogenum concentrating
initially on NRRL1951. Although small-scale rapid isolation can be
achieved by lysis and phenol extraction of protoplasts[24], it has been

found at PCL that extraction of large quantities of nucleic acid is best done by grinding lyophilised mycelium.

Using high-performance liquid chromatography, we have determined the base content of DNA extracted from P. chrysogenum, after acid hydrolysis. Reversed-phase chromatographic systems employing an anionic ion-pairing agent have been developed which enable the rapid separation and sensitive quantitation of all major nucleic acid bases[25]. The relative G+C content of DNA obtained from P. chrysogenum has been determined by this method to be 51.5% correlating with data we have obtained previously using density gradient centrifugation. Optimization of the chromatographic procedure for methylated bases, resulted in the detection of N^6-methyladenine and, using estimates obtained for molar proportions of the bases, was determined to be present at 0.1 mole percent. No 5-methylcytosine was detected in samples of the same DNA after either acid or enzymic hydrolysis. The fractionation of high molecular weight DNA can be achieved either by density gradient centrifugation or chromatography using RPC-5 analog[26,27]. Although ultracentrifugation provides good separation of nuclear from mitochondrial DNA, RPC-5 Analog is much better suited to the isolation of ribosomal RNA genes as a discrete part of nuclear DNA. Using RPC-5 Analog high molecular weight DNA was fractionated into the three distinct types expected[26]. Using DNA isolated and fractionated in this way a mitochondrial restriction enzyme map for NRRL1951 has been constructed[28]. In addition fragments of the ribosomal repeat unit[29] and most recently more than 90% of the mitochondrial genome[24] have been cloned in a yeast/E. coli chimaeric vector designed to permit the detection of autonomously replicating sequences (ars) in yeast[30].

We have also analysed the nucleic acid content of a range of wild type isolates of P. chrysogenum, kindly provided by the late Dr. Dorothy Fennel. In general although strain NRRL1951 contains considerable quantities of viral RNA[31] other wild isolates of the same species do not. In fact 95% of isolates we tested using a rapid extraction procedure, did not appear to contain viral RNA and those that did appeared to harbour different molecular weight species to those characteristically found in NRRL1951. Conversely restriction enzyme analysis of the mitochondrial DNA from 14 wild isolates has demonstrated identical patterns to that found for NRRL1951 except for two strains that show significant changes in their mitochondrial genome one having lost 30% and the other 56% by molecular weight[24]. To date no plasmid-like DNA elements, of either nuclear or mitochondrial origin, have been detected in any of the isolates examined in detail.

Characterization in a similar way of the mitochondrial DNA from a
number of strains with higher penicillin yields (including P1, P2 from
Panlabs Inc. and Wis54-1255[32]) show no gross changes in the
mitochondrial DNA.

To assist vector development extensive gene banks of NRRL1951 have
been constructed in the E. coli plasmid vector pBR328 using partial
digests of BamHI or HindIII and E. coli strain HB101[29] as recipient
(see Fig. 1). Several thousand colonies obtained were pooled from
plates and stored at -20°C. Aliquots of the pool were pelleted, washed

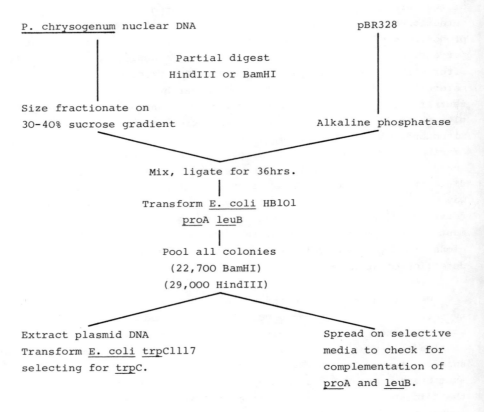

Figure 1. Construction of P. chrysogenum clone banks.

3X in liquid minimal medium and then plated on selective agar, selection being made for growth in the absence of proline or leucine. From the HindIII bank, isolates able to grow independently of a proline or leucine supplement were obtained. Subsequent investigations demonstrated the ability of these two recombinant plasmids (pPC-1 and pPC-2) to transform HB101 cultures to proline and leucine independence respectively. Curing of the HB101 plasmid-carrying strains resulted in the concomitant loss of the ability to grow without supplements.

In addition using the BamHI clone bank we have isolated a further recombinant plasmid able to complement the trpC mutation of E. coli. It will be realised that these are the essential prerequisites for successful transformation of P. chrysogenum.

In our studies involving the use of HPLC to investigate the bio-synthesis of β-lactam antibiotics, detection by UV absorption of intermediates such as isopenicillin N and 6-APA which possess no chromogenic moiety, was considered unsatisfactory due to high back-ground interferences from other sample constituents. Thus, two derivatization procedures were developed which allow the determination of β-lactam antibiotics at trace levels (0.5-1.0µg/ml) in complex samples with the minimum of pretreatment[33,34] (see Fig. 2). In one of these procedures, post-column reaction of β-lactams possessing a primary amino group with o-phthaldialdehyde permits fluorescence detection of the antibiotics following reversed-phase HPLC. Alternatively, imidazole-catalysed isomerism of penicillins to penicillenic acids has been used as a pre-column derivatization method allowing detection of the products at 325nm.

These HPLC techniques have been employed to investigate the production of hydrophobic penicillins and their biosynthetic precursors by strains of Penicillium chrysogenum, isolated in our laboratories after mutagenic treatment. Several of these strains, derived from the strain P1, appeared to be partially impaired in hydrophobic penicillin production. For example, P42 produced only 3.1% of penicillin V when compared to the parent strain P1 which produced 4.9mg/ml of this anti-biotic under the same fermentation conditions. However, no accumulation of the intermediates, 6-APA or isopenicillin N was detected in any of these strains and those that appeared impaired in hydrophobic penicillin production also produced lower titres of the intermediates.

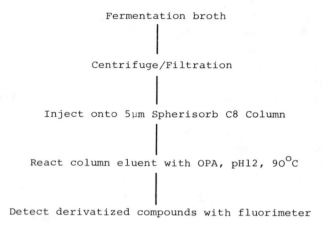

eg. amino acids, dipeptides, tripeptides, penicillin N, 6-APA, cephalosporins, cephamycins.

Post Column Derivatization Using o-Phthaldialdehyde
_____

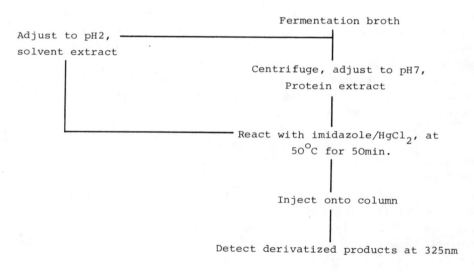

eg. Penicillins F, G, K, V, X

Pre-Column Derivatization of β-lactams with Imidazole/HgCl₂
_____

Figure 2.   Derivatization techniques for detection of β-lactams

The production of intermediates has been studied during the fermentation of P. chrysogenum in which side-chain precursor was omitted from the media, thus reducing yield of the final hydrophobic penicillin. These investigations have shown an initial accumulation of isopenicillin N in the media, followed by a decline in the concentration of this antibiotic after 3-4 days growth. Concomitantly, accumulation of 6-APA occurred at a slightly later stage in the fermentation, beginning after approximately 3 days growth and continuing throughout the 7 day fermentation period. In addition, we have analysed by HPLC a large number of Npe derivatives. Employing derivatisation techniques and radiolabelling of intermediates, no accumulation of either 6-APA or isopenicillin N has been observed. These data lend support to the proposal that a branched biosynthetic pathway occurs in the late stages of penicillin synthesis and in order to obtain such an accumulation at least two specific enzymic steps would have to be impaired.

Cephalosporin-producing organisms such as Acremonium chrysogenum produce both isopenicillin N and penicillin N intermediates[35]. Using the pre-column derivatization procedure previously described[36] which enables separation of these isomers, we have investigated the specific isomeric nature of the intermediate produced by P. chrysogenum. Following isolation by HPLC of the ^{14}C-labelled intermediate from a fermentation of strain Pl, the sample was analysed by pre-column derivatization with 2,3,4,6-tetra-O-acetyl- -D-glycopyranosyl isocyanate. Following HPLC, only isopenicillin N was detected using UV absorption and liquid scintillation counting of the fractions collected. This supports the claim[37] that P. chrysogenum is incapable of penicillin N production and thus is devoid of the necessary precursor for 'normal' cephalosporin biosynthesis.

In recent years, much attention has been focused on the bio synthesis of β-lactam antibiotics and in particular the specific enzymic steps involved in cephalosporin biosynthesis[3,4,38]. Although assays for certain of the enzymes involved in penicillin biosynthesis have been described[39,40,41] relatively little has appeared in the literature recently concerning these enzymes. Discrete vesicles, present in the cytoplasm of P. chrysogenum, have been isolated which are claimed to be capable of penicillin biosynthesis when supplied with certain cofactors and amino acid precursors[42] although we have failed to reproduce these findings.

Recently the ring closure enzyme (isopenicillin N synthetase) from

both A. chrysogenum[43] and P.chrysogenum[44] have been characterized and
purified to homogeneity. In both cases they appear to be stimulated
by ferrous ions and are present in a soluble fraction of the cell
constituents. Studies are underway in different labs to investigate
the possible occurrence of a previously described monobactam intermediate produced by P. chrysogenum[45].

In another context we have recently worked on the enzyme
β-lactamase which is produced under certain conditions by
P. chrysogenum[46]. These studies have involved an investigation of
purification techniques for β-lactamase including reversed-phase
HPLC[47], and high-performance liquid affinity chromatography in which
the ligand, cephalosporin C, was bound to a rigid polymer support
matrix (TSK4000PW) following activation with cyanogen bromide[48]. Since
low, medium and high penicillin yielding strains are capable of
producing β-lactamase this enzyme appears not to be directly related
to penicillin biosynthesis.

Much work remains to be done on the biosynthesis and regulation of
β-lactam production. Of the major groups of organisms producing such
antibiotics[12] the streptomycetes can already be studied using
appropriate cloning vectors[49,50]. In the case of the fungi,vectors
for use in Aspergillus, are already available[18,19]
and there is no doubt that such systems are now available for
Penicillium and Acremonium. The future therefore now looks bright to
unravel the structure and regulation of genes involved in β-lactam
biosynthesis. This has implications not only for immediate commercial
production but for the wider understanding of secondary metabolism.

REFERENCES

(1) J. F. Martin, P. Liras, Trends in Biotech. 3 (2) (1985) 39-44.

(2) S. W. Queener, S. Wilkerson, D. R. Tunin, J. R. McDermott, J. L.
    Chapman, J. L. Nash, C. Platt, J. Westpheling in E. Vandamme (Ed.),
    Biotechnology of Industrial Antibiotics, Marcel Dekker, 1984,
    pp. 141-170.

(3) D. J. Hook, L. T. Chang, R. P. Elander, R. B. Morin, Biochem.
    Biophys. Res. Commun. 87 (1979) 258-265.

(4) M. K. Turner, J. E. Farthing, J. J. Brewer, Biochem. J. 173 (1978)
    839-850.

(5) G. Pontecorvo, J. A. Roper, L. M. Hemmons, K. D. Macdonald, A. W. J. Bufton, Adv. in Genet. 5 (1953) 141–238.

(6) K. B. Raper, D. F. Alexander, J. Elisha Mitchell Scientific Soc. 61 (1947) 74–113.

(7) P. M. J. Normansell, I. D. Normansell, G. Holt, J. Gen. Microbiol. 112 (1979) 113–126.

(8) J. F. Makins, G. Holt, K. D. Macdonald, J. Gen. Microbiol. 119 (1980) 397–404.

(9) J. F. Makins, A. E. Allsop, G. Holt, J. Gen. Microbiol. 122 (1981) 339–343.

(10) C. M. Blake, G. Holt, unpublished data.

(11) K. N. Timmis in S. W. Glover, D. A. Hopwood (Eds.), Genetics as a Tool in Microbiology, Society for General Microbiology, 1981, pp. 49–109.

(12) G. Holt, M. W. Adlard, E. Lisboa, M. E. Rogers, S. D. Rogers, G. Saunders, T. M. Smith, Biochem. Soc. Trans. 12 (1984) 577–580.

(13) K. F. Chater, D. A. Hopwood, T. Keiser, C. J. Thompson in E. Hofschneider, S. Goebel (Eds.), Gene Cloning in Organisms Other than E. coli, 1982, pp. 69–107.

(14) D. A. Hopwood, M. J. Bibb, C. J. Bruton, K. F. Chater, J. S. Feitelson, J. A. Gil, Trends in Biotech. 1 (2) (1983) 42–48.

(15) M. E. Case, M. Scheweizer, S. R. Kushner, N. H. Giles, Proc. Natl. Acad. Sci. 76 (10) (1979) 5259–5263.

(16) L. L. Stohl, A. M. Lambowitz, Proc. Natl. Acad. Sci. 80 (1983) 1058–1062.

(17) D. M. Grant, A. M. Lambowitz, J. A. Rambosek, J. A. Kinsey, Mol. Cell. Biol. 4 (10) (1984) 2041–2051.

(18) D. J. Ballance, F. P. Buxton, G. Turner, Biochem. Biophys. Res. Commun. 112 (1983) 284–289.

(19) J. Tilburn, C. Scazzochio, G. G. Taylor, J. H. Zabicky-Zissman, R. A. Lockington, R. W. Davies, Gene 26 (1983) 205-221.

(20) M. M. Yelton, J. E. Hamer, W. E. Timberlake, Proc. Natl. Acad. Sci. 81 (1984) 1470-1474.

(21) M. A. John, J. F. Peberdy, Enz. Micro. Tech. 6 (9) (1984) 386-389.

(22) G. Saunders, M. F. Tuite, G. Holt, Trends in Biotech, in press.

(23) G. Banks, Curr. Genet. 7 (1983) 73-77.

(24) P. Ford, G. Saunders, G. Holt, unpublished data.

(25) S. D. Rogers, G. Saunders, G. Holt, Proc. NATO Adv. Study Inst., Recent Developments in Biotechnology, Plenum Press, 1985, in press.

(26) G. Saunders, M. E. Rogers, M. W. Adlard, G. Holt, Molec. Gen. Genet. 194 (1984) 343-345.

(27) G. Saunders, M. E. Rogers, M. W. Adlard, G. Holt, Trans. Biochem. Soc. 12 (1984) 692-693.

(28) T. M. Smith, G. Saunders, L. M. Stacey, G. Holt, J. Biotech. 1 (1984) 37-46.

(29) G. Saunders, G. Holt, unpublished data.

(30) J. F. Monteil, C. J. Norbury, M. F. Tuite, M. J. Dobson, J. S. Mills, A. J. Kingsman, S. M. Kingsman, Nucl. Ac. Res. 12 (2) (1984) 1049-1067.

(31) I. D. Normansell, G. Holt, Mycovirus Newsl. 6 (1978) 15.

(32) R. P. Elander in A. L. Demain, N. A. Solomon (Eds.), Antibiotics Containing the β-lactam Structure, Springer-Verlag, 1983, pp. 97-146.

(33) M. E. Rogers, M. W. Adlard, G. Saunders, G. Holt, J. Chromatogr. 257 (1983) 91-100.

(34) M. E. Rogers, M. W. Adlard, G. Saunders, G. Holt, J. Liquid

Chromatogr. <u>257</u> (1983) 91-100.

(35) T. Konomi, S. Herchen, J. E. Baldwin, M. Yoshida, N. A. Hunt, A.
     L. Demain, Biochem. J. <u>184</u> (1979) 427-430.

(36) N. Neuss, D. M. Berry, J. Kupka, A. L. Demain, S. W. Queener,
     D. C. Duckworth, L. L. Huckstep, J. Antibiot. <u>35</u> (1982) 580-584.

(37) A. L. Demain, N. A. Solomon (Ed.), Antibiotics Containing the
     β-lactam Structure, Springer-Verlag, Berlin 1983, p. 197.

(38) S. E. Jensen, W. S. Donald, W. S. Westlake, S. Wolfe, J.
     Antibiot. <u>37</u> (1985) 263-265.

(39) P. A. Fawcett, J. J. Usher, E. P. Abraham, Biochem. J. <u>151</u> (1975)
     741-746.

(40) R. Brunner, M. Roehr, M. Zinner, Z. Hoppe-Seylers, Physiol.
     Chem. <u>349</u> (1968) 95-103.

(41) B. Spencer, C. Maung, Proc. Biochem. Soc. <u>118</u> (1970) 39-40.

(42) W. Kurzatkowski, W. Kurylowicz, A. Penyige, Appl. Micro. Biotech.
     <u>19</u> (1984) 312-315.

(43) I. J. Hollander, Y.-Q. Shen, J. Heim, A. L. Demain, Science <u>224</u>
     (1984) 610-612.

(44) F. R. Ramos, M. J. Lopez-Nieto, J. F. Martin, Antimicrob. Agents
     Chemother. <u>27</u> (1985) 380-387.

(45) B. Meesschaert, P. Adriaens, H. Eyssen, J. Antibiot. <u>33</u> (1980)
     722-730.

(46) S. Whan Lee, K. Chung Hur, K. Soo Lee, W. S. Kim, Dor. J. Mycol.
     <u>8</u> (1) (1980) 63-68.

(47) M. E. Rogers, M. W. Adlard, G. Saunders, G. Holt, Analyst (in
     press).

(48) M. E. Rogers, M. W. Adlard, G. Saunders, G. Holt, J. Chromatogr.
     (in press).

(49) J. S. Feitelson, D. A. Hopwood, Molec. Gen. Genet. <u>190</u> (1983) 394-398.

(50) D. A. Hopwood, F. Malpartida, H. M. Kieser, H. Ikeda, J. Duncan, I. Fujii, B. A. M. Rudd, H. G. Floss, S. Omura, Nature <u>314</u> (1985) 642-644.

Enzymes Involved in Penicillin and Cephalosporin Formation

Sir Edward P. Abraham

University of Oxford, Sir William Dunn School of Pathology, South Parks Road, Oxford OX1 3RE, England

SUMMARY

Virtually all the biosynthetic reactions involved in the biosynthesis of penicillins and cephalosporins have now been demonstrated in cell-free systems. Some of them have parallels in other fields but those catalysed by isopenicillin N synthetase and the deacetoxycephalosporin C-forming ring expansion enzyme are of a new type. The synthetase has been isolated in an almost pure state. Cloning of the gene which mediates its production is within sight and cloning of other genes may follow. Advances in this area could throw light on the regulation of antibiotic production.

1 INTRODUCTION

Benzylpenicillin and other solvent-soluble penicillins are produced by Penicillium chrysogenum while cephalosporin C and other cephalosporins are formed by Cephalosporium acremonium, Streptomyces spp. and some species of eubacteria. The non-polar N-acyl side-chain of the penicillins from P. chrysogenum (RCO in 1) can be changed by the addition of appropriate precursors to a fermentation, but in general the D-α-aminoadipyl side-chain of the cephalosporins (2) is invariable.

There is now convincing evidence, based on studies with cell-free enzymes and blocked mutants, for the belief that both series of compounds are derived from the same three L-amino acids, which condense to form δ-(L-α-aminoadipyl)-L-cysteinyl-D-valine (LLD-ACV).

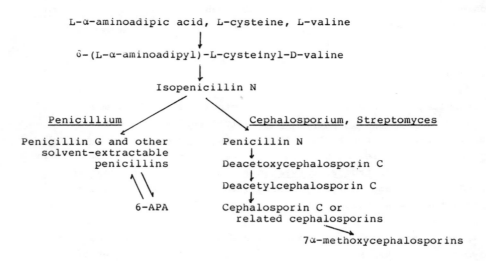

This tripeptide can undergo an oxidative cyclisation to yield
isopenicillin N, with an L-α-aminoadipyl side-chain. The zwitteronic
side-chain of isopenicillin N can be exchanged in <u>P</u>. <u>chrysogenum</u> for
side-chains such as phenylacetyl and phenoxyacetyl and can also be
removed to yield 6-aminopenicillanic acid (6-APA), but it is
epimerised in the <u>Cephalosporium</u> and <u>Streptomyces</u> spp. to the
D-α-aminoadipyl side-chain of penicillin N. The five-membered
thiazolidine ring of penicillin N then undergoes an oxidative
expansion to the six-membered dihydrothiazine ring of
deacetoxycephalosporin C. The latter is the precursor of other
cephalosporins, formed by oxidation of its exocyclic methyl group to
a hydroxymethyl group (<u>2</u>, R' = OH, X = H) which can be acylated. In
<u>Streptomyces</u> spp. a methoxy group can then be introduced into
the 7α-position of the β-lactam ring (<u>2</u>, X = OCH₃). These
biosynthetic pathways are summarised in Fig. 1.

L-α-aminoadipic acid, L-cysteine, L-valine

↓

δ-(L-α-aminoadipyl)-L-cysteinyl-D-valine

↓

Isopenicillin N

<u>Penicillium</u>   <u>Cephalosporium</u>, <u>Streptomyces</u>

Penicillin G and other   Penicillin N
  solvent-extractable
  penicillins   Deacetoxycephalosporin C

                                    Deacetylcephalosporin C

        6-APA   Cephalosporin C or
                                      related cephalosporins

                                              7α-methoxycephalosporins

Fig. 1. Biosynthetic pathways to penicillins and cephalosporins.

Virtually all the reactions leading to penicillin and cephalosporin biosynthesis have now been demonstrated in cell-free systems. Some of these reactions have parallels in wider fields. They include those which result in transacylation in P. chrysogenum and those which bring about epimerisation of the side-chain of isopenicillin N, and the oxidation of a methyl group at C-3 and the introduction of a methoxy group at C-7 in the cephalosporin series. However, the oxidative reactions catalysed by isopenicillin N synthetase, which converts LLD-ACV to isopenicillin N, and by a ring expansion enzyme, which converts penicillin N to deacetoxycephalosporin C, are of a new type.

What is the present state of our knowledge of this collection of at least eight different enzymes? The isolation of the enzymes can tell us nothing, in itself, about the regulation of the reactions that they catalyse. But the purification of an enzyme can be followed by the determination of some of its amino acid sequence and this in turn can lead to the cloning of the corresponding gene and to a knowledge of the regulation of its expression.

2 THE COMMON TRIPEPTIDE PRECURSOR

The situation is perhaps least satisfactory with respect to the synthesis of LLD-ACV. Following its isolation fourteen years ago from the mycelium of Cephalosporium acremonium (1) this peptide was found to be produced in small amount in ultrasonic extracts of the mycelium from δ-(L-α-aminoadipyl)-L-cysteine and [^{14}C] valine and it was concluded that its biosynthesis was analogous to that of glutathione (2). But the failure to obtain extracts with more than a very low activity appears to have hindered further study of the enzymes involved. This problem deserves further attention, since an inadequate production of the tripeptide would limit the rate at all the subsequent biosynthetic steps. In two cases the concentration of LLD-ACV in extracts of high-yielding strains of C. acremonium obtained from pharmaceutical companies appeared to be considerably higher than the strain available in our laboratory. Under some conditions the production of penicillin by P. chrysogenum can be limited by the supply of α-aminoadipic acid, which is controlled by lysine (3,4).

3   THE ACYLASE AND TRANSACYLASE IN PENICILLIUM SPECIES

Reports on the presence of an acylase in P. chrysogenum which
removes the side-chain of benzylpenicillin to yield 6-APA and of an
acyltransferase which catalyses an exchange of side-chains between
benzylpenicillin and other solvent-soluble penicillins, or between
such penicillins and 6-APA, have a long history (5,6,7,8). The
production of penicillins from 6-APA and acylcoenzyme A in
the presence of an acyltransferase was described in 1968; and later
a phenylacyl:CoA ligase was isolated (9). It was suggested that the
acylase and transferase activities were associated with a single
enzyme (10). The acylase was said to bring about no detectable
hydrolysis of penicillin N or isopenicillin N (11,12). But it was
shown later that an enzyme, or enzymes, in an extract obtained by
grinding the mycelium with sand would catalyse the formation of
benzylpenicillin ($\underline{5}$, R = $C_6H_5CH_2$) from isopenicillin N ($\underline{3}$), as well
as from 6-APA ($\underline{4}$), in the presence of phenylacetylCoA (13).

Preliminary attempts to isolate an isopenicillin N acylase from a
strain of P. chrysogenum were hampered by the extreme instability of
the enzyme in crude extracts of the mycelium obtained by grinding the
latter with glass beads at 4°C (14). This problem was largely
overcome by carrying out the early stages of purification, during
which some proteases were presumably removed, as rapidly as possible.
By conventional procedures a purification of more than a hundred fold
could then be achieved (15). The enzyme appeared to have a molecular
weight of less than 40,000. It catalysed the formation of 6-APA from
both isopenicillin N ($\underline{3}$) and benzylpenicillin ($\underline{5}$) at an initial rate
which was about 30% of the corresponding rate with
phenoxymethylpenicillin (5, R = $C_6H_5OCH_2$) as a substrate; since the
L-α-aminoadipyl side-chain of isopenicillin N was liberated as
α-aminoadipic acid the latter was presumably used again in the
synthesis of LLD-ACV. However, under the conditions used the
reaction virtually ceased after only a small proportion of substrate
had been hydrolysed. This could not be attributed simply to a
reversible reaction, because no formation of a penicillin was
detected when the enzyme was incubated with 6-APA and L-α-aminoadipic
acid. But 6-APA itself was found to be a powerful inhibitor of
the acylase. The inhibition was reversible, since activity was
regained when the inactivated acylase was passed through a column of
Sephadex G-25.

This active preparation showed transacylase as well as acylase
activity although there was no evidence for the presence of more than
one enzyme. It catalysed the transfer of a phenylacetyl group from

phenylacetylCoA to 6-APA. It also catalysed an exchange of the
ô-(L-α-aminoadipyl) group of isopenicillin N for the phenylacetyl
group of phenylacetylCoA. Whether free 6-APA is a obligatory
intermediate in the latter reaction and is acylated by the type of
ping-pong mechanism believed to operate in the acylation of
sulphanilamide (Fig. 2) remains to be determined. If so, its removal

by acylation would reduce the inhibition resulting from its own
formation. In the mycelial cell the accumulation of 6-APA could also
be reduced by its excretion into the surrounding medium. It was
thought at first that penicillin N, unlike isopenicillin N, was not
a substrate for the transacylase (13). But when more active
preparations of the enzyme could be tested it became evident that
the requirement for the L-isomer of a ô-(α-aminoadipyl) side-chain
was not absolute, since the initial rate of production of 6-APA from
penicillin N was about 5% of that from isopenicillin N. This is one
of a number of cases in which enzymes catalysing reactions in
the pathways shown in Fig. 1 can use modified substrates, although
less effectively than the natural ones. Recently it has been

reported that extracts of several mutant strains of P. chrysogenum
contain an acyltransferase which can bring about a detectable
exchange of the δ-(D-α-aminoadipyl) side-chain of cephalosporin C for
a phenoxyeacetyl side-chain and thus yield a cephalosporin analogue
of penicillin V (16).

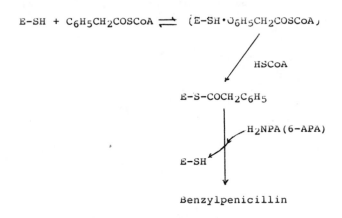

$$E-SH + C_6H_5CH_2COSCoA \rightleftharpoons (E-SH \cdot C_6H_5CH_2COSCoA)$$

HSCoA

$$E-S-COCH_2C_6H_5$$

H$_2$NPA(6-APA)

E-SH

Benzylpenicillin

Fig. 2. Possible mechanism for the formation of
benzylpenicillin from 6-APA.

4 EARLY AND LATE STAGES OF CEPHALOSPORIN BIOSYNTHESIS

The first reaction in the branch of the pathway that leads from
isopenicillin N via penicillin N to cephalosporins in Cephalosporium
and Streptomyces spp. is catalysed by an epimerase. The penicillin N
is partly excreted into the culture fluid and partly converted to
deacetoxycephalosporin C (2, R = X = H). The epimerase was shown to
be present in a lysate of protoplasts of C. acremonium (and later in
an extract obtained by mechanical disruption of the mycelium) by
measurement of the large increase in activity against Salm. typhi
which accompanies the isopenicillin N to penicillin N conversion
(17). The epimerase in these extracts was extremely unstable. The
corresponding enzyme in extracts of Streptomyces clavuligerus was
also unstable but was found to be protected sufficiently by pyridoxal
phosphate (which did not stimulate its activity) for a 35-fold
purification to be accomplished (18). The molecular weight of this
epimerase was estimated to be about 60,000. It has been reported to
be a racemase which produces a 1:1 mixture of epimers (19).

Transacylases are involved in reactions at the end of the
biosynthetic pathway to cephalosporins, as they are in the case of

the hydrophobic penicillins produced by P. chrysogenum. An acetyl group is transferred from acetylCoA to the hydroxyl group of deacetylcephalosporin C (2, R' = OH, X = H) in extracts of C. acremonium (20) and a carbamoyl group is transferred from carbamoyl phosphate to the hydroxyl group of deacetylcephalosporin C (2, R' = OH) in homogenates of Streptomyces clavuligerus (21). The specificity of the enzyme, or enzymes, involved in these transacylations does not appear to have been established.

Other enzymes which function on the pathways from deacetoxycephalosporin C to further cephalosporins are oxygenases. Mass spectrum analysis of cephalosporins produced by suspensions of the mycelium of C. acremonium and Streptomyces clavuligerus in the presence of $^{18}O_2$ showed that the oxygen atoms attached to the exocyclic methylene of cephalosporin C (2, R'$\approx$OCOCH$_3$) and to the β-lactam ring of a 7α-methoxycephalosporin (2, X = OCH$_3$) respectively were derived from molecular oxygen (22,23). It was then found that the oxidation of the methyl group at C-3 in deacetoxycephalosporin C was brought about by a dioxygenase (hydroxylase) requiring Fe^{2+}, ascorbate and α-ketoglutarate for activity (24) and subsequently that the incorporation of a 7α-methoxy group into cephalosporin C or into the carbamoyl derivative of deacetylcephalosporin C depended on a similar dioxygenase and the transfer of a methyl group from S-adenosylmethionine (25). Deacetoxycephalosporin C hydroxylase from C. acremonium (26) and S. clavuligerus (27) has been partially purified by chromatography on DEAE Sephacryl.

5   ISOPENICILLIN N SYNTHETASE

The failure of early attempts to demonstrate the biosynthesis of the penicillin or cephalosporin ring system in cell-free preparations can be attributed, at least in part, to a lack of knowledge of the co-factors required and to the instability of the enzymes concerned in crude extracts of mycelium. However, in a concentrated extract obtained by the lysis of protoplasts of C. acremonium LLD-ACV was found to be converted with its skeleton intact into a compound which behaved as either penicillin N or isopenicillin (28,29). Later a similar experiment revealed that the product was in fact isopenicillin and that little or no epimerisation of the α-aminoadipyl group had occurred under the conditions used (30,31). The conversion of LLD-ACV (6) to isopenicillin N (7) was also shown to occur in extracts of Streptomyces clavuligerus obtained by ultrasonic treatment (32).

The finding that isopenicillin N synthetase required Fe^{2+} and molecular oxygen for activity and that its activity was greatly stimulated by the presence of ascorbate and to a lesser extent by thiol compounds, such as DTT, and by catalase opened the way to further investigations (33). It was shown that the synthetase could

6

7

be extracted by grinding the mycelium of C. acremonium with glass beads on a larger scale than was feasible by the preparation and osmotic lysis of protoplasts. A partial purification of the enzyme was then accomplished by chromatography on DEAE-Sephadex. Additional purification by conventional methods led to material which appeared to be about 83% pure and which catalysed the formation of isopenicillin N at a rate of about 45 µmol/min/µmol protein (34). Modifications of the procedure used raised the specific activity to about 60µmol isopenicillin N/min/µmol protein (35). On SDS gel electrophoresis this product showed a major band and minor bands which were visible only at high loading. Proteins associated with some of the latter were removed by HPLC and the remainder may have been derived from the synthetase itself.

Isopenicillin N synthetase obtained from a different strain of C. acremonium by ultrasonic treatment was partially purified by analogous procedures (36) and the enzyme from a higher yielding strain has also been reported to have been obtained in a state approaching homogeneity as revealed by SDS gel electrophoresis (37). In the latter experiments the value of HPLC for rapid purification of the enzyme was stressed and the product of the reaction was shown to be isopenicillin N by chromatography of the derivative that it formed with a chiral D-glucopyranosylisothiocyanate (38).

Isopenicillin N synthetase in an extract of a strain of

P. chrysogenum was partially purified (34). A comparison of
extracts of several strains of P. chrysogenum indicated that
the activity of the synthetase that they contained paralleled the
amount of benzylpenicillin produced by them in fermentations (39).

The isopenicillin N synthetases from Cephalosporium, Penicillium
and Streptomyces spp. appear to resemble each other closely and to
have molecular weights of between 35,000 and 40,000. They all
require Fe^{2+} as a cofactor and their activity is stimulated by
ascorbate. Unlike the oxygenases that are involved in other
oxidative reactions in the penicillin and cephalosporin pathways,
they do not require α-ketoglutarate for activity. The
isopenicillin N synthetase from C. acremonium has at least two
cysteine residues. The thiol group of one of them is essential for
synthetase activity and is accessible to some thiol reagents but not
to others.

6   DEACETOXYCEPHALOSPORIN C SYNTHETASE

Experimental evidence for the view that penicillin N is
a precursor of a cephalosporin was first obtained in 1976 by use of
a protoplast lysate of C. acremonium (40). The product of the
reaction was subsequently shown to be deacetoxycephalosporin C (2,
R' = X = H) (41). The enzyme deacetoxycephalosporin C synthetase
requires the addition of Fe^{2+}, ascorbate and α-ketoglutarate for
maximum activity (42). A corresponding enzyme is present in
Streptomyces clavuligerus and the enzymes from both organisms have
been partly purified (26,27). The enzyme from Streptomyces
clavuligerus was estimated to have a molecular weight of 29,600 by
gel filtration (27). Deacetoxycephalosporin C synthetase and the
isopenicillin N synthetase can be separated from each other by ion
exchange chromatography and are clearly different enzymes (43,44).

Deacetoxycephalosporin C synthetase and deacetoxycephalosporin C
hydroxylase bring about sequential reactions in the biosynthetic
pathways (Fig. 1). In extracts obtained by ultrasonic treatment of
Streptomyces spp. these enzymes were readily separated from each
other by chromatography on DEAE-trisacryl and the hydroxylase
appeared to have a molecular weight of about 26,200 from its
behaviour on gel filtration through Sephadex G200 (27). On the other
hand, there was no separation under similar conditions of the enzymes
in an extract of C. acremonium (26). In view of this finding and the
similarity in co-factor requirements it was suggested that
the synthetase and hydroxylase activities were properties of a single

bifunctional enzyme (26). A more likely explanation, however, is
that the deacetoxycephalosporin C synthetase from C. acremonium binds
more strongly than that from S. clavuligerus to DEAE-trisacryl, and
is thus not separated from the hydroxylase (27).

7 SUBSTRATE PROFILES OF THE PENICILLIN AND CEPHALOSPORIN SYNTHETASES

   LLD-ACV is not the only substrate that is converted into
a penicillin by isopenicillin N synthetase but it is by far the best
of those tested. However, analogues of this tripeptide in which
certain changes have been made in its N-terminal δ-(L-α-aminoadipyl)
residue yield penicillins with the corresponding side-chains. Thus
the D-α-aminoadipyl analogue, which was at first thought to be
unacceptable to the enzyme, was shown to be converted into
penicillin N (in the absence of an epimerase) when more active
synthetase preparations became available. The adipyl analogue and
the S-carboxymethy-L-cysteinyl analogue (containing S in place of one
CH_2 in the α-aminoadipyl chain) also yielded the corresponding
penicillins (36,45,46,47). It is of interest that an
adipylpenicillin was found to be produced by fermentations of
P. chrysogenum to which adipic acid had been added (48) and that
a penicillin with a S-carboxymethyl-D-cysteinyl side-chain was
produced when the corresponding L-amino acid was added to
the fermentation of a lysine auxotroph of C. acremonium which was
unable to synthesise α-aminoadipic acid (49). In the latter case, at
least, the penicillin is presumably formed from the corresponding
tripeptide and not by the action of an acyl transferase on
isopenicillin N.
   In contrast, peptides in which the L-α-aminoadipyl residue of
LLD-ACV had been replaced by an L-glutamyl or a glutaryl residue were
not substrates, although cephalosporins with a glutaryl side-chain
have been reported to be produced by Cephalosporium mutants (50).
The failure of hexanoyl-L-cysteinyl-D-valine to yield a penicillin is
consistent with the assumption that there is no biosynthetic pathway
from such peptides to the penicillins with non-polar side-chains
produced by P. chrysogenum. δ-Aminovaleryl-L-cysteinyl-D-valine and
the tetrapeptide N-glycyl-LLD-ACV also failed to yield corresponding
penicillins in the presence of purified isopenicillin N synthetase
although the tetrapeptide was hydrolysed to LLD-ACV itself in crude
enzyme preparations and was thus converted to isopenicillin N (34).
In general, the acyl moiety of an N-acyl-L-cysteinyl-D-valine appears

to need a six carbon or equivalent chain ending in a carboxyl group
for it to function as a substrate (45).

The tripeptide LLL-ACV is not a substrate for isopenicillin N
synthetase. But peptides in which the valine residue of LLD-ACV has
been changed to D-isoleucine, D-alloisoleucine or D-α-aminobutyric
acid also yield the corresponding penicillins in the presence of the
enzyme and its co-factors (51). The use of ^{13}C, ^{1}H and ^{3}H n.m.r. to
follow such reactions has enabled new light to be thrown on the
stereochemistry of ring closures. It has also indicated that one
mole of oxygen is consumed per mole of the isopenicillin N formed
from LLD-ACV (52) and has shown that isopenicillin N synthetase can
catalyse the formation of cephams (dihydrocephalosporins) and related
compounds, as well as penams (isopenicillin N analogues), from
tripeptides with an appropriate C-terminal residue. For example,
when this residue is D-α-aminobutyrate the cepham (**8**) is formed in
addition to a desmethylpenicillin (53). Free radical mechanisms
appear to offer an acceptable explanation of these reactions (54).

In contrast to these findings all the changes made in
the L-cysteinyl residue of LLD-ACV have abolished the ability of
the resulting peptide to act as a substrate or to compete with
a substrate for the active site of isopenicillin N synthetase.
Analogues of LLD-ACV containing a serine in place of a cysteine
residue are produced by P. chrysogenum (55) but such peptides are
inert in the presence of the enzyme. A cysteine thiol group may be
involved in the binding of substrates or inhibitors to the enzyme.

Analogues of penicillin N that are obtained from modified
tripeptide substrates by the use of isopenicillin N synthetase and
the epimerase may be converted to the corresponding cephalosporins by
deacetoxycephalosporin C synthetase. In the bioconversion of
penicillin N to deacetoxycephalosporin C the β-methyl group of
the penicillin is incorporated into the endocyclic methylene of
the cephalosporin and the α-methyl group of the penicillin becomes
the exocyclic methyl group of the cephalosporin (56). In
the penicillins produced by isopenicillin N synthetase from
tripeptides with C-terminal D-α-aminobutyric acid, D-isoleucine and

D-alloisoleucine the normal gem dimethyl group is replaced by

and

respectively (51).

In the presence of the epimerase and deacetoxycephalosporin C synthetase from $\underline{S}$. $\underline{clavuligerus}$ these penicillins are converted to the corresponding cephalosporins ($\underline{9}$) in which $R_1 = R_2 = H$, $R_1 = R_2 = CH_3$ and $R_1 = H$, $R_2 = CH_2CH_3$ respectively (57). The deacetoxycephalosporin C synthetase also catalyses the ring expansion of penicillins with an S-carboxymethyl-D-cysteinyl side-chain.

9

8   PROBLEMS AND PROSPECTS

What can be expected from future studies of these eight or more enzymes? Only one of them, isopenicillin N synthetase, has so far been obtained in a pure state. The instability of others in mycelial extracts, due in part to proteolysis (34), has presented technical problems that remain to be solved. The introduction of more effective protease inhibitors and of a rapid and specific method of isolation, such as might be provided by the use of monoclonal antibodies, seems to be desirable.

Not surprisingly, the levels of penicillin acyl-transferase and isopenicillin N synthetase have been found to be higher in high yielding strains of $\underline{P}$. $\underline{chrysogenum}$ than in lower yielding strains. But which biosynthetic reactions are rate limiting in different strains of penicillin and cephalosporin-producing organisms appears to be unknown. Moreover, the rate of a reaction in mycelial cells may be controlled by factors which are absent, or more clearly defined, when the reaction is studied with a cell-free enzyme. Thus the isopenicillin N synthetase extracted from the mycelium of a relatively low-yielding strain of $\underline{C}$. $\underline{acremonium}$ could produce isopenicillin N, in the presence of optimum concentrations of LLD-ACV and co-factors, at a rate which was at least an order higher than the rate of production of penicillin N and cephalosporin C combined by the same amount of mycelium at the time of harvesting (34).

Suboptimal amounts of co-factors, an inadequate rate of production of the tripeptide substrate from amino acids, suboptimal oxygen transfer, or low epimerase activity might all contribute to the lower rate of production of extracellular antibiotics by the mycelium.

In crude extracts of mycelium a higher concentration of Fe^{2+} is required for maximum activity than in solutions of the purified enzyme, apparently because substances in these extracts compete for Fe^{2+} with the synthetase. The finding that the concentration of LLD-ACV was higher in high yielding strains of C. acremonium than in a low-yielding strain, raises the question whether synthesis of the peptide was rate-limiting in the latter. However, a further property of isopenicillin N synthetase is of interest in relation to its function in mycelial cells. The conversion of LLD-ACV to isopenicillin N by the isolated synthetase is accompanied by inactivation of the enzyme, apparently mechanism-based, which becomes evident after the latter has turned over a limited number of times (35). If this occurs in vivo it must be balanced by synthesis of the enzyme de novo during the productive phase of a fermentation.

Four different oxygenases each requiring ferrous iron are involved in the biosynthesis of penicillins and cephalosporins. Efficient oxygen transfer into the mycelium is therefore needed for maximum antibiotic production by a given set of biosynthetic enzymes. Two oxidative stages occur during the conversion of penicillin N to cephalosporin C. With suspensions of C. acremonium an increase in aeration could be used to increase the ratio cephalosporium C/penicillin N without changing significantly the total antibiotic production (58).

In view of the medical and commercial importance of the penicillins and cephalosporins it is natural to ask whether studies of the enzymes that bring about their biosynthesis may lead to results with practical application as well as of scientific interest. Several ways in which they might do so can be envisaged. The finding that the substrate specificities of isopenicillin N synthetase and deacetoxycephalosporin C synthetase are not absolute enables penicillins and cephalosporins with modified ring systems to be made by the use of isolated enzymes. Such substances cannot be obtained by fermentation because the appropriate peptide precursor is not synthesised by the organism, or cannot compete effectively as a substrate with LLD-ACV itself. It is possible that new compounds that are valuable in themselves, or as starting points for further chemical synthesis, will be obtained in this way. Secondly, an understanding of the efficient biosynthetic mechanisms by which the penicillin and cephalosporin ring systems are made could lead to

new and more effective methods of entirely chemical synthesis. The
availability of pure biosynthetic enzymes will facilitate the cloning
of the corresponding genes. This in turn will reveal the complete
amino acid sequences of the enzymes and thus bring nearer the
determination by X-ray analysis of their three-dimensional
structures, at high resolution, if suitable crystals can be obtained.
Thirdly, the cloning of genes might also open the way to
the construction of higher yielding organisms or of organisms
containing new combinations of genes that endowed them with new
biosynthetic abilities.

Cloning of the gene that encodes the isopenicillin N synthetase in
C. acremonium is about to be accomplished. It may well be that the
cloning of this and the other genes that code for the series of
enzymes in the biosynthetic pathways to penicillins and
cephalosporins will lead to major advances in this field during
the next decade.

9 REFERENCES

(1)   P. B. Loder, E. P. Abraham, Biochem. J. 123 (1971) 471-476.

(2)   P. B. Loder, E. P. Abraham, Biochem. J. 123 (1971) 477-482.

(3)   C. G. Friedrich, A. L. Demain, J. Antibiot. 30 (1972) 760-761.

(4)   J. M. Luengo, G. Revilla, M. J. Lopez-Nieto,
      J. R. Villanueva,J. F. Martin, J. Bacteriol. 144 (1980) 869-876.

(5)   K. Sakaguchi, S. Murao, J. Agr. Chem. Soc. Japan 23 (1950) 411.

(6)   W. H. Peterson, W. E. Wideburg, Proc. 4th Inter. Congr.
      Biochem. Vienna 15 (1960) 136.

(7)   S. Gatenbeck, U. Brunsberg, Acta Chem. Scand. 22 (1968)
      1059-1061.

(8)   R. Brunner, M. Röhr, M. Zinner, Hoppe-Seyler's Z. Physiol. Chem.
      349 (1968) 95-103.

(9)   R. Brunner, M. Röhr, Methods Enzymol. 43 (1975) 476-481.

(10) B. Spencer, C. Maung, Biochem. J. 118 (1970) 29P-30P.

(11) M. Cole, Appl. Microbiol. <u>14</u> (1966) 98-104.

(12) H. Vanderhaeghe, M. Claesen, A. Vlietnick, G. Parmentier, Appl.
     Microbiol. <u>16</u> (1968) 1557-1563.

(13) P. A. Fawcett, J. J. Usher, E. P. Abraham, Biochem. J. <u>151</u>
     (1975) 741-746.

(14) A. Fisher, E. P. Abraham, unpublished experiments.

(15) P. Whiteman*, E. P. Abraham, unpublished experiments.

(16) R. B. Frederiksen, C. Emborg, Biotechnol. Lett. <u>6</u>(<u>9</u>) (1984) 549.

(17) G. S. Jayatilake, J. A. Huddleston, E. P. Abraham, Biochem. J.
     <u>194</u> (1981) 645-647.

(18) S. E. Jensen, D. W. S. Westlake, S. Wolfe, Can. J. Microbiol. <u>29</u>
     (1983) 1526-1531.

(19) S. Wolfe, A. L. Demain, S. E. Jensen, D. W. S. Westlake, Science
     <u>226</u> (1984) 1386-1392.

(20) M. Liersch, J. Nuesch, H. J. Treichler, In Proceedings of the
     2nd International Synposium on the Genetics of Industrial
     Microorganisms, K. D. MacDonald (Ed.), Academic Press London
     1976, pp. 179-195.

(21) S. J. Brewer, T. T. Boyle, M. K. Turner, Biochem. Soc. Trans. <u>5</u>
     (1977) 1026-1029.

(22) C. M. Stevens, E. P. Abraham, F.-C. Huang, C. J. Sih, Fed. Proc.
     <u>34</u> (1975) 625.

(23) J. O'Sullivan, R. T. Aplin, C. M. Stevens, E. P. Abraham,
     Biochem. J. <u>179</u> (1979) 47-52.

(24) M. K. Turner, J. E. Farthing, S. J. Brewer, Biochem. J. <u>173</u>
     (1978) 839-850.

(25) J. O'Sullivan, E. P. Abraham, Biochem. J. <u>186</u> (1980) 613-616.

* Formerly P. A. Fawcett(26)

(26) A. Scheidegger, M. T. Küenzi, J. Nüesch, J. Antibiotics 37 (1984) 522-531.

(27) S. E. Jensen, D. W. S. Westlake, S. Wolfe, J. Antibiotics 38 (1985) 263-265.

(28) P. A. Fawcett, P. B. Loder, M. J. Duncan, T. J. Beesley, E. P. Abraham, J. Gen. Microbiology. 79 (1973) 293-309.

(29) P. A. Fawcett, J. J. Usher, J. A. Huddleston, R. C. Bleaney, J. J. Nisbet, E. P. Abraham, Biochem. J. 157 (1976) 651-660.

(30) J. O'Sullivan, R. C. Bleaney, J. A. Huddleston, E. P. Abraham, Biochem. J. 184 (1979) 421-426.

(31) T. Konomi, S. Herchen, J. E. Baldwin, M. Yoshida, Biochem. J. 184 (1979) 427-430.

(32) J. O'Sullivan, E. P. Abraham, In Antibiotics IV "Biosynthesis" J. W. Corcoran Ed. Springer-Verlag Berlin Heidelberg 1981, pp. 101-122.

(33) E. P. Abraham, J. A. Huddleston, G. S. Jayatilake, J. O'Sullivan, R. L. White, In Recent Advances in the Chemistry of β-Lactam Antibiotics. Roy. Soc. Chem. Special Publication No 38, 1981, pp. 125-134.

(34) C.-P. Pang, B. Chakravarti, R. M. Adlington, H.-H. Ting, R. L. White, G. S. Jayatilake, J. E. Baldwin, E. P. Abraham, Biochem. J. 222 (1984) 789-795.

(35) D. Perry, E. P. Abraham, unpublished experiments.

(36) J. Kupka, Y.-Q. Shen, S. Wolfe, A. L. Demain, Can. J. Microbiol. 29 (1983) 488-495.

(37) I. J. Hollander, Y.-Q. Shen, J. Heim, A. L. Demain, S. Wolfe, Science 224 (1984) 610-612.

(38) N. Neuss, D. M. Berry, J. Kupka, A. L. Demain, S. W. Queener, D. C. Duckworth, L. L. Huckstep, J. Antibiotics 35 (1982) 580-584.

(39) F. R. Ramos, M. J. Lopez-Nieto, J. F. Martin, Antimicrob. Agents
     Chemother. 27 (1985) 380-386.

(40) M. Kohsaka, A. L. Demain, Biochem. Biophys. Res. Commun. 70
     (1976) 465-473.

(41) J. E. Baldwin, J. W. Keeping, P. D. Singh, C. A. Vallejo,
     Biochem. J. 194 (1981) 649-651.

(42) D. J. Hook, L. T. Chang, R. P. Elander, R. B. Morin,
     Biochem. Biophys. Res. Commun. 87 (1979) 258-265.

(43) J. Kupka, Y.-Q. Shen, S. Wolfe, A. L. Demain, Microbiology
     Letters 16 (1983) 1-6.

(44) B. Chakravarti, unpublished work.

(45) J. E. Baldwin, E. P. Abraham, R. M. Adlington, G. A. Bahadur,
     B. Chakravarti, B. P. Domayne-Hayman, L. D. Field,
     S. L. Flitsch, G. S. Jayatilake, A. Spakovskis, H.-H. Ting,
     N. J. Turner, R. L. White, J. J. Usher, J. Chem. Soc.
     Chem. Commun. (1984) 1225-1227.

(46) J. E. Shields, C. S. Campbell, S. W. Queener, D. C. Duckworth,
     N. Neuss, Helv. Chim. Acta 67 (1984) 870-875.

(47) R. J. Bowers, S. E. Jensen, L. Lyubechansky, D. W. S. Westlake,
     S. Wolfe, Biochem. Biophys. Res. Commun. 120 (1984) 607-613.

(48) A. Ballio, F. Dentici di Accadia, M. Francesco,
     M. Pietro-Cancellieri, G. Morpurgo, G. Serlupi-Crescenzi,
     G. Sermonti, Nature 185 (1960) 97-99.

(49) H. Troonen, P. Roelants, B. Born, J. Antibiot. 29 (1976)
     605-606.

(50) K. Kitano, Y. Fujisawa, K. Katamoto, K. Nara, Y. Nakao,
     J. Ferment. Technol. 54 (1976) 712-719.

(51) G. A. Bahadur, J. E. Baldwin, J. J. Usher, E. P. Abraham,
     G. S. Jayatilake, R. L. White, J. Amer. Chem. Soc. 103 (1981)
     7650-7651.

(52) R. L. White, E.-M. M. John, J. E. Baldwin, E. P. Abraham,
     Biochem. J. <u>203</u> (1982) 791-793.

(53) J. E. Baldwin, E. P. Abraham, R. M. Adlington, B. Chakravarti,
     A. E. Derome, J. A. Murphy, L. D. Field, N. Green, H.-H. Ting,
     J. J. Usher, J. Chem. Soc. Chem. Commun. (1983) 1317-1319.

(54) J. E. Baldwin, T. S. Wan, Tetrahedron <u>37</u> (1981) 1589-1595.

(55) N. Neuss, R. D. Miller, C. A. Affolder, W. Nakatsukasa, J. Mabe,
     L. L. Huckstep, N. De La Higuera, J. L. Occolowitz,
     J. H. Gilliam, Helv. Chim. Acta <u>63</u> (1980) 1119-1129.

(56) H. Kluender, C. H. Bradley, C. J. Sih, P. Fawcett,
     E. P. Abraham, J. Amer. Chem. Soc. <u>95</u> (1973) 6149-6150.

(57) S. Wolfe, A. L. Demain, S. E. Jensen, D. W. S. Westlake, Science
     <u>226</u> (1984) 1386-1392.

(58) P. A. Fawcett, D.Phil. Thesis, University of Oxford, 1975.

The Integration of Cyclopenin-Cyclopenol Biosynthesis into the Developmental Program of Penicillium cyclopium

*Martin Luckner, *Werner Lerbs and Werner Roos*

Martin-Luther-University Halle-Wittenberg, Section of Pharmacy, Weinbergweg 15, DDR-4020 Halle, GDR

*Academy of Sciences of GDR, Institute of Plant Biochemistry, Weinbergweg 3, DDR-4020 Halle, GDR

SUMMARY

The most important regulatory events in the development of P. cyclopium proceeded immediately after spore germination in the trophophase and in the early idiophase. At the transition from trophophase to idiophase the trophophase-specific protein pattern changed into an idiophase-specific pattern. However, most of the mRNA species encoding idiophase-specific proteins were present already at the beginning of the trophophase. At this period the cells were competent to respond to signals influencing the expression of idiophase processes, like conidiospore and alkaloid biosynthesis (determination phase). One of these signals is the P-factor, a developmental hormone produced in P. cyclopium.

Among the idiophase-specific events expression of cyclopenin-cyclopenol biosynthesis held a special position. In contrast to most idiophase-specific mRNA species those encoding the enzymes of cyclopenin-cyclopenol biosynthesis were formed and translated at the beginning of the idiophase. Alkaloid biosynthesis reached its maximum at the late idiophase. It continued for several weeks, if nutrients were available.

Abbreviations: d p.i. days after inoculation

1 THE DEVELOPMENTAL PROGRAM OF P. CYCLOPIUM

P. cyclopium is a mold growing on the surface of rotting fruits, vegetables etc. Its development may be divided into the phase of conidiospore germination (germination phase), the phase of hyphal growth (trophophase), and the phase of cell specialization (idio-phase) (for a summary cf. ref. 1). The most prominent idiophase processes are the formation of different types of specialized cells including the conidiospores, and the biosynthesis of alkaloids of the cyclopenin-viridicatin group (Fig. 1).

If conidiospores of P. cyclopium germinate in large distance from each other macrocolonies will develop. These colonies contain tropho-phase hyphae at the rim and idiophase hyphae and newly formed conidiospores towards the center of the colonies (9). If conidio-spores germinate in high density near each other a mycelial mat con-sisting of a large number of microcolonies is formed whose hyphae develop more or less synchronously. The synchronization of develop-ment can be improved by reduction of the nutrients (10) (Fig. 2). All experiments described in the following were carried out using these cultures with synchronized development.

2 THE EXPRESSION OF ALKALOID BIOSYNTHESIS

The enzymes of cyclopenin-cyclopenol biosynthesis became mea-surable in vitro at the transition from the trophophase to the idio-phase (Fig. 2). The activity increase of cyclopeptine dehydrogenase, dehydrocyclopeptine epoxidase, and cyclopenin m-hydroxylase mea-surable in vitro was stopped by 5-fluorouracil and cycloheximide, inhibitors of RNA and protein biosynthesis, respectively (1, 11). This inhibition strongly indicated that the amount of the enzymes present in the cells was regulated by control of transcription of the respective genes and that the mRNA species formed were immedi-ately translated. Transcription and translation of the nucleic acids encoding the enzymes of cyclopenin-cyclopenol biosynthesis were transient processes proceeding during a restricted period of develop-ment only.

The activities of anthranilate adenylyltransferase, which is part of the cyclopeptine synthetase system (2), and of cyclopenase were regulated posttranslationally (12, 13). With anthranilate adenylyl-

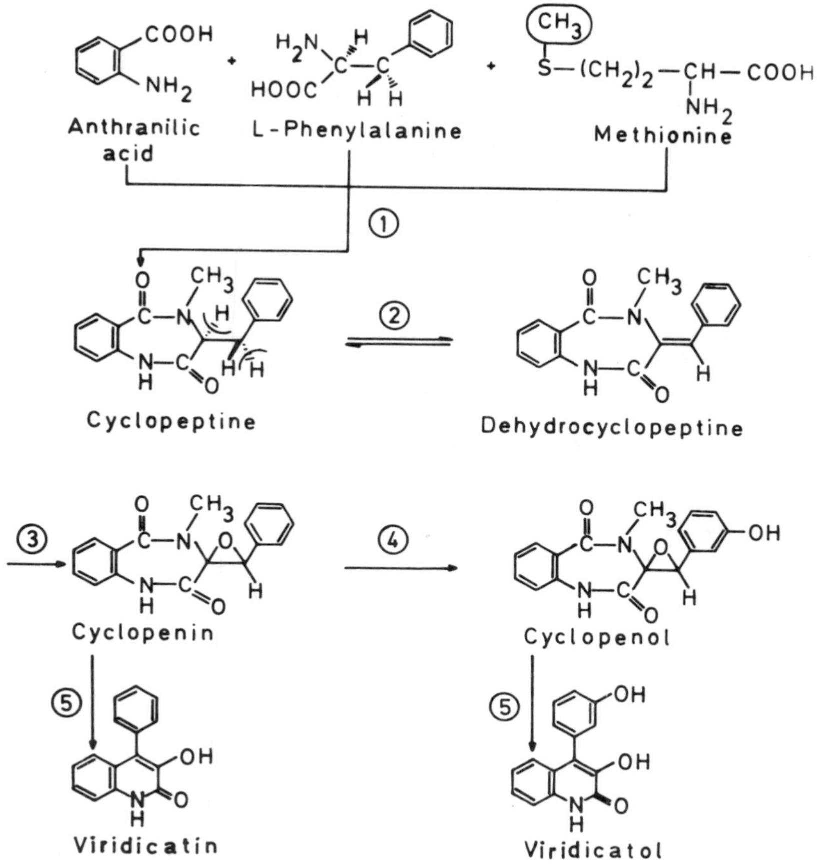

Fig. 1. Pathway of alkaloid biosynthesis in P. cyclopium

1 Cyclopeptine synthetase system (2), 2 cyclopeptine dehydrogenase
(3,4), 3 dehydrocyclopeptine epoxidase (5), 4 cyclopenin m-hydroxylase (6), 5 cyclopenase (7,8)(present in the conidiospores, but not
in the hyphae)

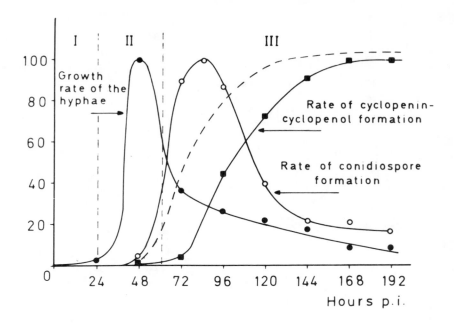

Fig. 2. Growth and cell specialization in surface cultures of
        P. cyclopium (1, 11, 12)

● —— ● Growth rate of the hyphae (100 = 79 /ug); o —— o Rate of
conidiospore formation (100 = 400 000 conidia;) ■ —— ■ Rate of cyclopenin-cyclopenol formation by the hyphae (100 = 12 pmol/sec.);
– – – Enzymes of cyclopenin-cyclopenol biosynthesis (anthranilate
adenylyltransferase 100 = 5.6 pkat, cyclopeptine dehydrogenase
100 = 40 pkat, dehydrocyclopeptine epoxidase 100 = 0.42 pkat, cyclopenin m-hydroxylase 100 = 12 pkat). All values are given in units/cm^2
culture area.

Synchronization of the transition of the cultures from the trophophase to the idiophase was brought about by removal of surplus
nutrients 2 d p.i. (cf. Experimental).

I Germination phase; II Trophophase; III Idiophase

transferase it was shown (12) that beginning 2.5 d p.i. the in vitro
measurable activity increase was resistant to inhibition by 5-fluoro-
uracil and cycloheximide, i.e., did not depend directly on RNA and
protein biosynthesis. This indicated that in the trophophase hyphae a
proenzyme exists whose activation during further development of the
mycelium is independent from the de novo formation of proteins. The
synthesis of this preprotein should proceed within a short period
(2 - 2.5 d p.i.) because at earlier stages the activity increase was
inhibited by cycloheximide and fluorouracil, indicating that at this
time the cells were still devoid of the preprotein.

In addition to enzyme amount enzyme activity was shown to regulate
the intensity of alkaloid biosynthesis. The rates of cyclopenin-
cyclopenol biosynthesis in hyphal cells, for instance, did not increase in parallel to the enzyme activity measurable in vitro during
the transition from the trophophase to the idiophase indicating that
the enzyme activity is controlled in vivo (1, 11) (Fig. 2). As the
increase of the rate of alkaloid formation during this period depended on mRNA and protein biosynthesis (shown by inhibition with
5-fluorouracil and cycloheximide), synthesis of an as yet unknown
protein limited the rate of cyclopenin-cyclopenol biosynthesis. This
protein probably influenced the spatial organization of cell metabolism, since compartmentation and channeling of precursors, intermediates and products were shown to be of great significance in the
regulation of alkaloid metabolism in P. cyclopium (1, 14 - 17).

In summary these results pointed out that the regulation of
enzyme synthesis and activity were the most important means in the
phase-dependent expression of the alkaloid metabolism in P. cyclopium. Both processes were integrated in the developmental program of
the mold and triggered by internal signals (cf. section 3.3). It was
therefore of interest to characterize the general pattern of protein
biosynthesis during the development of P. cyclopium and to examine
its relation to the expression of alkaloid formation.

3 <u>THE MOLECULAR BACKGROUND OF THE INTEGRATION OF ALKALOID</u>
  <u>BIOSYNTHESIS INTO THE DEVELOPMENTAL PROGRAM OF P. CYCLOPIUM</u>

3.1 mRNA and protein biosynthesis during trophophase and idiophase

DNA and protein biosynthesis in hyphal cells were at maximum in
the trophophase (2 d p.i.), but later on decreased rapidly (18).
Accordingly, the absolute amount and the concentration of the
membrane-bound RNA present in the hyphae went through a maximum 2 d
p.i. The free polysomes reached their maximum amount 3 d p.i., and
their highest relative concentration 1.5 d p.i. (Table 1). A detailed
analysis showed that their size, i.e., the number of ribosomes bound
per mRNA molecule, was reduced strongly beginning at the end of the
trophophase (2.5 d p.i.) (Fig. 3).

Table 1. Free and membrane-bound polysomes in the hyphae of P.
         cyclopium at different developmental stages

Age of the mycelium (d p.i.)	Polysomes		% of the total	
	free	membrane-bound	free RNA	membrane-bound RNA
1.5	5.1	2.1	56	48
2.0	9.4	5.5	37	78
2.5	9.0	2.6	25	24
3.0	12.6	2.7	26	18
3.5	8.2	3.2	17	20
4.0	7.4	3.1	14	20

The amount of polysomes was calculated from the OD_{260} after
redissolving in homogenization buffer and is given per mycelial area.

By two-dimensional gel electrophoresis it was shown that different
pattern of protein biosynthesis characterize trophophase and idiophase mycelium (Fig. 4). The differences included several hundreds
of polypeptides. A massive breakdown of trophophase proteins 2 d p.i.
was accompanied by the appearance of large amounts of low molecular
polypeptides. Relative to the rate of biosynthesis during the
development of the mold several groups of polypeptides may be

Free polysomes

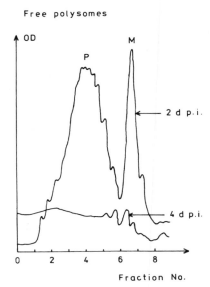

Membrane – bound polysomes

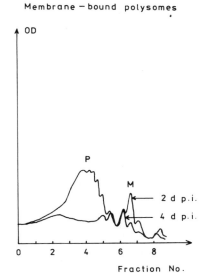

Fig. 3. Ratio of polysomes and monosomes during the development of
        P. cyclopium

P. cyclopium strain SM 72 was cultivated as described in Fig. 2. At
the time points given the polysomes and microsomes were isolated
according to (19), cf. Experimental.

P polysomes, M monosomes

The polysomes containing high numbers of ribosomes appear at low
fraction numbers. They are present 2 d p.i., but vanish untill 4 d
p.i. in correspondence with the strongly reduced rate of mRNA
translation.

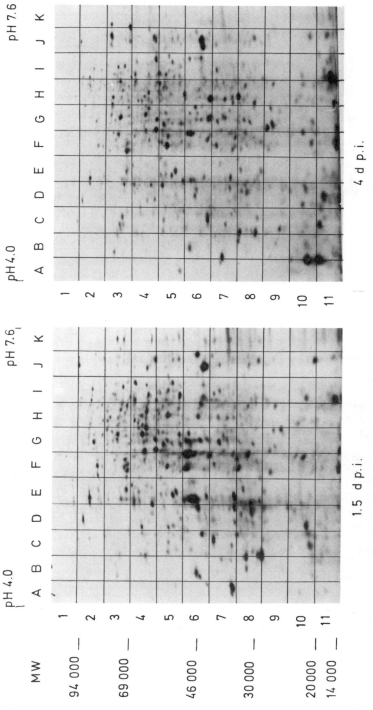

Fig. 4. Protein pattern characteristic for trophophase and idiophase hyphae after two-dimensional separation according to (20).

P. cyclopium was grown as given in Fig. 2. At the time points indicated the cultures were harvested and the protein solutions prepared. 10 /ul of the sample were spotted at the upper left corner of the chromatogram.

distinguished. Fig. 5 shows that only a small amount of the polypeptides is formed during the whole life cycle of the mold, whereas
the biosynthesis of the vast majority is restricted to certain
developmental phases.

In order to facilitate the identification of the idiophase-
specific proteins an antiserum was raised against the proteins
present in hyphal cell 4 d p.i. (cf. 21). The specificity of this
antiserum to the idiophase-specific proteins was tested in reactions
with a) the proteins extracted from surface cultures of the wild
type strain at different developmental stages, and b) the proteins
derived from cultures of the wild type strain grown under submerged
conditions at which the typical idiophase processes are not expressed. Extracts from surface-grown trophophase mycelium 2 d p.i.
and to a smaller extend 2.5 d p.i., from hyphae grown submerged
4 d p.i., as well as from mutants with disturbed development, e.g.,
mutant dev 379 (22), left definite fractions of the antibodies
unreacted. This demonstrated the absence of the corresponding
idiophase-specific proteins in these preparations.

With the technique of line-immunoelectrophoresis (23) using the
antiserum mentioned above it was demonstrated that the accumulation
of the idiophase-specific proteins started already between 1.5 - 2 d
p.i. and lasted till about 3.5 d p.i. (Fig. 6). In contrast the
trophophase-specific proteins went through a maximum 2 d p.i. and
then decreased. Only a few of the proteins were present in trophophase as well as in idiophase mycelium (phase-nonspecific proteins).
Certain trophophase-specific and phase-nonspecific proteins of
surface cultures were also present in the mycelium grown submerged
(subm.). Idiophase-specific proteins, however, were absent or
occured in very small quantities only.

3.2 Stable mRNA pattern during the development of P. cyclopium

In contrast to the different pattern of proteins formed the
amount and composition of extractable poly$(A)^+$RNA remained stable
during the development of P. cyclopium. Fig. 7 shows that the in
vitro translation of the mRNA isolated at different developmental
stages (1.5 - 4 d p.i.) in the wheat germ system (cf. 24) yielded
polypeptide pattern which showed only small differences. After two-
dimensional chromatography more than 300 polypeptides were detected.

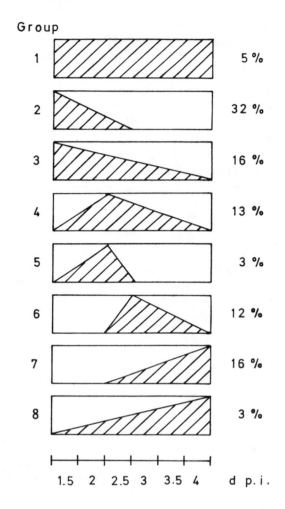

Fig. 5. Schematic representation of the rate of biosynthesis of different types of polypeptides during the development of P. cyclopium

Relative to the time course of biosynthesis during the development of surface cultures the following groups of polypeptides may be distinguished: group 1: biosynthesis phase independent. Group 2 - 8: biosynthesis phase dependent.

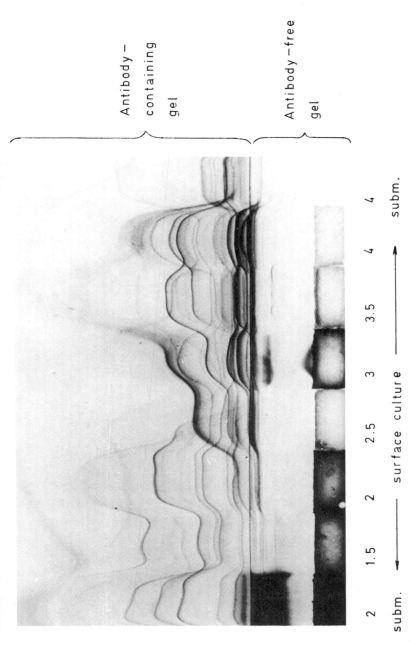

Fig. 6. Line-immunoelectrophoresis of proteins obtained from cultures of P. cyclopium at different developmental stages.

Identical proteins give continuous precipitation lines. The position of the line within the antibody-containing gel corresponds to the amount of protein present. High amounts of proteins result in a long distance between starting point and precipitation line.

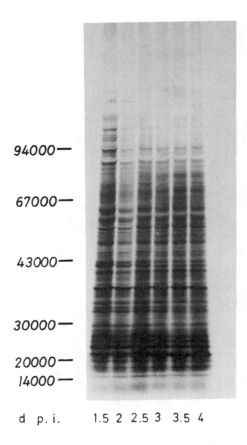

Fig. 7. Polypeptides formed by the in vitro translation of
poly(A)$^+$RNA in the wheat germ system after SDS
electrophoresis

The polypeptide mixtures formed were adjusted to equal radioactivity, precipitated with acetone and solved in a solution
containing 64 mM TRIS, 2.3 % SDS, 10 % sucrose and 5 % C_2H_5SH.

Only 12 of them were not present already 1.5 d p.i. and only 60 of
those formed in the sample obtained from mycelium 1.5 d p.i. were
absent in the samples prepared with the mRNA from older cultures
(Table 2).

Table 2. Polypeptides detected by two-dimensional SDS-PAGE
chromatography after in vitro translation of the poly(A)$^{+}$RNA

Age of the mycelium (d p.i.)	1.5	2	2.5	3	3.5	4
Polypeptides detected	364	354	335	333	330	301
Polypeptides not detected in the preceding sample		1	10	1	0	0
Polypeptides detected in the preceding sample, but absent in the sample examined		11	29	3	3	20

P. cyclopium was grown as given in Fig. 2.

These results indicated:
- that most mRNA species which can be translated in vitro under the
  experimental conditions used were present already in the early
  trophophase, i.e., 1.5 d p.i.
- that the pattern of translatable genetic information was stable
  and
- that the mRNA population present in the cells was selectively
  transcribed during the development of P. cyclopium.

Thus most of the idiophase-specific mRNA species obviously
remained untranslated till the synthesis of the homologous proteins
really began. Regulation of protein biosynthesis during the idiophase,
unlike that of the developmental proteins of Dictyostelium discoideum
(25), occurred therefore primaryly at the level of translation of
preexisting mRNA.

A special position within the group of idiophase-specific proteins held, however, the enzymes of alkaloid biosynthesis present in
the hyphae of P. cyclopium. With respect to cyclopeptine dehydrogenase, dehydrocyclopeptine epoxidase and cyclopenin m-hydroxylase
simultaneous transcription and translation was shown to occur at the
beginning of the idiophase. Likewise for anthranilate adenylyltrans-

ferase no indications exists for a separation in time of transcription and translation (cf. section 2). These results indicate that
the mRNA species endoding the enzymes of cyclopenin-cyclopenol biosynthesis are part of those mRNAs responsible for the small changes
in the polypeptide pattern obtained by in vitro translation at
different development stages (Table 2).

3.3 Influence of signals on idiophase processes during the early
    trophophase (determination phase)

    As discussed above most of the mRNA species characteristic for the
later developmental stages of P. cyclopium are formed in the early
trophophase, i.e., before 1.5 d p.i. Hence at this phase the expression of the characteristics of later development is determined
(determination phase). During this period hyphal cells are competent
to respond to signals which influence the intensity of idiophase
processes (including alkaloid formation). A typical effector acting
as signal in this respect is the P-factor, a hormone-like principle
isolated from the cells of P. cyclopium (26). Its influence on
alkaloid formation is shown in Fig. 8.

    The P-factor may be obtained from surface cultures of different
developmental stages, but also from mycelium grown submerged under
conditions which depress the formation of conidiospores and alkaloids.
It has a molecular weight of about 5000 D, is hydrophil, heat stable
and resistant to acid and alkali at room temperature. There are indications that the P-factor or part of it is derived from amino acids.

    The addition of P-factor preparations to surface cultures during
the determination phase stimulates mRNA and protein synthesis resulting in an increase of the protein content of the cells as well
as in an accelleration of spore germination and hyphal growth
(Fig. 9).

    The general stimulation of protein synthesis involves that of
permeases responsible for the accumulation of amino acids. A more
detailed analysis showed that the synthesis of L-phenylalanine and
L-leucine permeases was stimulated twice as much as that of the bulk
proteins. In contrast transport of L-glutamic acid and L-arginine
was stimulated only proportionally to the increase of the protein
content (Table 3). L-Phenylalanine and analogs of this amino acid
administered to cultures during the determination phase exerted

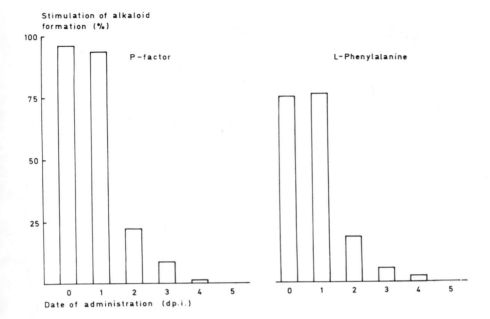

Fig. 8. Influence of P-factor and L-phenylalanine on
cyclopenin-cyclopenol biosynthesis

Cultures of P. cyclopium were grown as given in Fig. 2. A P-factor
preparation or L-phenylalanine (3 mM) were added to the nutrient
solution at the time points indicated. The formation of alkaloids
started 4 d p.i. Alkaloid accumulation was measured 7 d p.i. The
P-factor and L-phenylalanine exert their stimulating effects only
if added during the germination phase or the early growth phase.

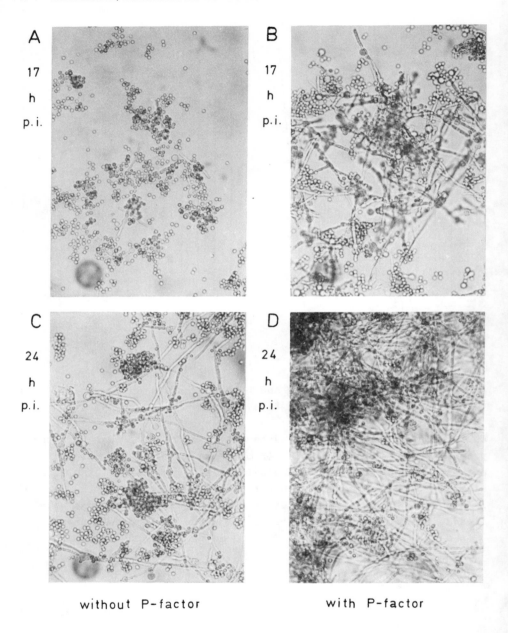

without P-factor   with P-factor

Fig. 9. Accelleration of spore germination and hyphal growth upon the influence of P-factor

effects on the idiophase processes similar to those of the P-factor (27). It might thus be speculated that the hormone-like effect of the P-factor is mediated via the uptake and/or intracellular compartmentation of L-phenylalanine. Uptake of L-phenylalanine into the vacuole has been found to be the rate limiting step during the accumulation of this amino acid in hyphal cells of P. cyclopium (15) which holds true also for P-factor treated cells. Probably the vacuolar accumulation of endogenously produced L-phenylalanine is increased after P-factor treatment as this was shown for exogenous L-phenylalanine, which under natural conditions is a constituent of the complex substrates used by P. cyclopium.

Table 3. Uptake of amino acids by hyphae of P. cyclopium. Influence of the P-factor

Amino acids	Control (C)	P-factor added (P)	C/P	Control (C)	P-factor added (P)	C/P
		Rates of uptake				
	$\left[\dfrac{pmol}{Mio.\ conidia\ .\ min}\right]$			$\left[\dfrac{pmol}{\mu g\ Protein\ .\ min}\right]$		
Arg	1.2	4.8	4.0	0.11	0.12	1.0
Glu	2.4	9.3	3.9	0.23	0.22	1.0
Phe	0.19	1.6	8.3	0.018	0.037	2.0
Leu	0.56	5.5	10.5	0.052	0.140	2.7

4 CONCLUSIONS

The results described demonstrate that the events most important for the developmental program of surface cultures of P. cyclopium proceed within a relatively short period at the beginning of the molds life cycle (Fig. 10). Characteristic is the synthesis of idiophase-specific mRNA species at the determination phase and their selected translation during later developmental stages. Similar determination phases may occur also in the development of other microorganisms (cf. 28). Transcription of idiophase-specific DNA at the beginning of development and the programmed translation of the corresponding mRNA at later stages might therefore be widespread in microorganisms.

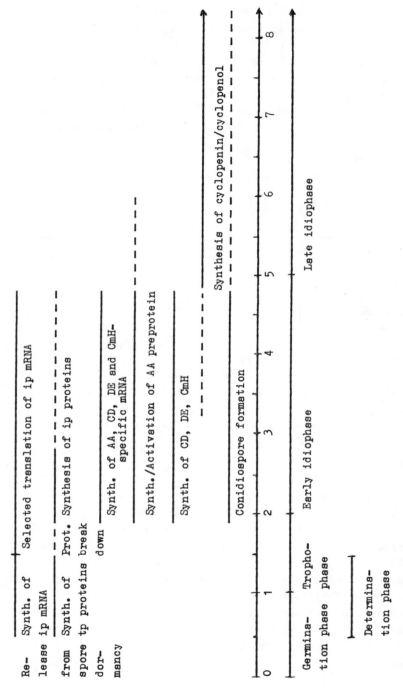

Fig. 10. Developmental program of surface cultures of P. cyclopium

ip idiophase-specific; tp trophophase-specific; AA anthranilic acid adenylyltransferase;
CD cyclopeptine dehydrogenase; DE dehydrocyclopeptine epoxidase;   CmH cyclopenin m-hydroxylase.

The expression of cyclopenin-cyclopenol formation is embedded into
this regulatory matrix. The mRNA species coding for the enzymes of
alkaloid biosynthesis and the enzymes themselves are formed between
the 2nd and 5th d p.i. (early idiophase), i.e., during a stage of
development at which the general biosynthesis of mRNA and proteins
is already strongly reduced. It is of interest that different regulatory principles control the amount of the alkaloid producing
enzymes (transcriptional control: cyclopeptine dehydrogenase, dehydrocyclopeptine epoxidase, cyclopenin m-hydroxylase; posttransla-
tional control: anthranilate adenylyltransferase, cyclopenase).
Regulation of the synthesis of the enzymes differs from that of most
other idiophase-specific proteins by tight coupling of formation and
translation of the respective mRNA species.

After the breakdown of the trophophase metabolism at the transition to the idiophase originated by as yet unknown endogenous signals
a new metabolic state is established which is characterized by the
flow of metabolites towards processes of cell specialization. The
formation of new specialized cells (biosynthesis of the penicilli and
the conidiospores) ceases at the end of the early idiophase. The late
idiophase is characterized by the formation of the alkaloids cyclopenin and cyclopenol which reaches maximum activity not before 10 d
p.i. and may last at least another 10 d if there is a continuous
supply of nutrients.

5 EXPERIMENTAL

Cultivation of P. cyclopium

Surface cultures of Penicillium cyclopium strain SM 72 were grown
on a nutrient solution containing 5 % glucose, 0,12 % ammonium, and
0.025 % phosphate (NL I). 2 d p.i. and then every 24 h   the culture
browth was replaced by a nutrient solution containing only 20 % of
the original carbon and nitrogen amounts and 2 % of the phosphate
content, respectively (NL II) (10).

Isolation of polysomes and monosomes

Before harvest the biosynthesis of proteins in the mycelium was
blocked by cycloheximide (0.1 mg/ml nutrient solution). The mycelium
was frozen with liquid nitrogen. The frozen mycelium was homogenized
with buffer (0.2 M HEPES pH 8.8, 0.1 M KCl, 0.05 M $MgCl_2$, 0.2 M

sucrose,   containing 0.1 mg cycloheximide, 0.05 mg dithioerythrol
and 2 mg heparin/ml). After removal of cellular debris the homogenate
was centrifuged at 5000 x g/5 min. The OD_{260} of the supernatant containing the free ribosomes was adjusted to 1.6 mg RNA. The sediment
was treated with the homogenization buffer containing 3 % triton
X-100 for the solubilization of membrane-bound polysomes and re-
centrifuged (22 000 x g/30 min). The polysomes were sedimented
through a 10 ml sucrose cushion (60 % sucrose w/v in 25 % homogenization buffer without cycloheximide) at 190 000 x g/5 h. The polysomal
pellet was redissolved in homogenization buffer. Size distribution of
the polysomes was determined by centrifugation over a 15 - 50 % w/v
sucrose gradient (122 000 g avg. in an SW-40 rotor/75 min). The
amount of polysomes is given in percent of the total RNA in the
22 000 x g supernatant (estimated from the material sedimenting at
190 000 x g).

Two-dimensional separation of proteins

   The mycelium was labelled for 6 h with radioactive amino acids.
Discs were homogenized in 30 mM TRIS-HCl pH 7.5 containing 0.3 % SDS
and 1 % C_2H_5SH. After centrifugation (10 000 g/3 min) 4 parts of the
supernatant were precipitated with 1 part 50 % TCA over night at $0^{\circ}C$.
The precipitate was washed with EtOH 80 % and EtOH 80 % containing
20 mM TRIS-base. It was solubilized in 100 mM TRIS-base containing
2.3 % SDS, 10 % sucrose, and 5 % C_2H_5SH. The solution was boiled for
3 min and used for isoelectric focussing as described by (29) with
ampholines pH 5-8 and a 10 % linear gel in the second dimension.
After electrophoresis the gels were fixed and silver stained according to (30). For autoradiography the dry gels were covered with ORWO
HS-11 X-ray film.

Production of antiserum against the idiophase-specific proteins
of P. cyclopium SM 72

   Protein extracts: P. cyclopium was grown as given in Fig. 2. At
the time points indicated the washed mycelium was lyophilized,
homogenized with sand and a buffer containing 0.05 M tricin pH 8.0,
0.01 M $MgSO_4$ and 1.5 % triton X-100. The protein extracts used were
obtained by centrifugation (5000 x g/15 min) at $0^{\circ}C$.

   Antiserum against idiophase-specific proteins: The protein extract from cultures 4 d p.i. (representing 4 mg protein in PBS) was

administered to rabbits by subcutanous injection (4 times within 4 months, first injection with complete adjuvans). The serum obtained from the blood of the rabbits was tested against the protein extract used for immunization by the Ouchterlony test in 2 week intervals beginning 1 month after the last injection.

To 0.2 ml of the antiserum the protein solution in question was added successively in small quantities untill no further precipitate was formed. The precipitations were removed by centrifugation (10 000 x g/15 min). In the supernatant remained the antibodies which did not find a partner protein (as well as the proteins not reacting with the antibodies). To the supernatant small amounts of a protein **extract from the wild type strain** P. cyclopium SM 72 was added prepared 4 d p.i. after labelling the mycelium with a pulse of radioactive amino acids. The proteins of this extract reacted with the antibodies left in the supernatant, but formed no precipitations due to their low concentration. The protein-antibody complexes were bound to protein A-Sepharose and analysed by SDS-PAGE (31). In the chromatogram those proteins gave radioactive spots which were absent in the protein solutions tested, i.e., for which free antibodies were left in the supernatant after reaction with the antiserum.

Examination of protein solutions by line-immunoelectrophoresis (23)

The lower part of a glass plate was covered with agarose gel in a buffer pH 8.6 containing 72 mM TRIS, 24 mM barbital, 13 mM NaN_3 and 0.01 % calcium lactate. Holes cut into the gel were filled with the protein extracts obtained from cultures of P. cyclopium at different developmental stages and mixed with the gel forming agarose solution. Equal amounts of proteins were used. The upper part of the plate was covered with a mixture of 1.2 ml of the idiophase-specific antiserum in 9.0 ml of the agarose solution. The electrophoresis was carried out in the buffer given in Fig. 7 (2 V/cm^2, 16 h). After the electrophoresis nonprecipitated proteins were eluted from the gel. The gel was dried and the precipitates of proteins with the antibodies stained with Coomassie blue in alcohol-acetic acid-water.

Determination of amino acid uptake by germinating conidiospores

Conidiospores of P. cyclopium strain SM 72 were cultivated submerged in NL I (10) (shaken flasks; 120 rpm). After 19 hours the germinating spores were removed by centrifugation, washed with water and cultivated in NH_4^+-free nutrient solution for 6 hours. They were

then collected by centrifugation and resuspended in maleate buffer
(60 mM, pH 3.5). To the aerated suspension radioactive-labelled
amino acids were added. The uptake of these amino acids was determined after washing the germinating spores with water (20 sec) and
resuspending them in dioxan scintillator. The uptake of the amino
acids was linear for more than 4 min.

In vitro translation of mRNA

Cell-free RNA translation by the wheat germ system (translation
of poly(A)$^+$RNA) and sample processing was carried out as described
by (24) except that the buffer for RNA extraction contained 100 mM
TRIS-HCl pH 8.8, 200 mM NaCl, 1 mM EDTA, and 1 % SDS. Samples containing 20 μg total RNA were incubated 80 min at 25°C in a test
mixture containing $\int^{35}S$ methionine. To determine total incorporation and kinetics 3 μl aliquots of the translation mixture were
transferred to filter-paper discs, washed with cold and hot (90°C)
trichloroacetic acid and counted for radioactivity. The remaining
assay was stopped by addition of an equal volume of a solution of
136 mM TRIS-HCl, pH 6.8, containing 5.0 % SDS, 20 % glycerol, 0.05 %
bromophenol blue, 10 % 2-mercaptoethanol, boiled for 2 min, and used
for SDS-gel electrophoresis or 2D PAGE.

6 REFERENCES

(1) M. Luckner, J. Natl. Prod. **43** (1980) 21.

(2) M. Gerlach, N. Schwelle, W. Lerbs, M. Luckner,
    Phytochemistry, in press.

(3) S. A. Aboutabl, M. Luckner, Phytochemistry **14** (1975) 2573.

(4) S. A. Aboutabl, A. El Azzouny, K. Winter, M. Luckner,
    Phytochemistry **15** (1976) 1925.

(5) S. Voigt, M. Luckner, Phytochemistry **16** (1977) 1651.

(6) I. Richter, M. Luckner, Phytochemistry **15** (1976) 67.

(7) S. Wilson, I. Schmidt, W. Roos, W. Fürst, M. Luckner,
    Z. Allg. Mikrobiol. **14** (1974) 515.

(8) S. Wilson, M. Luckner, Z. Allg. Mikrobiol. <u>15</u> (1975) 45.

(9) M. Luckner, in: Cell Differentiation in Microorganisms, Plants and Animals, L. Nover, K. Mothes (Eds.), p. 538, Fischer Verlag, Jena 1977.

(10) L. Nover, M. Luckner, Biochem. Physiol. Pflanzen <u>166</u> (1974) 293.

(11) S. Voigt, S. El Kousy, N. Schwelle, L. Nover, M. Luckner, Phytochemistry <u>17</u> (1978) 1705.

(12) W. Lerbs, M. Luckner, Z. Allg. Mikrobiol. (J. basic microbiol.), in press.

(13) S. El Kousy, E. Pfeiffer, G. Ininger, W. Roos, L. Nover, M. Luckner, Biochem. Physiol. Pflanzen <u>168</u> (1975) 79.

(14) L. Nover, W. Lerbs, W. Müller, M. Luckner, Biochim. Biophys. Acta <u>584</u> (1979) 270.

(15) M. Luckner, W. Roos, in: Overproduction of Microbial Products, V. Krumphanzl, B. Sikyta, Z. Vanek (Eds.), p. 111, Academic Press, London 1982.

(16) W. Roos, M. Luckner, Biochem. Physiol. Pflanzen <u>171</u> (1977) 127.

(17) W. Roos, W. Fürst, M. Luckner, Nova Acta Leopoldina, Suppl. 7, p. 175.

(18) L. Nover, M. Luckner, Nova Acta Leopoldina, Suppl. 7, p. 229.

(19) B. A. Larkins, E. Davies, Plant Physiol. <u>55</u> (1975) 749.

(20) P. H. O'Farrell, J. Biol. Chem. <u>250</u> (1975) 4007.

(21) R. P. Legocki, D. P. S. Verma, Cell <u>20</u> (1980) 153.

(22) I. Schmidt, L. Nover, G. Ininger, M. Luckner, Z. Allg. Mikrobiol. <u>18</u> (1978) 219.

(23) H. Friemel, Immunologische Arbeitsmethoden, Fischer Verlag, Jena 1980.

(24) S. Lerbs, W. Lerbs, N. L. Klyachko, E. G. Romanko, O. N. Kulaeva, R. Wollgiehn, B. Parthier, Planta 162 (1984) 289.

(25) T. H. Alton, H. F. Lodish, Develop. Biology 60 (1977) 180.

(26) Z. Zendem, S. Khalil, M. Luckner, Phytochemistry 21 (1982) 839.

(27) R. Dunkel, W. Müller, L. Nover, M. Luckner, Nova Acta Leopoldina, Suppl. 7, p. 281.

(28) M. Luckner, L. Nover, H. Böhm, Secondary Metabolism and Cell Differentiation, Springer, Berlin 1977.

(29) J. I. Garrels, J. Biol. Chem. 254 (1979) 7961.

(30) C. R. Merril, M. L. Dunau, D. Goldman, Anal. Biochem. 110 (1981) 201.

(31) U. K. Laemmli, Nature 227 (1970) 680.

Ergot Peptide Alkaloid Synthesis in Claviceps purpurea

Ullrich Keller

Technical University of Berlin, Institute of Biochemistry and Molecular Biology, Franklinstr. 29, D-1000 Berlin 10 (West)

SUMMARY

A survey is given of recent physiological and biochemical work on the formation of ergot peptide alkaloids in Claviceps purpurea. The development of a protoplast system from this fungus in this laboratory has enabled to establish a technique for efficient mutagenesis of the aconidial C. purpurea strain ATCC 20102 by regenerating cells from protoplasts which had been prepared from mycelium of mutagenized cultures. Protoplasts of C. purpurea also proved to be useful for studies of precursor relationships in the biosynthesis of the peptide alkaloids and the physiological factors affecting the synthesis within the cells. Techniques were established for isolation of organelles such as the vacuoles, which were shown to contain hydrolytic enzymes and free amino acids. It could be demonstrated that sclerotia-like cells of C. purpurea strain 1029 display a characteristic compartmentation of the free amino acid pool which differs from that found in non-differentiated (sphacelial) mycelium from this organism. Evidence is presented for an induction effect of tryptophan on ergot peptide synthesis in C. purpurea similar to that observed in Claviceps fusiformis. Furthermore, amino acids such as valine, leucine or proline had an influence in increasing the amount of ergot peptide formed and also overcame the growth-linked repression of the alkaloid synthesis through phosphate. The data indicate a control of peptide alkaloid synthesis through α-amino nitrogen sources which differs from that observed in clavine

producing <u>Claviceps</u> species. Data from biochemical work in this laboratory indicate the presence of a D-lysergic acid activating enzyme in
<u>C</u>. <u>purpurea</u>. The enzyme has been shown to be present in various <u>C</u>.
<u>purpurea</u> strains at a high level when these had been grown in alkaloid
production media, but was present at a much lower level in cells grown
in media, where alkaloid production is low.

1   INTRODUCTION

The ergot peptide alkaloids represent a family of important metabolites produced by the ergot fungus <u>Claviceps</u> <u>purpurea</u>. They consist of
an unusual cyclic arrangement of three different amino acids having
both lactam and lactone structures as shown in Figure 1. The tetracyclic D-lysergic acid is attached to the amino terminus of such cyclol
peptides via an amide bond. The amino acids present in the peptide
chains characterize the different ergot peptide alkaloids. The ergot
peptide alkaloids, for convenience-sake also named ergopeptines, have
as penultimate precursors the corresponding ergopeptams with similar
structures but missing the cyclol bridge. These latter compounds represent a novel group of ergot peptides, which are becoming more and
more discovered in natural alkaloid mixtures (1).

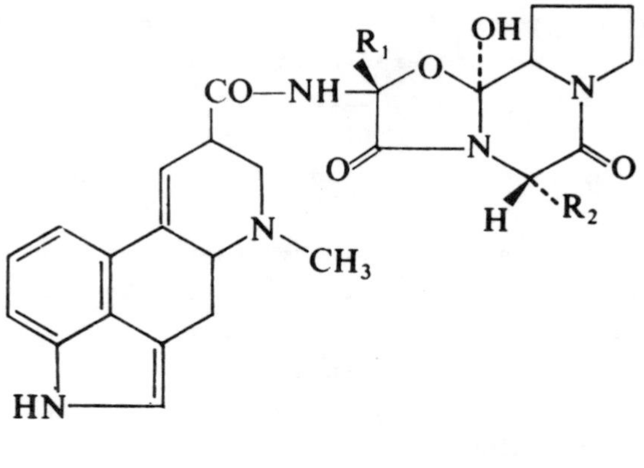

<u>Fig. 1</u>   Structural formula of ergot peptides
Ergotamine: R_1=-CH_3, R_2=-CH_2-C_6H_5; ergocryptine: R_1=-CH(CH_3)$_2$,
R_2=-CH(CH_3)-C_2H_5; ergosine: R_1=-CH_3, R_2=-CH_2-CH(CH_3)$_2$;
ergocornine: R_1=-CH(CH_3)$_2$, R_2=-CH(CH_3)$_2$.

D-lysergic acid is the common building block of ergot peptides and

it is synthesized from tryptophan and dimethylallyl pyrophosphate via
the chanoclavine-I pathway. This pathway also operates for the biosynthesis of the simpler clavine alkaloids produced by various Claviceps
species. Most clavines have in common with D-lysergic acid the tetracyclic ergoline nucleus but are missing the 8-carboxyl group. Accordingly, these compounds are restricted from forming more complex structures. Their importance as therapeutic agents is much less than that
of D-lysergic acid derived compounds.

The history of cultivation of the ergot fungus Claviceps purpurea
and ergot fungi producing clavines or simple D-lysergic acid derivatives is an impressive example of the development of biotechnological
exploitation of microbial organisms (2,3,4). Growing under natural
condition as a parasite on a variety of grasses and cereals, ergot
fungi such as C. fusiformis or C. paspali can be exploited in high
yield fermentations for industrial production of D-lysergic acid via
D-lysergic acid methylcarbinol amide (4) and paspalic acid (5), respectively. Production of ergopeptines by fermentation of C. purpurea
strains with considerable yields is also possible (2). However, due to
the instability of various C. purpurea strains used, ergopeptines are
still mostly produced by agricultural exploitation (6). Laboratory cultures of Claviceps sp. actively synthesizing ergot alkaloids show a
high level of oxidative metabolism (7) resulting in the synthesis of
reserve materials such as lipids, carbohydrates etc. A specific cellular morphology of producing strains is a prerequisite for high alkaloid yields (8). This morphology is characterized by the appearance of
a mycelium mainly consisting of short, branched hyphae with more or
less isodiametric cells similar to the plectenchymatic tissue that is
present in the sclerotia. The formation of cells with this morphology
in submerged culture is strongly influenced by the composition of the
nutrient media. Such media are characterized by an unusual high concentration of a sugar and by the presence of an acid from the tricarboxylic acid cycle. Low levels of phosphate provide the basis of growth
under substrate limitation in the later stages of cultivation when alkaloids are synthesized. Strains which develop in such media a mycelium
of the sphacelial (or non-differentiated) type scarcely produce alkaloid. Such sphacelial mycelia consist of long and thin hyphae (9).

2 STUDIES WITH PROTOPLASTS OF CLAVICEPS PURPUREA

Protoplasts of fungi and yeasts are widely used for physiological
studies, organelle isolation and genetic manipulations such as proto-

plast fusions (10). <u>Claviceps</u> <u>purpurea</u> protoplasts can be prepared by
treatment of mycelia with snail gut enzyme or enzyme from <u>Cyptophaga</u>
(11,12). Good results in preparation of <u>Claviceps</u> <u>purpurea</u> protoplasts
were achieved by using snail gut enzyme alone or in combination with a
cellulase preparation of <u>Trichoderma</u> <u>viride</u> in a medium with 0.8 M sucrose and the additional presence of earth alkaline ions such as Ca^{2+}
and Mg^{2+} (13,14).

A) MUTAGENESIS OF THE ERGOT FUNGUS

Protoplasts of <u>C</u>. <u>purpurea</u> were used for the mutagenesis of <u>Clavi-</u>
<u>ceps</u> <u>purpurea</u> strain ATCC 20102 (15). This strain does not form conidia
under laboratory conditions. It was grown in submerged culture in the
presence of mutagens such as N-methyl-N'-nitro-N-nitrosoguanidine (NTG)
or ethylmethane sulfonate (EMS). Protoplasts from such cultures were
prepared and regenerated on solid medium to obtain colonies mostly derived from single cell units. Frequencies of auxotrophs and variants
among the samples tested with improved alkaloid yields were on the order of 1 to 2%. Remarkably, in one mutagenic step variants could be obtained with peptide alkaloid levels up to 700 mg/l corresponding to a
ca. 50-fold improvement of the parent strain. Strains with increased
yields of alkaloids displayed a brownish-violet pigmentation and had
sclerotia-like cell morphology. Several strains with intermediary levels of alkaloid synthesis showed sectors of white, cotton-like morphology when grown as giant colonies. However, sector formation was not
found to be correlated with higher levels of alkaloid production in
the strains. This was shown by growing strain 1029 (400-700 mg/l) or
1029/10 (up to 900 mg/l) as giant colonies on solid media where they
did not show sectors. In addition, strains were isolated which had requirements for vitamins such as nicotinic acid or pyridoxine. Also
these auxotrophs did not show segregation and were stable in respect of
the production of a relatively high amount of alkaloid (200-400 mg/l).
This indicates that heterokaryosis is not a prerequisite for alkaloid
production in this aconidial <u>Claviceps</u> <u>purpurea</u> strain. The fact that
amino acid auxotrophs generally were low producers (< 25 mg/ml ergot
peptide) therefore seems to be merely an effect of the mutation rather
than be caused by homokaryosis (16,17).

One further round of mutagenesis of strain 1029 with NTG or EMS did
not result in the isolation of strains with a significant additional
increase of alkaloid production (16). By contrast the majority (up to
80%) of regenerated colonies from mutagenised protoplasts and even the

mutagen-free controls had lost the dark pigmentation, the sclerotia-like cell morphology and produced only low levels of ergot peptides. Apparently the process of protoplasting and/or protoplast regeneration has a labilizing influence on the stability of the sclerotia-like morphology and alkaloid production. Such instability was not observed when fragmented hyphae were plated on the same media.

B) BIOCHEMICAL AND PHYSIOLOGICAL STUDIES OF ERGOT PEPTIDE SYNTHESIS

Protoplasts were also useful for studying ergot alkaloid synthesis on a biochemical and physiological level. Clavine alkaloid synthesis was demonstrated previously in protoplasts of Claviceps strain SD 58 (18). Ergotamine synthesis in protoplasts of Claviceps purpurea could be measured during short term experiments by following the incorporation of [^{14}C]phenylalanine and [^{14}C]proline into the peptide chain of the alkaloid (13). The conditions of protoplast preparation had a stimulatory effect on the synthetic activity of these cells probably due to N-starvation. Experiments with control mycelium revealed an increase of radioisotope incorporation rates into ergotamine when compared to freshly harvested mycelium, which is due to the lack of N-sources in the medium used for protoplast preparation (19).

The short term incorporation experiments with protoplasts of C. purpurea indicated isotope dilution of radioactive precursors such as [^{14}C]phenylalanine and [^{14}C]proline by the presence of the unlabeled amino acids in the internal pool of protoplasts. In addition, a possible control of the extent of alkaloid synthesis by amino acids was indicated by the finding that addition of tryptophan or methionine to protoplasts or control mycelium of Claviceps purpurea actively synthesizing ergotamine reduced [^{14}C]phenylalanine incorporation into ergotamine during short term experiments significantly. This was surprising in view of the role of these two amino acids as precursors of the ergoline nucleus. In experiments with other amino acids such as glutamate, asparagine or cysteine a similar effect was observed (19). Although the mechanism of inhibition of ergotamine synthesis in these short term experiments is still unclear, it may be assumed that addition of an N-source such as an amino acid to the N-starved protoplasts or control mycelium activated vegetative functions resulting in an inhibition or repression of alkaloid synthesis. This effect of tryptophan and the other amino acids in such short term experiments indicates a careful balance in the metabolic pools of the cells.

The addition of D-lysergic acid to protoplast suspensions and control mycelia of Claviceps purpurea significantly stimulated ergotamine synthesis. It was argued that the internal D-lysergic acid concentration is a rate-limiting factor in ergopeptine synthesis. Thus, a high rate of ergoline ring synthesis in the cells results in a high level of ergopeptine synthesis. This assumption was further substantiated by experiments which indicated a stimulation of ergosine synthesis in Claviceps purpurea by the addition of elymoclavine or agroclavine (20).

C) ISOLATION OF VACUOLES FROM PROTOPLASTS

It was noted that protoplasts from Claviceps purpurea actively synthesizing ergopeptines were strongly vacuolated. This is not surprising since the extent of vacuolation in fungi is age dependent and alkaloid production takes place in the later stages of cultivations. In the case of other ascomycetes such as Neurospora and Saccharomyces species vacuolar compartmentation of metabolites such as amino acids and polyphosphates was demonstrated (21,22,23). In the light of the above findings, it was interesting to investigate the role of such vacuoles in intracellular compartmentation of free amino acids. Attempts concentrated on the development of techniques for vacuole preparation from the ergot fungus. Initially, the preparation of vacuoles from protoplasts of sclerotia-like cells proved to be difficult (24). Therefore, for comparative purposes Claviceps purpurea strain 1029 was first grown in Vogel medium in which this strain grows as a sphacelial (non-differentiated) mycelium. Accordingly, it does not produce alkaloids. Protoplasts were prepared by an improved method from this type of mycelium. These strongly vacuolated protoplasts can be easily lysed under isotonic conditions in the absence of earth alkaline ions by treatment with the detergent Triton X-100 (14). By stabilization with Ficoll 400 and subsequent mannitol-sucrose gradient centrifugation a pure vacuole preparation can be obtained. A biochemical characterization of such vacuoles is shown in Table 1. The comparative analysis of several hydrolytic enzymes and the free amino acid pool in vacuoles and whole protoplasts revealed copurification of these enzymes and the basic amino acids. This indicated that these compounds had been copurified with vacuoles and thus the hydrolytic enzymes such as α-mannosidase, acid phosphatase and β-glucosidase could serve as vacuolar markers of Claviceps purpurea vacuoles as in the case of those of other fungi.

Vacuoles from sclerotia-like cells of strain 1029 producing alkaloid were prepared by short low speed centrifugations of protoplast lysates.

Biochemical analysis of this kind of vacuoles is shown in Table 2. Also here the three hydrolytic enzymes had been purified together with the vacuoles and could be taken as vacuolar markers. However, the enrichment of the basic amino acids and also that of the other amino acids is much less than that observed in vacuoles from non-differentiated cells of Claviceps purpurea. From these data, it appears that sclerotia-like cells show a characteristic compartmentation with a large portion of the free (particularly basic) amino acids in the cyptoplasm. Whether this fact has significance in respect of peptide alkaloid synthesis remains to be seen.

Enzyme/amino acid	Activity or content per 10^{10} proto-plasts[b]	Activity or content in vacuoles prepared from 10^{10} protoplasts[b]	Yield in vacuoles (% protoplasts)
Enzyme			
α-Mannosidase	230	25.2	10.9
Acid phosphatase	61	6.8	11.1
β-Glucosidase	11.3	1.05	9.3
Glucose 6-phosphate dehydrogenase	1,100	3.57	0.32
Phosphoglucoisomerase	3,187	25.7	0.8
Total protein	3,053	101	3.3
Amino acid			
Proline	1,518	56	3.7
Glycine	477	28	5.8
Valine	458	20	4.4
Methionine	20	0.8	4.1
Isoleucine	129	4	3.1
Leucine	387	14	3.6
Tyrosine	160	11	6.9
Phenylalanine	278	1.6	5.8
γ-Amino butyrate	599	20	3.3
Ornithine	1,193	133	11.1
Lysine	1,483	166	11.2
Arginine	595	75	12.6
β-Alanine	90	3.4	3.8

Table 1   Distribution of various enzyme activities and amino acids in vacuoles and whole protoplasts derived from non-differentiated (sphacelial) mycelium of Claviceps purpurea. From (14).

Preliminary data from work in our laboratory with several low and high alkaloid yielding strains of Claviceps purpurea including methionine and tryptophan auxotrophs indicate identical composition and compartmentation of amino acid pools when grown in Vogel medium (Table 1). No increase of intracellular methionine or tryptophan (which generally is absent) in the cells of the auxotrophs was noted despite the fact that these cells had been grown in the presence of these two amino acids. On the other hand, under growth conditions where alkaloid production can take place only the sclerotia-like cell forming strains

1029 and 1029/10 showed the characteristic increased level of all amino acids in the cytoplasm as shown in Table 2, whereas the other strains with the tendency of forming long and thin hyphae did resemble the non-differentiated pattern observed in cells grown in Vogel medium (Table 1). These findings would strengthen the relationship of alkaloid production in C. purpurea with a particular morphology and metabolic state of the producing cell.

Enzyme/amino acid	Activity or content per 10^{10} proto-plasts[b]	Activity or content in vacuoles prepared from 10^{10} protoplasts[b]	Yield in vacu-oles (% proto-plasts)
Enzyme			
α-Mannosidase	51.2	3.1	6.05
Acid phosphatase	84.5	5.5	6.5
β-Glucosidase	10.9	0.65	5.9
Glucose 6-phosphate dehydrogenase	1,408	0.6	0.04
Phosphoglucoisomerase	4,250	4.2	0.1
Total protein	3,874	23.4	0.6
Amino acid			
Proline	438	2.2	0.5
Glycine	262	5.7	2.2
Valine	226	2.4	1.1
Methionine	23	0.3	1.3
Isoleucine	101	0.9	0.9
Leucine	270	2.3	0.8
Tyrosine	60	1.1	1.8
Phenylalanine	138	1.1	0.8
γ-Amino butyrate	465	4.2	0.9
Ornithine	1,009	35	3.5
Lysine	983	26	2.6
Arginine	541	20	3.6
β-Alanine	47	0.2	0.4

Table 2   Distribution of various enzyme activities and amino acids in vacuoles and whole protoplasts derived from sclerotia-like mycelium of Claviceps purpurea. From (14).

3   CONTROL OF ERGOT PEPTIDE SYNTHESIS IN CLAVICEPS PURPUREA BY AMINO ACIDS

Tryptophan acts as an inducer of clavine alkaloid synthesis in Claviceps fusiformis strain SD 58 (25). Several analogs and bioisosters of tryptophan were found to have a similar effect (26,27). Such effects were not observed in strains of Claviceps purpurea producing ergot peptide alkaloids (28). For investigating the effect of tryptophan inhibition of ergotamine synthesis in protoplasts of Claviceps purpurea ATCC 20102 during short term incubations, tryptophan (3 mM) was

added to a culture of <u>Claviceps purpurea</u> strain 1029/6 at the eighth
day of fermentation (Figure 2).

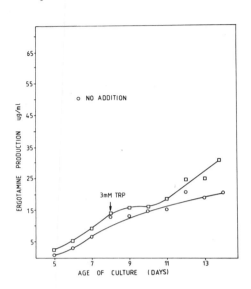

Figure 2   Effect of adding tryptophan at 3 mM concentration to an
ergotamine producing culture of <u>Claviceps purpurea</u> strain
1029/6. From (29).

As could be expected from the results obtained in the short term experiments with protoplasts, ergotamine synthesis of the culture strongly slowed down after addition of tryptophan for about two days. After
this period ergotamine synthesis began to continue and at the 14th day
of cultivation the amount of ergotamine formed was even significantly
higher than that in the control culture without tryptophan.

The transient cessation of ergotamine synthesis in the culture clearly correlates with the observed inhibition of ergotamine synthesis in
protoplasts of <u>C</u>. <u>purpurea</u> during short term experiments. However,
after prolonged incubation in a production culture this inhibitory effect apparently is overcome and the presence of the amino acid has a
clear stimulatory effect on ergotamine production. In order to test
whether tryptophan may play a similar role as an inducer of ergot peptide alkaloid synthesis in <u>C</u>. <u>purpurea</u> as in the case of clavine alkaloid synthesis in <u>C</u>. <u>fusiformis</u> in another set of experiments the
influence of tryptophan on ergotamine synthesis in strain 1029/6 was

measured. In these experiments tryptophan was present at the beginning of the fermentations. Data presented in Fig. 3 clearly reveal that
tryptophan at 3 mM concentration stimulates ergotamine synthesis by a
factor of 2. In addition, tryptophan also had the effect to overcome
the low level of ergotamine formation in the presence of 1 g/l KH_2PO_4,
which is due to growth-linked repression. These findings indicate a
similar role of tryptophan as an inducer of ergot peptide alkaloid
synthesis as has been shown in the case of clavine alkaloids in Claviceps fusiformis strain SD 58 (26,27).

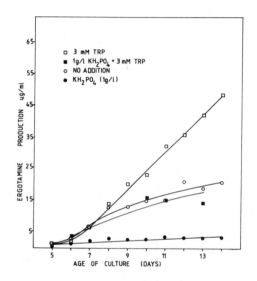

Figure 3   Influence of tryptophan on ergotamine synthesis in
             Claviceps purpurea strain 1029/6. From (29).

Other amino acids such as valine, leucine, proline or asparagine
also had a significant stimulatory effect on ergotamine synthesis in
Claviceps purpurea strain 1029/6 (Table 3). Some of these (valine, proline) could also overcome the growth-linked repression through phosphate as was observed in the case of tryptophan. In C. fusiformis the
presence of amino acids such as leucine had a clear effect of decreas-
ing alkaloid formation most probably due to overcoming the nitrogen
starvation in the medium used (25). Therefore, the mechanism of control
of alkaloid synthesis through amino acid nitrogen sources must be a
different one in C. purpurea strain 1029/6. Whether the stimulatory effect of the various amino acids depends on induction phenomena as in
the case of tryptophan is not known. Therefore, more experiments are

necessary to elucidate the mechanisms of control of ergot peptide synthesis, e.g. by measuring enzyme activities involved in alkaloid synthesis at various stages of cultivation.

Compound added	ergotamine mg/l	ergocryptine mg/l	dry weight mg/ml
No	20.7	< 1	17.3
TRP 3 mM	48.5	< 1	20.7
1g/l KH_2PO_4	3.5	< 1	26.5
TRP 3 mM+1g/l KH_2PO_4	14.1	< 1	25.9
Val 10 mM	63.9	< 1	-
Val 25 mM	82.5	34.2	17.7
Val 50 mM	80.3	50.7	16.8
Val 50 mM+1g/l KH_2PO_4	29.6	8.9	37.2
Leu 10 mM	39.6	< 1	-
Pro 50 mM	125.4	< 1	17.2
Pro 50 mM+1g/l KH_2PO_4	23.7	< 1	32.6
Asparagine 50 mM	51	< 1	-
Asparagine 50 mM+ 1g/l KH_2PO_4	3.9	< 1	-
Phenylalanine 50 mM	14.2	< 1	16.7
Phenylalanine 50 mM+ 1g/l KH_2PO_4	3.5	< 1	32.7

Table 3   Influence of various amino acids on ergot peptide synthesis
in Claviceps purpurea strain 1029/6. From (29).

4   ENZYMATIC STUDIES ON ERGOT ALKALOID SYNTHESIS

Enzymes involved in ergot alkaloid synthesis are dimethylally pyrophosphate: tryptophan dimethylallyl transferase which catalyzes the
first reaction in the biosynthetic pathway of the ergoline ring (30)
and chanoclavine-I cyclase catalyzing the cyclization of chanoclavine-I
to tetracyclic ergolines (31). Recently, a cell-free system of ergopeptine synthesis has been described (20). Starting with a crude extract
from an ergosine producing Claviceps that catalyzes the incorporation
of [^{14}C]leucine into ergosine at the expense of ATP, the system was re-
fined during further studies and the synthesis of ergotamine by an ammonium sulphate fractionated enzyme extract was demonstrated (32). In-

terestingly, agroclavine rather than D-lysergic acid was effective as
the precursor of peptide bound D-lysergic acid. Studies of ergopeptine
synthesis in this laboratory concentrated on   studies in respect to
the activation of the constituents of ergot peptides in partially purified protein fractions. The observation that D-lysergic acid when added
to protoplasts stimulated ergotamine synthesis (13) led to the screening for a D-lysergic acid activating enzyme in such fractions. Support
for this hypothesis came from previous work where the efficient conversion of dihydrolysergic acid into dihydroergotamine by Claviceps purpurea PCCE1 was demonstrated (33). Thus if D-lysergic acid or dihydrolysergic acid are free intermediates in ergot peptide synthesis, prior
to amide bond formation activation of the free carboxy group of the er-
golinic acid must take place. Such activation is likely to proceed via
the corresponding adenylate, as known in other cases of the enzymatic
biosynthesis of peptides (Fig. 4) (34).

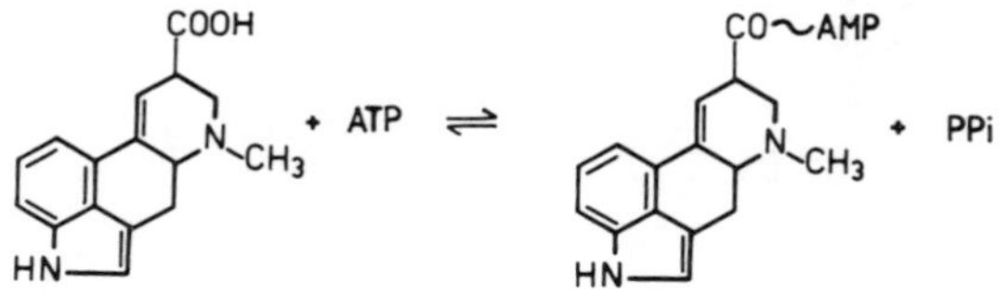

Figure 4   Reaction scheme for D-lysergic acid activation

By means of the D-lysergic acid dependent ATP pyrophosphate exchange reaction a D-lysergic acid activating enzyme was purified 145-
fold (35). Although not yet purified to homogeneity, analysis of the
enzyme revealed a native M_r in the range of 130-140 kDa and a nearly
absolute specificity for D-lysergic acid. Dihydrolysergic acid gave a
much lower ATP-pyrophosphate exchange (1-2%). Amino acids present in
the peptide chain of ergopeptines were not activated. Attempts were
made to demonstrate the formation of D-lysergic acid adenylate or dihydrolysergic acid adenylate by using [^{14}C]ATP as the radiolabel. However, the formation of such adenylates could not be demonstrated. On
the other hand, the enzyme was significantly effective in converting
[^{32}P]pyrophosphate and chemically synthesized D-lysergic acid adenylate
into [^{32}P]ATP. Conversion of dihydrolysergic acid adenylate to ATP

could also be detected although to a much lower extent as in the case
of D-lysergic acid. Measurements of specific activities of the enzyme
in cell extracts obtained from various Claviceps cultures (Table 4)
show that the enzyme is much less present in cells grown in Vogel medium where alkaloid production is very low. By contrast, specific activity is high in cells obtained from culture media which favour alkaloid production. The data also show that the specific activity of the
original C. purpurea ATCC 20102 is nearly the same as in strain 1029
with a much higher yield of ergot peptide. The enzyme was also detected at a high level in an ergocristine producing C. purpurea Ecc 93.
The fact that the enzyme is present at the same level in the original

Strain	Synthetic capacity mg/l	Medium (Age of mycelium)	Sp. activity nkat/mg
1029	100-150	Inoculum Medium (8 d)	0.108
1029	< 1	Vogel Medium (2 d)	0.0009
1029	< 1	Vogel Medium (3 d)	0.0040
1029	< 1	Vogel Medium (4 d)	0.0047
WT	0.5-2	Inoculum Medium (8 d)	0.094
Ecc 93	30-60	Ammonium-oxalate Production-Medium (8 d)	0.23

Table 4   Specific activity of D-lysergic acid activating enzyme in
           partially purified enzyme fractions from various Claviceps
           purpurea strains grown in different media.

ATCC strain and strain 1029 does not necessarily contradict its involvement in ergot alkaloid synthesis because as noted earlier the internal D-lysergic acid concentration is a rate limiting factor in ergot peptide alkaloid synthesis (13). Moreover, strain 1029 is known to
possess a higher level of ergoline ring synthesis than its parent strain

ATCC 20102 (19). Further evidence for the most certain involvement of a D-lysergic acid activating enzyme comes from data concerning the cell-free conversion of elymoclavine to paspalic acid by a particulate fraction from Claviceps purpurea PCCE1 (36). These data suggest evidence of the presence of free paspalic acid, the precursor of D-lysergic acid, within the cells of C. purpurea. Interestingly enough the enzyme activity was absent in clavine alkaloid producing Claviceps strain SD 58 which may explain the absence of D-lysergic acid derived alkaloid in this organism (36). Exactly how the D-lysergic acid activating enzyme is involved in the overall biosynthetic process as part of a multifunctional cyclol synthetase is still unknown and we must therefore await more data on the total enzymatic synthesis of ergopeptines.

5   ACKNOWLEDGEMENTS

I wish to thank Dr. H. Kobel, Sandoz AG (Basel, Switzerland) for providing me with Claviceps purpurea strain Ecc93 and Dr. R. Zocher, Institute of Biochemistry and Molecular Biology, for valuable discussions.

6   REFERENCES

(1) Stadler, P.A. (1982) Planta medica 46, 131-144.
(2) Mantle, P.G. (1975) In "The Filamentous Fungi, Vol. I" (Smith, I. E. and D.R. Berry, eds.) p. 281-300, Arnold London.
(3) Arcamone, F. (1977) In "Biologically Active Substances-Exploration and Exploitation" (Hems, D.A. ed.) p. 49-77, Wiley London.
(4) Arcamone, F., Chain, E.B., Feretti, A., Minghetti, A., Penella, P., Tonolo, A., Vero, L. (1961) Proceedings of the Royal Society Series B 155, 26-54.
(5) Kobel, H., Schreier, E., Rutschmann, J. (1964) Helvetica Chimica Acta 47, 1052-1064.
(6) Floss, H.G. (1976) Tetrahedron 32, 873-912.
(7) Spalla, C., Fillipini, S., Grein, A. (1978) Folia Microbiologia 23, 505-508.
(8) Mantle, P.G., Tonolo, A. (1968) Transactions of the British Mycological Society 51, 499-505.
(9) Kobel, H., Sanglier, J.J. (1978) In "Antibiotics and Other Secondary Metabolites, Biosynthesis and Production", FEMS Symposium No. 5 (Hütter, R. ed.) p. 233-242, Academic Press New York and London.

(10) Peberdy, J.F. (1979) Annual Review of Microbiology 33, 21-39.

(11) Stahl, Ch., Neumann, P., Schmauder, H.-P., Gröger, D. (1977) Biochemie und Physiologie der Pflanzen 171, 363-368.

(12) Spalla, C., Marnati, M.P. (1978) In "Antibiotics and Other Secondary Metabolites, Biosynthesis and Production", FEMS Symposium No. 5 (Hütter, R. ed.) p. 219-232, Academic Press New York and London.

(13) Keller, U., Zocher, R., Kleinkauf, H. (1980) Journal of General Microbiology 118, 485-494.

(14) Keller, U., Madry, N., Kleinkauf, H., Glund, H. (1984) Applied and Environmental Microbiology 47, 710-714.

(15) Keller, U. (1983) Applied and Environmental Microbiology 46, 580-584.

(16) Spalla, C., Amici, A.M., Scotti, T., Tognoli, L. (1969) In "Fermentation advances" (D. Perlman, ed.) New Brunswick N.J.

(17) Srikrai, S., Robbers, J.E. (1983) Applied and Environmental Microbiology 45, 1165-1169.

(18) Robbers, J.E., Cheng, L.-J., Anderson, J.A., Floss, H.G. (1979) Journal of Natural Products (Lloydia) 42, 537-539.

(19) Keller, U., Zocher, R., Kraepelin, G. (1982) In "Peptide Antibiotics-Biosynthesis and Functions" (Kleinkauf, H., von Döhren, H. eds.) p. 161-168 Walter de Gruyter Berlin-New York.

(20) Maier, W., Erge, D., Schumann, B., Gröger, D. (1981) Biochemical and Biophysical Research Communications 99, 155-162.

(21) Cramer, C.L., Vaughn, L.E., Davis, R.H. (1980) Journal of Bacteriology 142, 945-952.

(22) Urech, K., Dürr, M., Boller, T., Wiemken, A., Schwencke, J. (1978) Archives of Microbiology 116, 275-278.

(23) Messenguy, F., Colin, P., Ten Have, J.-P. (1980) European Journal of Biochemistry, 108, 439-447.

(24) Keller, U., Zocher, R., Kleinkauf, H. (1982). In "Advances in Biotechnology, vol. III" (Vezina, C., Singh, K.,eds.) Pergamon Press Inc. Toronto.

(25) Robbers, J.E., Robertson, L.W., Hornemann, K.M., Jindra, A., Floss, G.H. (1972) J. Bacteriol. 112, 791-796.

(26) Krupinski, V.M., Robbers, J.E., Floss, H.G. (1976) J. Bacteriol. 125, 158-165.

(27) Robbers, J.E., Skikrai, S., Floss, H.G., Schlossberger, H.G. (1982) J. Nat. Prod. 45, 178-181.

(28) Erge, D., Schumann, B., Gröger, D. (1984) Z. Allg. Mirkobiol. 10, 667-678.

(29) Han, M., Keller, U. (to be published).

(30) Heinstein, P.F., Lee, S.-L., Floss, H.G. (1971) Biochem. Biophys. Res. Commun. 44, 1244-1251.

(31) Erge, D., Maier, W., Gröger, D. (1973) Biochem. Physiol. Pflanzen 164, 234-247.

(32) Maier, W., Erge, D., Gröger, D. (1981) FEMS Microbiol. Lett. 12, 143-146.

(33) Anderson, J.A., Kim, I.-S., Lehtonen, P., Floss, H.G. (1978) J. Nat. Prod. 42, 271-273.

(34) Kleinkauf, H. (1974) Planta Med. 35, 1-18.

(35) Keller, U., Zocher, R., Krengel, U., Kleinkauf, H. (1984) Biochem. J. 218, 857-862.

(36) Kim, S.-U., Cho, Y.-J., Floss, H.G., Anderson, J.A. (1983) Planta med. 48, 145-148.

Enzyme Systems Synthesizing Peptide Antibiotics

Horst Kleinkauf and Hans von Döhren

Technical University of Berlin, Institute of Biochemistry and Molecular Biology, Franklinstr. 29, D-1000 Berlin 10 (West)

SUMMARY

In the enzymatic formation of peptide antibiotics, generally multienzymes serve as protein templates. Experimental strategies for the detection of such multienzyme systems by immunological cross reactions and the use of analogs of ATP in amino acid activation assays are presented. Expression of a lacZ fused ornithine activating fragment of gramicidin S synthetase in E. coli is discussed. From structural considerations, mechanisms of multigene rearrangements are proposed to operate in the construction of these multienzyme systems.

Examples of recently cloned single step enzymes catalyzing peptide bond formation are considered, namely glutathione and the iron chelator aerobactin.

Concerning regulation of multienzyme expression, the induction of gramicidin S synthetase by decoynine has been reported, however, no stabilization has been achieved. In chemostat experiments with B. brevis ATCC 9999, limiting conditions for the production of this multienzyme system have been determined. Oxygen uptake proved to be of primary importance in the attainment of high levels of enzyme. Both low and high levels of oxygen uptake lead to a decrease.

Recent examples of directed biosynthesis are discussed: The precursor directed formation of arphamenines by Chromobacterium

violaceum, the production of novel quinomycins by Streptomyces
echinatus, and the accumulation of half actinomycins in Streptomyces
antibioticus by feeding with analogs of 4-methyl-3-hydroxy-anthranilate.

1   INTRODUCTION

The current developments in biotechnology have opened up new perspectives in the production of metabolites. The characterization of
enzymes catalyzing metabolic conversions has been aided by the introduction of new separation techniques. Thus, in the last few years, remarkable progress has taken place in the description of enzymes involved in secondary metabolism. This step will be followed by cloning
efforts and the elucidation of primary structures. Structural genes
and their control elements may then be manipulated to improve the production and properties of metabolites (Table 1).

In the following survey, current and future applications, as well as
recent applications of the traditional techniques, will be discussed
in the fields of peptide antibiotics and bioactive peptides.

Table 1 : Current Approaches in Metabolite Production

Genetic (internal)	Environmental (external)
overproduction directed by regulatory mutation or gene copy number	fermentation control chemostat culture precursor direction
manipulation of the enzymic outfit in composition and design	immobilisation

In a recent compilation (1) of such compounds, we have listed some
400 peptides, most of them produced by microorganisms. Although they
were the first type of antibiotics to be discovered, increasing interest
is being noted again, the number of known compounds almost doubling
within the last decade. To recall the basic features of their biosynthesis, three major routes have been described so far (Fig. 1):
the ribosomal pathway, peptide formation on multienzyme templates, and
sequences of enzymes catalyzing single reaction steps.

Fig. 1: **Biosynthetic Mechanisms of Peptide and Protein Formation**

SYSTEM	PRODUCT
nucleic acid dependent	**ribosomal**

TYPE 1
choice of program
assembly line

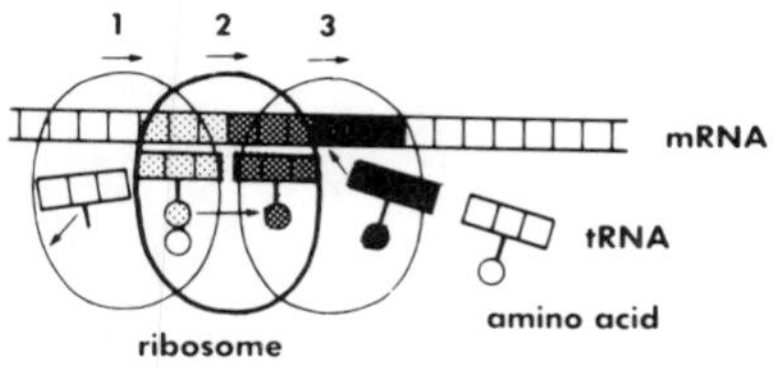

mRNA
tRNA
amino acid
ribosome

complex mechanism
- up to 180 components participating -

ribosomal
- linear polypeptides of any sequence and length from 20 proteinogenic amino acids
- activation as aminoacyladenylates
- high specificity
- high energy requiring
- proof reading mechanisms
- processing of propeptides

nucleic acid independent

TYPE 2
fixed program
assembly line

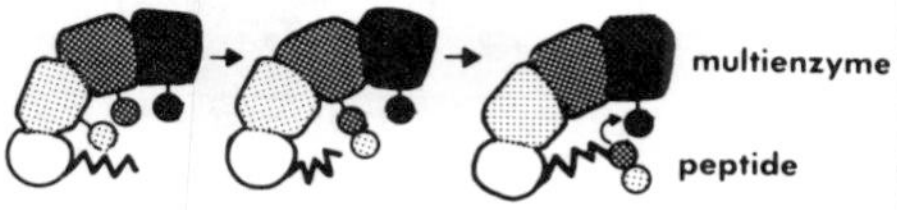

multienzyme
peptide

all intermediates remain enzyme-bound
the sequence is determined on the multifunctional enzyme-chain
4'-phosphopantetheine is cofactor
enzymes identified so far only in bacteria or fungi

enzymatic
- linear, branched and cyclic peptides and depsipeptides, e. g. gramicidin S
- activation as aminoacyladenylates
- low specificity
- incorporation of analogs
- non-protein amino acids (D-configuration, ornithine, diaminobutyrate)
- modification, e. g. N-methylation
- length of peptides up to about 30 amino acids

TYPE 3
supply process

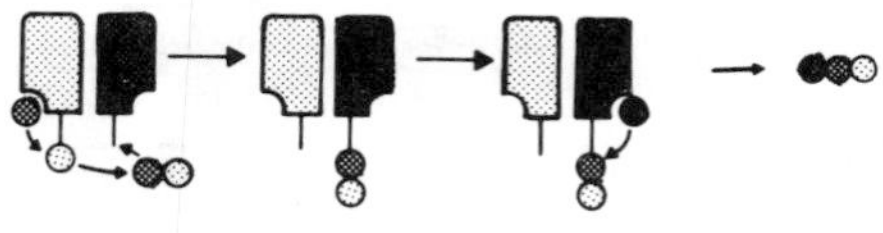

intermediates are soluble
- only one component is activated -

- linear peptides, e. g. glutathione
- activation as phosphates or as aminoacyladenylates
- synthesis of short peptides (approximately 5 amino acids)
- non-protein amino acids are components
- low specificity

2   RIBOSOMAL PATHWAYS

The ribosomal pathway is used to form antitumor polypeptides such as neocarzinostatin, but requires the addition of a chromophore (Fig. 2). The well known food preservative nisin and its close relative subtilin, formed by <u>Streptococcus</u> <u>lactis</u> and <u>Bacillus</u> <u>subtilis</u> are also presumably derived from larger precursor polypeptides (5), and then highly modified by enzymic conversions (Fig. 3).

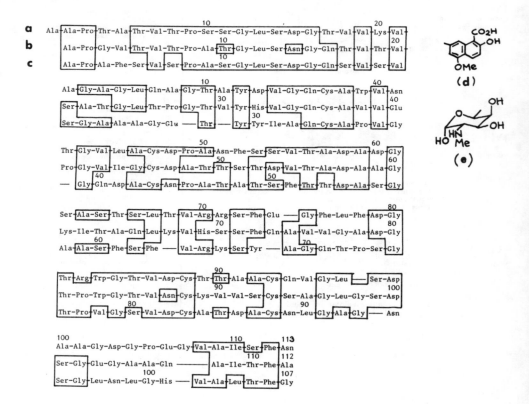

<u>Fig. 2:</u> Structures of neocarzinostatin (a), macromomycin (b) and actinoxanthin (c), antitumor polypeptides of ribosomal origin produced by strains of Streptomyces (3). Structures (d) and (e) are components of the essential chromophore (4).

Some evidence has been obtained that nisin production is located on a 30 MDa plasmid together with nisin resistance and sucrose fermentation (6). The information required for the primary structure is thus easily accessible, while modifying enzymes have not been characterized.

The similarities of transformation of the subtilin and nisin precursors, as well as the many known examples of structural homologies of metabolites from unrelated organisms have been interpreted in terms of extrachromosomal location of genes, or transposon like transfer of information. Genes coding for structural elements or modifying enzymes may be carried on transposable elements, and by mixing and reassortment lead to novel products (7).

This is an hypothesis quite attractive in the field of peptide antibiotics originating by the second pathway on multienzyme templates.

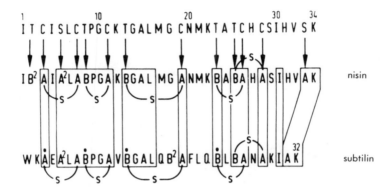

Fig. 3: Structures of the ribosomally derived peptides nisin and subtilin, and the so far predictable precursor structure of nisin. Dehydroalanine (A^2) and dehydrobutyrate (B^2) are derived from serine and threonine upon dehydration. Formation of thioether (-S-) bridges leads to an unusually fixed structure.

3   MULTIENZYME SYSTEMS

The first two peptide antibiotics characterized, tyrocidine and gramicidin S from <u>Bacillus</u> <u>brevis</u>, show remarkable sequence homologies (Fig. 4). The protein templates directing the formation of these cyclic decapeptides have been partially characterized.

These are multifunctional polypeptides containing up to 6 amino acid activating functions, and, if catalyzing elongation, the enzyme-bound cofactor 4'-phosphopantetheine. Such an assembly for multifunctional polypeptides reduces the number of genes of each pathway considerably.

Table 2: Current State of Research of Enzyme Systems Forming Peptides and Peptide-like Structures

compound	organism / source	activation of precursors adenylate	activation of precursors phosphate	total enzymatic synthesis	enzyme studies prelim.	enzyme studies advanced	genetic studies (cloning)
actinomycin	Streptomyces antibioticus	+		–	+		
aerobactin	Escherichia coli			+	+		+
alamethicin	Trichoderma viride	+		+	+		+
bacitracin	Bacillus licheniformis ATCC 10716	+		+		+	(+)
beauvericin	Beauveria bassiana	+		+	+		
bleomycin	Streptomyces verticillus			–			
carnosine	Chick muscle / rat brain		+			+	
cyclosporine	Tolypocladium inflatum	+		–	+		
edeine	Bacillus brevis Vm4	+		(+)	+		
enniatins	Fusarium oxysporum	+		+		+	
enterochelin	Escherichia coli K-12 Salmonella typhimurium	+		+		+	
ergot-peptides	Claviceps purpurea	+		(+)			
ferrichrome	Aspergillus quadricinctus			+	+		
folyl-poly- γ-Glu	Corynebacterium sp. Escherichia coli rat liver / chinese hamster ovary cells			+		+	
glutathione	Escherichia coli K-12 bovine erythrocytes		+	+		+	+

Table 2: Current State of Research of Enzyme Systems Forming Peptides and Peptide-like Structures

compound	organism / source	activation of precursors		total	enzyme studies		genetic studies
		adenylate	phosphate	enzymatic synthesis	prelim.	advanced	(cloning)
gramicidin (linear)	Bacillus brevis ATCC 8185	+		(+)	+		
gramicidin S	Bacillus brevis ATCC 9999	+		+	+	+	+
leupeptin	Streptomyces roseus	+		+		+	
mycobacillin	Bacillus subtilis B 3		+	+	+	+	
penicillin	Cephalosporium acremonium			+	+		+
	Penicillium chrysogenum						
	Streptomyces clavuligerus						
4'-phospho-pantetheine	Escherichia coli B		+	+		+	
	rat liver						
	Brevibacterium ammoniagenes						
poly-γ-D-Glu	Bacillus licheniformis			+	+		
polymyxin	Aerobacillus polyaerogenes	+		+	+		
	Bacillus polymyxa						
tyrocidine	Bacillus brevis ATCC 8185	+		+		+	(+)

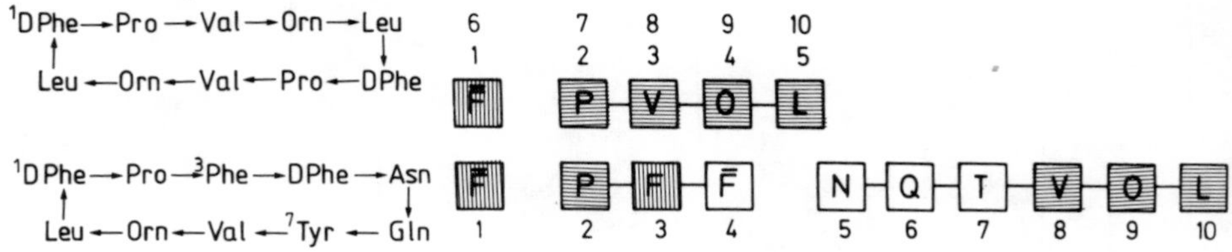
1DPhe → Pro → Val → Orn → Leu
Leu ← Orn ← Val ← Pro ← DPhe
6 7 8 9 10
1 2 3 4 5
F P V O L
1DPhe → Pro → 3Phe → DPhe → Asn
Leu ← Orn ← Val ← 7Tyr ← Gln
F P F F N Q T V O L
1 2 3 4 5 6 7 8 9 10

Fig. 4: Structures of gramicidin S and tyrocidine (left), and their protein templates (right). The possible structural homologies of the multienzymes have been indicated. Squares symbolize amino acid activating units. Peptide carrier protein region containing pantetheine is not shown (2).

The fungal depsipeptides enniatin and beauvericin are thus formed by single multienzymes (Fig. 5). The dodecapeptide bacitracin is formed by a set of three multienzymes (Fig. 6). Other examples of less well characterized enzyme systems are linear gramicidin, alamethicin, polymyxin, edeine, and cyclosporin (9) (Table 2).

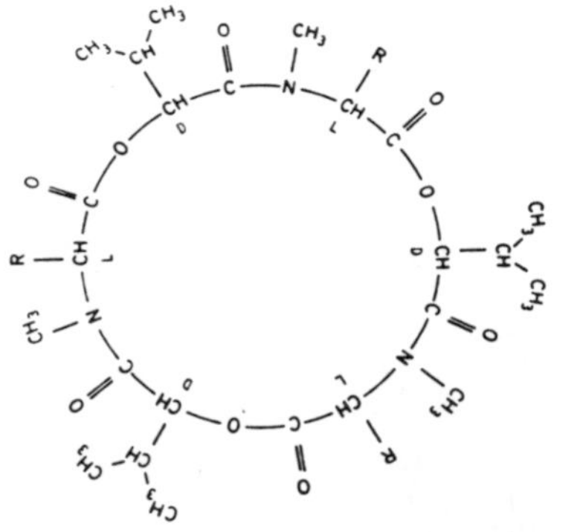

Fig. 5:

Structures of enniatin A (R= $-CH(CH_3)CH_2CH_3$), enniatin B (R= isopropyl), enniatin C (R= $CH_2CH(CH_3)_2$), and beauvericin (R= phenyl). These depsipeptides are formed on single multienzymes from amino acid, hydroxy acid, S-adenosyl-methionin and $MgATP^{2-}$ (7,8).

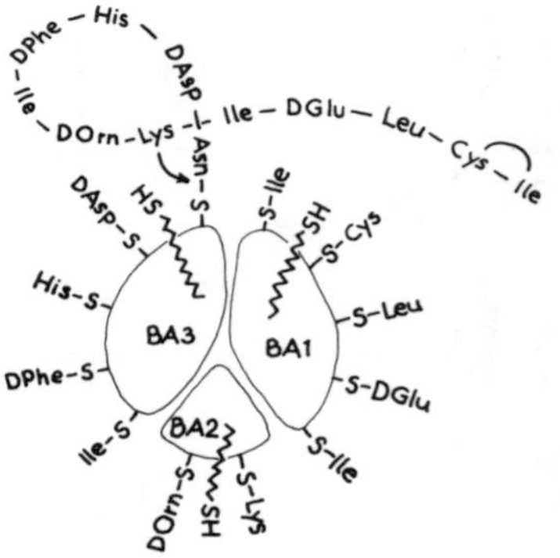
BA3
BA1
BA2

Fig. 6:

Structure of bacitracin, illustrated by the terminating step on the symbolized multienzyme system with BA1 (330 KDa, steps 1-5), BA2 (210 KDa, steps 6, 7), and BA3 (380 KDa, steps 8-12) (12, 13).

Remarkable sequence homologies within the peptaibol family of linear
aminoisobutyrate containing peptides with a C-terminal hydroxyl function can be noted (Table 3). On the basis of the above hypothesis, such
homologies can be interpreted by multigene rearrangements (Fig. 7).
Primary sequences of peptide made nonribosomally would then be fixed
by the assembly of amino acid activating units on the DNA level.

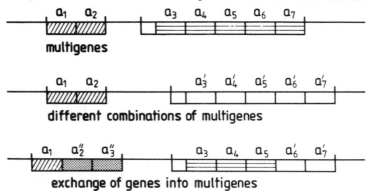

Fig. 7:   Hypothetical multigene rearrangements, leading to various
structures, sequential pathways fused to multigenes lead
to multienzymes containing fused functional units. Single
units or sequences of units can be integrated in different
pathways into multifunctional structures   (18).

Such models now call for verification to more clearly define activating units and the functional principle of this thiotemplate mechanism.
As a first approach, antibodies directed against gramicidin S synthetase 2, a multienzyme activating proline, valine, ornithine, and
leucine, were assayed for their interaction with other multienzymes.
By blotting techniques cross-reactions of various multienzymes have
been demonstrated (19). A quite unexpected reaction with enniatin
synthetase has been studied in more detail. Comparing both multienzymes
(Table 4), one of *Bacillus brevis*, the latter of *Fusarium oxysporum*,
an eucaryote, they are of similar size, both containing 4'-phospho-
pantetheine, and display similar images on negatively stained electron
micrographs (20, 21).

Sheep antibodies produced against enniatin synthetase cross-react
with gramicidin S synthetase (Fig. 8). Both antibodies lead to inhibition of enzyme activity of amino acid or hydroxy acid activation
reactions (Fig. 9). Comparing the valine sites of both enzymes, a less
pronounced inhibition is found with the heterologous antibodies, compared to a stimulation in case of hydroxy acid activation.

Table 3: Peptaibols and Related Peptides

Name	Producer	Structure [4]
antiamoebins [1]	Emericellopsis poonensis / Emericellopsis synnematicola / Cephalosporium pimprine	AcPheAib$_2$IvaGlyLeuAib$_2$HypGlnIva[13]HypAibProPhol
alamethicins	Trichoderma viride	AcAibProAibAlaAib[6]AlaGlyAibValAibGlyLeuAibProValAib$_2$GluGlnPhol
emericins [2]	Emericellopsis microspora	AcPheAib$_3$ValGlyLeuAib$_2$HypGlnIvaHyp[14]AibPhol
gliodeliquescin A	Gliocladium deliquescens	Ac(AibAla)$_3$GlnAibValAibGlyLeuAibProValAib$_2$Gln$_2$Phol
hypelcins	Hypocrea peltata	AcAibProAibAlaAib$_2$GlnAib[15]LeuAibGlyAib$_2$ProValAib$_2$Gln$_2$Leuol
leucinostatin B [3]	Paecilomyces lilacinus	MheMeProAhmodHyLeuAibLeu$_2$Aib$_2$βAlaDpd
paracelsins	Trichoderma reesei	Ac(AibAla)$_3$GlnAib[8]LeuAibGlyAib$_2$ProValAib$_2$GlnPhol
suzukacillin	Trichoderma viride	Ac(AibAla)$_3$GlnAib$_3$GlyLeuAibProValAibIvaGluGlnPhol
trichopolyn	Trichoderma polysporum	MedaAlaAib$_2$IleAlaAib$_2$Tda
trichotoxins	Trichoderma viride	AcAibGlyAibLeuAibGlnAib$_2$AlaAib$_2$ProLeuAib[16]Iva[17]GlnValol
zervamycins	Emericellopsis salmosynnemata	AcTrp[2]Ile[3]Gln Iva[4]Val[5]ThrAib[8]LeuAibHypGlnAibHypAibProPhol

1) identical with TÜ165,   2) samaosporin or stilbellin,   3) P168 or antibiotic 1907,   4) known replacements are

[2]Ile-Val, [3]Glu-Gln, [4]Iva-Aib, [5]Val-Ile, [6]Ala-Aib, [8]Leu-Val, [13]Hyp-Pro, [14]Aib-Ala, [15]Leu-Ile, [16]Iva-Aib, [17]Glu-Gln

abbreviations are: Ahmod: 2-amino-6-hydroxy-4-methyl1-8-oxodecanoic acid, Aib: α-aminoisobutyric acid,
Dpd: (2S)-N^1-methylpropane-1,2-diamine, HyLeu: hydroxy-Leu, Hyp: [4]-hydroxy-Pro,
Iva: isovaline (α-ethylalanine), Meda: (R)-2-methyldecanoic acid, Mhe: (4S)-(2E)-4-methylhex-2-enoic acid,
-ol: carboxyl reduced to alcohol, Tda: trichodiaminol

Table 4: Comparison of Enniatin Synthetase and
Gramicidin S Synthetase 2

	GS 2	EN
organism	Bacillus brevis	Fusarium oxysporum
size	280 KDa	250 KDa
pantetheine	+	+
activates	Pro,Val,Orn,Leu	Val,DHiv (Leu,Ile)
other reactions	initiation with	N-methylation
	GS 1, cyclization	cyclization

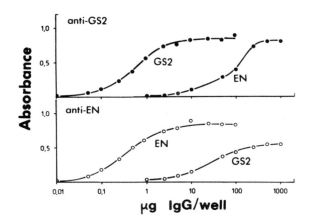

Fig. 8: Cross reaction of GS 2 with anti-EN-IgG (bottom) and EN
with anti-GS 2-IgG (top) as studied by ELISA with per-
oxidase labelled anti-sheep IgG. The sensitivity of the
heterologous system is about 100-fold lower than that of
the homologous systems GS 2 / anti-GS 2-IgG or EN/anti-
EN-IgG, respectively.

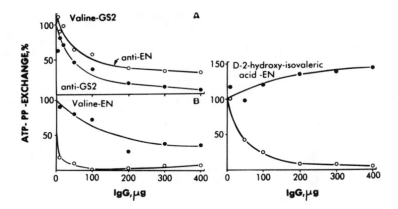

<u>Fig. 9:</u>   Inhibition of activation reactions of multienzymes by sheep-
IgG.   A: top, valine activation site of GS 2, open circles
anti-EN-IgG, full circles anti-GS 2-IgG.   Bottom, valine
activation site of EN, symbols as above.   B: hydroxyisovale-
rate activation site of EN, symbols as above.

This apparent structural homology can be used in identifying unknown
peptide synthetases or multienzyme fragments derived by cloning procedures.

     Another sensitive assay for this purpose has come from the analysis
of substrate analogs in amino acid activation reactions. In probing
analogs of ATP for a possible classification scheme of activation sites,
as was reported for aminoacyl-tRNA-synthetases (22) (Fig. 10), there
were only minor differences between the activation sites of gramicidin
S synthetases. An extension of the ATP-site architecture to other
multienzymes again indicates similarity of structures. Twenty-two sites
on 11 different multienzymes accept 2'-deoxy-ATP. This quite sensitive
assay permits differentiation at most aminoacyl-tRNA synthetases not
accepting 2'-deoxy-ATP as substrate in crude extracts. We thus arrive
at a second useful procedure for the analysis of nonribosomal peptide
synthetase functions which has been applied in recent genetic studies
of the gramicidin S system.

     The first genetic approaches to gramicidin S formation attempted
to trace an extrachromosomal location of antibiotic synthetase genes,
since intercalating agents lead to nonproducer mutants at a high frequency (Table 5). A plasmid (27, 28) and a defective phage (29) have
been characterized, but have not been associated with peptide formation.

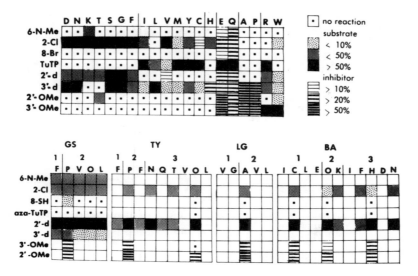

<u>Fig. 10:</u>   Detection of families of aminoacyl-tRNA-synthetases in
Escherichia coli by analogs of ATP in tRNA aminoacylation
(22), top. Bottom: interaction of various peptide synthetases with analogs of ATP in amino acid activation reactions
detected by amino acid dependent ATP-PPi-exchange. The
following compounds were used: 6-N-Me = 6-N-methyl-ATP,
2-Cl = 2-chloro-ATP, 8-SH = 8-SH-ATP, TUTP = tubercidine-
triphosphate, 2' or 3'd = 2' or 3' deoxy-ATP, or 3'OMe
= 2' or 3'o-methyl-ATP (23). Enzyme nomenclature is as
introduced by us (24): GS, gramicidin S snythetase,
TY, tyrocidine synthetase, LG (linear) gramicidin synthetase, BA, bacitracin synthetase; the numbers 1-3 indicate
the sequence of multienzymes.

<u>Table 5:</u>   Effectiveness of Mutagens in the Production of Gramicidin
S-negative Strains

mutagen	number of colonies	GS⁻ mutants	references
NTG	6000	20	Saito et al. (25)
NTG	2100	4)	
EB	200	16)	Marahiel et
AO	200	17)	al. (26)

NTG : N-methyl-N'-nitro-N-nitrosoguanidine

EB : ethidium bromide

AO : acridine orange

Other observations demonstrate that these curing agents may also be
directed against certain chromosomal DNA regions (Table 6).

Table 6:   Some Effects of DNA-Intercalating Drugs on
            Gene Expression or Developmental Events

organism	repression of	agent	source	
S. alboniger	o-demthylpuromycin-transferase	EB	Sankaran & Pogell	(30)
E. coli	ß-galactosidase	AO	ibid.	
E. coli	acid hexose phospha-tase	AO	ibid.	
B. subtilis Marburg	early sporulation functions (T_o-T_1)		Rogolsky & Nakamura	(31)
B. subtilis	stops sporulation process (T_o-T_4)	PR	Burke & Spizizen	(32)
	stops sporulation process (T_o-T_2)	AO	ibid.	
B. subtilis 168	stops sporulation process until stage IV	AO	Takahashi & MacKenzie	(33)
Xenopus laevis	transcription initiation	EB	Pruit & Reeder	(67)

EB: ethidium bromide,   AO: acridine orange,   PR: promethazine

   In the following studies it proved to be quite difficult to adapt
genetic procedures established for B. subtilis to B. brevis ATCC 9999.
From a gene bank constructed with the cosmid pQB 79-1, which has been
selected according to the expected DNA size of up to 10 kilobases for
these multienzymes, no expression of proteins cross-reacting by immu-
noblotting has been found. However, with the expression vector pUR2-
Bam, which has been derived from pBR 322, a 3.9 kilobase insert of
B. brevis ATCC 9999, has been cloned under lac promoter control
(Fig. 11). In presence of IPTG, a 150 KDa-protein is expressed in
E. coli activating ornithine. The fragment is unstable, and degraded
to fragments ranging from 70 to 140 KDa. Partial purification revealed
that binding and kinetics of ATP, ornithine, and 2'-deoxy-ATP were unchanged compared to the wild type multienzyme.

   This DNA is now being used as a probe for the detection for the
remaining DNA of gramicidin S synthetase 2 as well as other synthetases.

Back in 1973, Sankaran and Pogell proposed that such intercalating dyes have an affinity for certain (30) conformations of promoter regions. The catabolite-sensitive expression of enzymes like the transferase catalyzing the final methyl transfer in puromycin biosynthesis, or ß-galactosidase proved to be inhibited. This inhibition could be reversed by cyclic AMP. Although of doubtful specificity, a number of sporulation specific events are also thought to be inhibited by acridine orange or promethazine. These results may be related so some pitfalls in relating plasmids to secondary product formation by the use of curing agents.

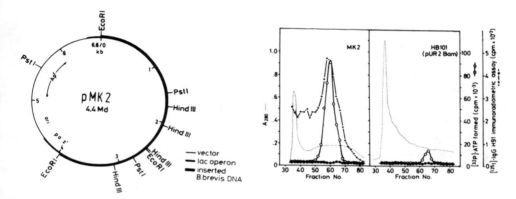

Fig. 11: Cloning and IPTG induced expression of the ornithine activation site of GS 2 in E. coli (34, 35). Left: map of a 3.9 kb insert of B. brevis ATCC 9999-DNA. Right: in presence of IPTG a protein cross reacting with anti-gramicidin S synthetase 2 IgG can be detected (AcA 34) in MK2 containing cells. When the total protein is applied to gel filtration, the activation of ornithine can be correlated with the antibody binding. In the control experiment with E. coli HB 101, a small ornithine-dependent activation reaction has also been detected (right), this activity has been assigned to lysyl-tRNA synthetase. Note that the size of this enzyme is 100 KDa, and that the MK2 preparation also contains a shoulder at the right site. The lys-tRNA-synthetase accepts, however, at a poor rate, ornithine as well as 2'-deoxy-ATP as substrates. It can be completely separated from the MK2 fragment activating ornithine on DEAE-cellulose.

From cloning and sequence studies of multienzymes and their fragments, the following results and information are available:

(1) Single amino acid activating units can be studied separately and prepared in quantity. Such fragments will be of use in enzymatic peptide synthesis (amino acid addition) and amino acid analysis (detection of amino acids);

(2)   gene segments of defined active units usually being constituents
      of multifunctional polypeptides will be used in the construction
      of new enzyme templates;

(3)   information on the linkage of such units will be used to ascer-
      tain if rearrangements, as observed with transposable elements,
      are involved in the construction of these enzyme systems; and

(4)   information on promoter regions and the possible involvement of
      RNA polymerase-associated polypeptides will be used to study regu-
      latory events.

4   SINGLE STEP ENZYMES

The third type of peptide biosynthesis is the stepwise addition
of components by individual enzymes. Well known systems are reaction
sequences leading to pantetheine, glutathione, or peptidoglycans.
This type of enzyme may be of particular interest in the study of
peptides with immunomodulating properties, such as FK-156 (Fig. 12).
The enzymes involved in formation of glutathione, which actually is not

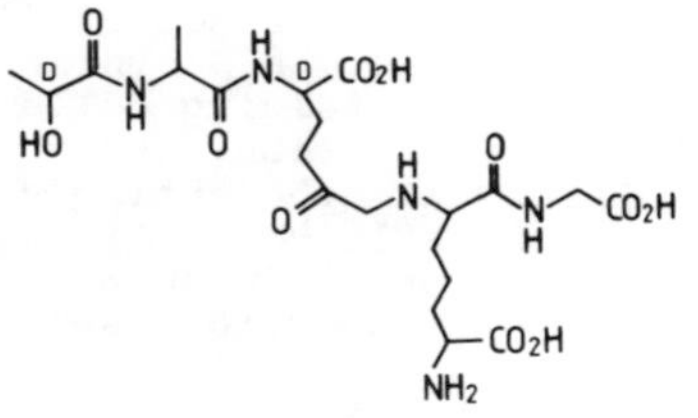

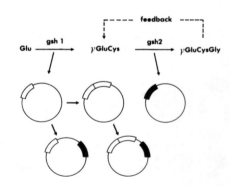

Fig. 12:

Structure of FK-156 a peptide
with immunomodulating properties produced by Streptomyces
violacens   (36)

Fig. 13:

Schematic illustration of cloning of
Y -glutamyl-cysteine synthetase and
glutathione-synthetase into pBR 322
derivatives by Kimura et al. (37-39).
For discussions see text.

considered a secondary metabolite, have been cloned to improve production (17, 18, 19)   (Fig. 13). We include this example since a clear
distinction between primary and secondary metabolites cannot always be

drawn (40). The γ-glutamylcysteine synthetase gene from E. coli strain B desensitized to feedback inhibition by reduced glutathione was introduced into pBR 322 by a Pst I chromosomal digest. The gene does not contain any Pst I susceptible sites. Selection was then carried out with a mutant deficient in production of the synthetase. Transformations were detected by a thiol-specific nitroprusside colour reaction. These methods permit only a prescreening, since the reaction is not specific. It was observed later that mainly thiol compounds other than GSH were responsible for positive reactions. This mutant was then used to insert the glutathione synthetase gene into the same vector. Both plasmids or constructions with pBR 325 containing both genes were used in the continuous production of glutathione with carrageenan immobilized E. coli B. This example illustrates the improvement of catalytic efficiency by removal of a control element and increase of the gene copy number. An equally important contribution came from studies on immobilization, the precursor supply, and ATP regeneration.

A system yet to be characterized that may well be related to peptide antibiotics are the enzymes synthesizing aerobactin (Fig. 14). For this peptide-related iron (III) chelator, the following pathway has been proposed (40):

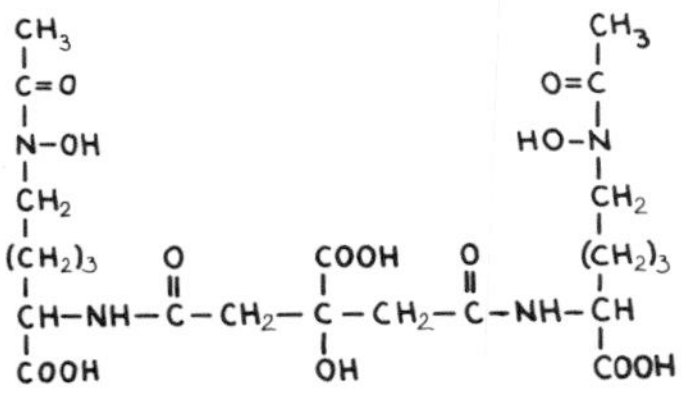
CH3
C=O
N-OH
CH2
(CH2)3
O
COOH
O
CH3
O=C
HO-N
CH2
(CH2)3
CH-NH-C-CH2-C-CH2-C-NH-CH
COOH
OH
COOH

Fig. 14: Structure of aerobactin

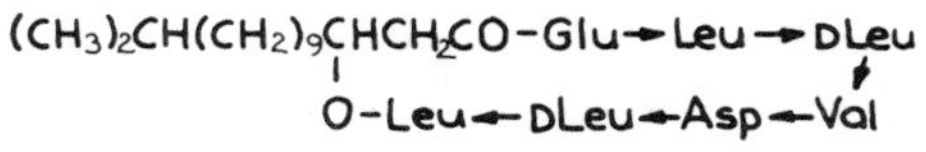
(CH3)2CH(CH2)9CHCH2CO-Glu→Leu→DLeu
O-Leu←DLeu←Asp←Val

Fig. 16: Structure of surfactin

First N-hydroxylation of lysine, followed by N-acetylation, then coupling to citrate with peptide bond formation. Aerobactin release has been traced to certain CoIV plasmids in E. coli K 12 (42), and the aerobactin region has been cloned into derivatives of pMR 322 (43, 44). As is the case with the well-known enterochelin synthetase from E. coli K 12 (45), the enzyme system is under control of extracellular iron. Thus 10 μM Fe^{3+} suppresses synthesis of the three enterochelin enzymes by 95 %. Several new structures of chelators have been des-

Table 7:   Iron Carrier Compounds

Compound	Producer Organisms	Structure[1] (→ peptide, — ester bond)
aerobactin	Aerobacter aerogenes enteric species	AcOHLys ← Cit → AcOHLys
albomycins	Streptomyces griseus, Streptomyces subtropicus	C(3MUSer → Ser → Ser → AcOHorn$_3$)
coprogen	Penicillium, Aspergillus, Neurospora, Ustilago	αActransHMPOHorn—C(transHMPOHorn$_2$)
dimerum acid	Fusarium dimerum	C(transHMPOHorn$_2$)
enterobactin	Escherichia coli, Salmonella typhimurium enteric species	Dhb → Ser ⟍ Ser / Dhb → Ser - Ser ← Dhb
ferramidochloromycin	Streptomyces AS 13	C(Gly$_3$ → AcOHorn$_3$)
ferrichrome	Penicillium, Aspergillus, Neurospora, Ustilago	C(Ser → Ser → Gly → AcOHorn$_3$)
ferrichrome A		C(Ser → Ala → Ser → AcOHorn$_3$)
ferrichrome C		
ferrichrysine	Aspergillus sp.	C(Ser → Ser → Gly → AcOHorn$_3$)
ferricrocine		C(Gly → Ser → Gly → AcOHorn$_3$)
ferrimycin A1	Streptomyces griseoflavus, Streptomyces galileus, Streptomyces lavendulae	3A5HBX → 1A5HP ← Suc → 1A5HP ← Suc → 1A5HP
ferrioxamin B	Streptomyces sp.	1A5HP ← Suc → 1A5HP ← Suc → 1A5HPAC
ferrioxamin E	Pseudomonas stutzeri	C(1A5HP ← Suc →)3
ferrirhodin	as ferrichromes	C(Ser → Ser → Gly → cisHMPOHorn$_3$)
ferrirubin		C(Ser → Ser → Gly → transHMPOHorn$_3$)

Table 7: Iron Carrier Compounds

Compound	Producer Organisms	Structure[1] ($\rightarrow$ peptide, — ester bond)
fusarinines	Fusarium roseum / Fusarium sp.	$(\text{cisHMPOHorm} -)_{1,2,3}$ or Cyclo $(\ )_3$
malonichrome	Fusarium roseum	$C(\text{Ala, Gly, Gly} \rightarrow \text{MaOHorm}_3)$
mycobactins	Mycobacteria	$^1SA \rightleftharpoons {}^2Ser \rightarrow FA(\varepsilon)\text{OHLys-3HyBu} \rightarrow \text{cOHLys}^2$
pseudobactin	Pseudomonas B10	$\text{ASuc} \rightarrow \text{DADNQ}(\varepsilon)\text{Lys} \rightarrow \text{D}\beta\text{THASp} \rightarrow \text{Ala} \rightarrow \text{DaThr} \rightarrow \text{Ala} \rightarrow \text{cDOHorm}$
pyoverdin Pa	Pseudomonas aeruginosa	$\text{ASuc} \rightarrow \text{DADNQ} \rightarrow \text{fDSer} \rightarrow \text{Arg} \rightarrow \text{fOHorm} \rightarrow \text{Thr} \rightarrow$ $\text{Lys} \rightarrow \text{cDOHorm}$
rhodotorulic acid	Rhodotorula sp.	$C(\text{AcOHorm}_2)$
tetraglycylferrichrome	Neovossia indica	$C(\text{Gly}_4 \rightarrow \text{AcOHorm}_3)$
thoricin	Epicoccum purpurescens	$\text{Ac}_2\text{OHorm} - C(\text{transHMPOHorm}_2)$

[1] Abbreviations used are: 1A5HP = 1,5-diaminopentan, 3A5HBX = a substituted 3-amino-hydroxy-benzoic acid
AcOHLys = N(σ)acetyl-N(σ)hydroxy-Lys, AcOHorm = N(σ)acetyl-N(σ)hydroxy-Orn, Ac$_2$OHorm = N(α,σ)diacetyl-N(δ)hydroxy-Orn,
aThr = allo-Thr, C = cyclo, Cit = citric acid, D = D-configuration, DADHQ = 2,3-diamino-6,7-dihydroxyquinoline,
Dhb = dihydroxybenzoic acid, f = formyl, HMP = 5-hydroxy-3-methyl-pent-2-enoic acid, MaOHorm = N(σ)malonyl-N(σ)hydroxy-Orn,
3MUSer = 3-methyl-uracil sulfon-attached to Ser, OHorm = N(σ)hydroxy-Orn, Suc-succinyl, THASp = β-threo-β-hydroxy-ASP

[2] Amino acid replacements in mycobactins are ^{2}Ser = ^{2}Thr and ^{3}HyBu = ^{3}3HyBu = ^{3}3H2MPA; the abbreviations are SA: salicylic acid,
may be replaced by 6-methyl-salicylic acid; the bentconnection between SA and Ser indicates an oxazoline ring formation;
the fatty acid (FA)-moiety varies, the main species is an n-cis-octadec-2-enoyl chain; the β-hydroxy acids are either
3-hydroxybutyric or 3-hydroxy-2-methylpentanoic acid (3H2MPA).

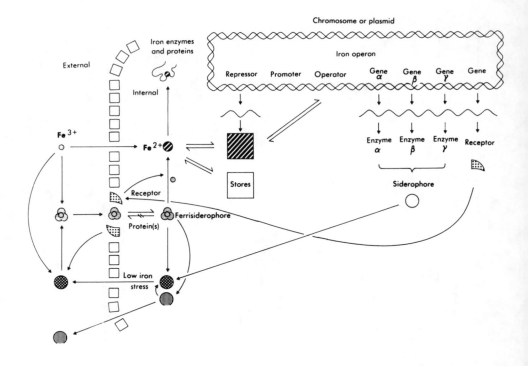

Fig. 15:   Schematic model of low- and high affinity iron transport
(44)

The siderophore, like aerobactin, or enterochelin (1) is
produced by the coordinate action of several enzymes. For
aerobactin, these are N-hydroxylase (α), N-acetyl-trans-
ferase (ß) and the synthetase (citrate activation and
coupling (γ). Transcription of the polycistronic mRNA is
under the control of a ferrous (Fe^{2+}) binding repressor
(3). Under low iron stress, when the low affinity transport (4) is insufficient, transcription is initiated. The
iron carrier synthesized is excreted (5), binds ferric
(Fe^{3+}) ions, attains the fixed conformation of the Fe^{3+}-
siderophore complex (6), and is taken up by at least one
receptor protein (7). The intracellular release of tightly
bound Fe^{3+} (8) occurs either by reduction to Fe^{2+}, or in
some cases, by modification of the carrier structure (9).

cribed within the last years (Table 7). The unique control mechanism, although not understood at present in detail, may significantly aid the molecular genetic approach of the biosynthetic mechanism (Fig. 15).

Contrary to iron chelators, the production of surfactin (Fig. 16) by B. subtilis ATCC 21332 is enhanced by the addition of Fe^{3+} in the mmolar range (46) (Fig. 17). This has been attributed to either a defective transport system, or a possible complex formation with the product, which upon removal by foam fractionation would lead to a gradual washout. Surfactin is the most powerful biosurfactant known so far, reducing the surface tension of water from 72 mN/m to 27 mN/m.

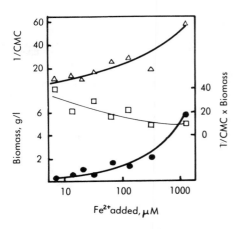

Fig. 17:

Enhancement of surfactin production by Fe^{2+} (46). Concentration
of surfactin is expressed in re-
ciprocals of critical micelle
concentration (1/CMC).

5   FERMENTATION PROCEDURES

Concerning the regulation of peptide production in fermentation procedures, many observations of simple improvements have been reported. The largest body of literature concerns gramicidin S. The fermentation of gramicidin S, however, has never reached the sophistication of penicillin production. An efficient process design would require detailed physiological studies of the producer, which have not yet been done in sufficient depth. Some general observations, that are in accord with other antibiotic fermentations or of general interest will be given.

Gramicidin S is produced in simple batch fermentations in the transition state as a typical idiolite. The original strain had been isolated from soil in Moscow in the early forties by Gauze and Brazhnikova. The antibiotic was industrially produced until the early sixties. When research on the enzyme system was taken up in 1967 and later in 1975, the yields of the strain obtained from the American Type Culture

Collection was far from what had been achieved in the past. Despite extensive nutritional studies most fermentations never reached 10 % of the 5 g/l that had been reported. A breakthrough was the approach of Vandamme et al., who by controlling the pH at the production phase level prolonged this phase, and thus achieved the required yield (41) (Fig. 18).

During this prolonged production phase, a second slow growth phase is observed. A similar phase and improvement have been reported in the

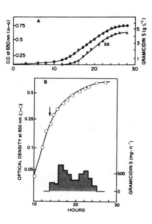

Fig. 18:

Controlled pH-fermentation of gramicidin S by Bacillus brevis ATCC 9999 (47,24). A: presentation according to Vandamme illustrates production during "active growth" when grown in a complex yeast extract/peptone medium at pH 7.3.
B: a semi log replot shows that the production starts at the end of the logarithmic growth phase, and continues during a period of slower growth.

fermentation of triostins (48) by Streptomyces sp. employing pH-control by buffering with 50 mM HEPES, or by the inclusion of high phosphate concentrations in the fermentation of gramicidin S synthetases. Although it had been shown before that gramicidin S formation is suppressed at high phosphate, and in chemostat experiments in a fumarate minimal medium an optimal phosphate concentration of 1 mM had been detected, we observed production of the synthetase at high phosphate concentrations (Fig. 19). While the in vivo productivity of the antibiotic parallels the enzyme concentration, the overall gramicidin S production is low. The extracted enzyme system has a higher antibiotic productivity than the growing cells. This, however, is not the usual case when high producing cells of other systems are extracted. Usually in vitro activities of only a few percent of high producer in vivo rates have been achieved. Similar enzyme concentrations as described above with high phosphate have been achieved at low phosphate with more efficient oxygen control. In chemostat experiments, oxygen limitation proved to be most important in production of gramicidin S

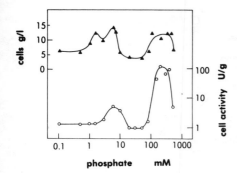

Fig. 19:

Phosphate dependence of gramicidin S
synthetase production in glutamate
minimal medium   (49).

synthetases. In his studies, Chiu designed a fumarate medium, that has
been improved to yield similar enzyme concentrations as obtained in
batch procedures (50). In continuous cultures, there is apparently
no specificity regarding the induction of gramicidin S synthetases
(Fig. 20). Under carbon source limitation, it can be seen that sporulation and enzyme production are unlinked processes. At low fumarate
concentration (18.8 mM), no enzyme activity was detected, while sporulation occured. At both carbon (81.2 mM fumarate) and nitrogen limitation, sporulation was observed at low dilution rates, enzyme activity at high dilution rates. At other limiting conditions (sulfur,
nitrogen, or oxygen) favouring enzyme formation, no sporulation was
found. These observations are in accord with the existence of sporu-
lating gramicidin S-nonproducer mutants. The yields, however, were
well below optimized batch procedures (Table 8). The inclusion of
glycerol, and, most important, oxygen limitation, lead to excellent
enzyme yields in the chemostat. Note that a rather high dilution rate
corresponding to a high rate of growth is required. The yield of
enzyme is 10 to 100 fold increased compared to fumarate alone (Fig. 20,
bottom graph). Both carbon sources, fumarate and glycerol, are metabolized at the same time.

If the specific oxygen uptake of the cells is related to the growth
rate (μ = dilution rate 1/h), it is evident that the glycerol supplemented culture requires less oxygen for efficient growth (Fig. 21).
The reason for this is not clear.

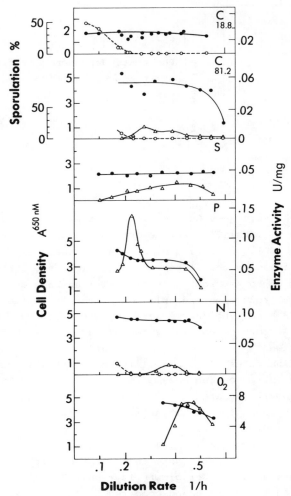

Fig. 20: Production of gramicidin S synthetases by continuous fermentation in fumarate based minimal medium. Optimal dilution rates for production at various limiting conditions (C 18.8-fumarate limitation, initial concentration s_0= 18.8 mM, C 81.2 : s_0= 81.2 mM; S-sulfate limitation, s_0= 20 mg/l; P-phosphate limitation, s_0= 1 mM, N-nitrogen limitation, s_0= 9 mM; O_2 - oxygen limitation in a medium containing glycerol and fumarate, limitation was 2.5 l air/min. at 250 rpm, corresponding to an O_2-transfer coefficient of 115 h^{-1}).

Table 8: Mixed Carbon Sources in Fermentation of Bacillus brevis ATCC 9999 and the Production of Gramicidin S Synthetases (50)

	source (g/l)		final OD$_{620}$	final pH	age of culture (h)	GS-synthetase (nmol GS/min) (DCW)
1.	Na-Acetate 22,0	+ Na-Succinate 2,2	0,50	7,8	34	0,76
2.	Na-Acetate 22,0	+ Na-Succinate 4,4	0,78	8,2	34	1,64
3.	Na-Acetate 22,0	+ Na-Glutamate 1,2	0,57	7,7	44	0,36
4.	Glycerin 10,0	+ Na-D,L-Malate 2,1	0,71	6,5	27	4,32
5.	Glycerin 10,0	+ Na-Fumarate 1,3	0,56	6,8	25	4,28
6.	Glycerin 10,0	+ Na-Fumarate 2,6	0,61	7,6	12	22,92
7.	Glycerin 10,0	+ Na-Succinate 2,2	0,62	6,65	12	27,00
8.	Glycerin 10,0	+ Na-Succinate 4,4	0,63	6,8	10	22,40
9.	Glycerin 10,0	+ Na-Glutamate 2,4	0,63	7,0	14	6,0
10.	Glycerin 10,0	+ Na-Citrate 1,6			no growth	
11.	Na-Lactate 16,7	+ Na-Fumarate 1,3	0,8	7,3	24	0,4
12.	Na-Fumarate 13,0	+ Na-Glutamate 1,2	0,55	7,69	12	1,88
13.	Na-Fumarate 13,0	+ Glycerin 2,0	0,62	7,03	7	26,48
14.	Na-Fumarate 13,0	+ Na-Pantothenate 1,7	0,66	7,95	11	14,40
15.	Fructose 9,8	+ Na-Succinate 4,4			no growth	
16.	Glucose 9,8	+ Na-Succinate 4,4	0,45	7,9	24	0,52
17.	Na-Glutamate 12,2	+ Na-Fumarate 2,6	0,63	7,65	10	17,80
18.	Na-Glutamate 12,2	+ Na-Succinate 4,4	0,62	7,62	12	16,24

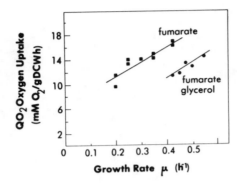

Fig. 21:

Rate of oxygen uptake of
B. brevis ATCC 9999 as a
function of the specific
growth rate μ in oxygen-
limited chemostat cultures
(50)

If production of synthetase is related to oxygen uptake (Fig. 22), it
follows that oxygen limited growth is required for enzyme production.
So far a possible induction by oxygen limitation has not been investigated.

To obtain more information on the oxygen requirement for enzyme
production, the oxygen uptake was manipulated by impeller speed at the
constant optimal dilution rate of 0,45 h^{-1}. Best enzyme production
was obtained when the oxygen uptake was limiting growth. However, there
is clearly a defined region of oxygen requirement with an oxygen transfer coefficient ß$_f$a between 150 and 250 h^{-1}.

Decoynine (Fig. 23), an inducer of sporulation in B. subtilis
was shown to induce formation of gramicidin S synthetase in

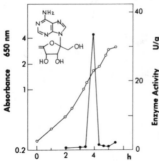

Fig. 23:

Induction of gramicidin S synthetase in B. brevis ATCC 9999 by
decoynine. High level induction
is followed by immediate inactivation in this experiment
using 250 mg/l   (49).

glutamate minimal medium. Addition of decoynine to a logarithmic phase
culture was followed by an immediate rise of enzyme activity (within
10 minutes), and rapid decline within 10 minutes. Thus a high level
of enzyme is synthesized, but the state of the cell cannot be stabili-
zed. At half the concentration of decoynine, no effect was observed.

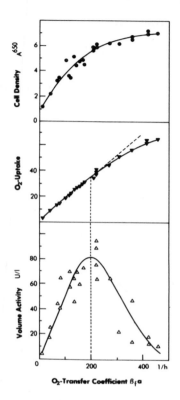

<u>Fig. 22:</u>   Gramicidin S synthetase production in chemostat culture of
B. <u>brevis</u> ATCC 9999. Top: cell concentration, middle: oxygen
uptake rate, bottom: activity of gramicidin S synthetase
(in units/l broth) as function of the oxygen transfer coefficient $\beta_f a$ (50).

Decoynine, as an inhibitor of GMP-formation, causes a partial deprivation of GDP and GTP   (51-53), as well as disappearance of ppGpp
(54) in B. <u>subtilis</u> vegetative cells.

A well-known study (55) of secondary metabolite expression during
strict exponential growth has been performed with <u>B</u>. <u>licheniformis</u>
NCIB 8874 on poorly utilized carbon and nitrogen sources (Fig. 24).
Cells were growing on a medium containing glucose and NH_4Cl with a
doubling time of 1.0 h.   Replacement of glucose by glycerol, pyruvic
acid, citric acid, or lactic acid, or of NH_4Cl by nitrate, alanine or
glutamate was followed by an exponential phase with doubling times of

up to 4 h. During these growth phases, production of bacitracin, protease, and sporulation was observed. The whole picture, however, may be quite complicated. Comparing bacitracin formation and multi-enzyme activity in B. licheniformis ATCC 10716, soluble and particulate forms are observed, either of which can be correlated with peptide production (56) (Fig. 25).

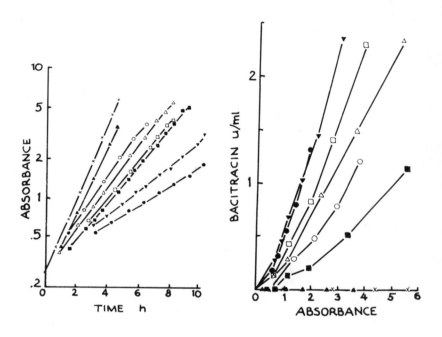

(✗) glucose and ammonium, (▲) glycerol, (■) pyruvic acid, (▼) citric acid
(●) lactic acid, (O) sodium nitrate, (△) alanine, (□) glutamic acid

Fig. 24:   Growth and bacitracin production in B. licheniformis
            in different defined media (55).

6   DIRECTED BIOSYNTHESIS

The production of peptides should easily be manipulated by amino acid addition. In case of gramicidin S synthetase, addition of phenylalanine led to a twofold stimulation of peptide production without affecting the enzyme level (57). Addition of lysine led to a partial replacement of ornithine by directed biosynthesis (58). High stimulations have recently been found for arphamenine production by Chromobacterium violaceum BMG 361-CF 4. Addition of the precursors tyrosine and phenylalanine led to a 3 to 10 fold increase of product concentration (59) (Fig. 26).

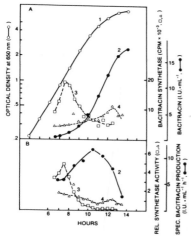

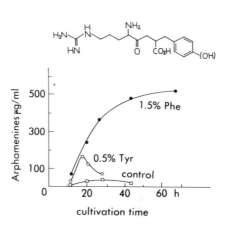

Fig. 25:

Fig. 26:

(A) Growth (1), bacitracin production (2), and the activity of bacitracin synthetase (3, soluble and 4, particular) in B. licheniformis ATCC 10716 when grown in a glutamate minimal medium containing 2 % phosphate.
(B) A replot showing specific activities. Enzyme content and peptide productivity are related to the absorbance of the culture. Redrawn from (56).

Improvement of arphamenine production in Chromobacterium violaceum by the addition of precursor amino acids (59).

Directed biosynthesis with acyl replacements are well known. A recent example is the production of chromophore analogs of the peptolides echinomycin and actinomycin, both produced by strains of Streptomyces. Twenty-two quinoxaline analogs have been fed to Streptomyces echinatus yielding four new compounds (Fig. 27) (60-63).

Biosynthesis of actinomycins is thought to involve coupling penta-
peptide lactones attached to 4-methyl-3-hydroxyanthranilic acid
(MHA) by phenoxazinone synthetase, which has recently been cloned by
Jones and Hopwood (64, 65). Analogs of MHA fed to Streptomyces
chrysomallus, that cannot form the phenoxazinone chromophore, lead to
the accumulation of actinomycin halves (66) (Fig. 28).

7   CONCLUSION

Regarding the state of enzymology, the field of peptide antibiotics is still leading in secondary product formation. Single step
as well as multistep reaction sequence enzymes are now in the progress
of primary structure elucidation. Regulatory sites are within direct
reach of DNA sequencing. The biosynthetic process of individual steps
permits direct access to different regions of complex structures
via feeding or enzymatic procedures. In fermentation procedures,
aspects of limiting conditions have been illustrated (growth rate,
pH, oxygen control).

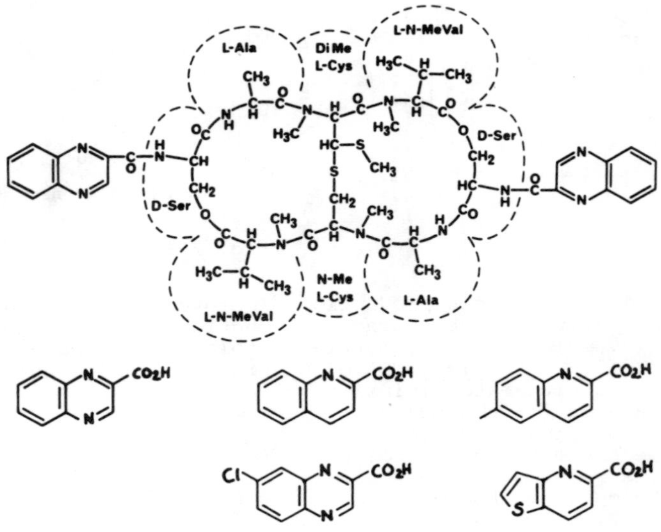

Fig. 27: New quinoxalines have been obtained by Gauvreau and Waring
(60-63) when feeding the producer S. echinatus with various
analogs of the chromophore.

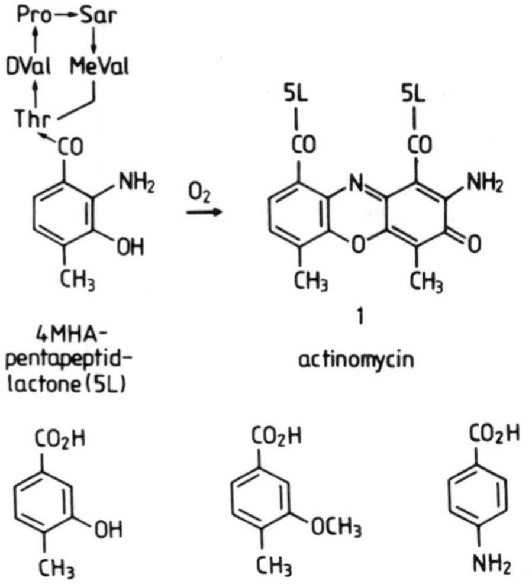

<u>Fig. 28:</u> The final reaction in actinomycin biosynthesis is the
formation of the phenoxazinone chromophore (1). If
analogs of 4-methyl-3-hydroxyanthranilic acid, that
are not substrates of phenoxazinone synthetase are fed,
half actinomycins are accumulated by <u>S</u>. <u>chrysomallus</u>
(66).

8   Acknowledgements:

This review contains work originating from collaboration with
Hansjürgen Aust, Dagmar Bothe, Chung-wai Chiu, Hanswerner Dellweg,
Wolfgang Freist, Michael Krause, Mohamed Marahiel, Bei-Fen Shen,
Marianne Simonis and Rainer Zocher.
We thank our colleagues for their cooperation and enthusiasm in
tacking unsolved problems.
The work in our laboratory was supported by the Bundesministerium
für Forschung und Technologie (BMFT) and the Deutsche Forschungs-
gemeinschaft, Sonderforschungsbereich 9 (DFG).

9   REFERENCES

(1) H. Kleinkauf and H. v. Döhren: Peptide Antibiotics. In: Comprehen-
     sive Biotechnology (M. Moo-Young, ed.), Vol. 3 (S. Drew, ed.),
     Pergamon Press, Oxford 1985, in press.

(2) H. Kleinkauf and H. v. Döhren, Current Topic Microbiol. Immunol.
     92, 129 (1981).

(3) B. W. Gibson, W. C. Herlihy, T. S. A. Samy, K.-S. Hahm, H. Maeda,
     I. Meienhofer, K. Biemann, J. Biol. Chem. 259, 10801 (1984).

(4) K. Edo, M. Ito, N. Ishida, Y. Koide, A. Ito, M. Haga, T. Takahashi,
     Y. Suzuki, G. Kusano, J. Antibiot. 35, 106 (1982).

(5) C. Nishio, S. Komura and K. Kurahashi, Biochem. Biophys. Res. Comm.
     116, 751 (1983).

(6) M. J. Gasson, FEMS Lett. 21, 7 (1984).

(7) V. S. Malik, Adv. Appl. Microbiol. 28, 27 (1982).

(8) R. Zocher, U. Keller and H. Kleinkauf, Biochem. 21, 43 (1982).

(9) H. Peeters, R. Zocher, N. Madry, P. B. Oelrichs, H. Kleinkauf and
     G. Kraepelin, J. Antibiot. 36, 1762 (1983).

(10) H. Kleinkauf and H. v.Döhren, Trends in Antibiotic Research,
     p. 220, Japan Antibiotics Res. Ass. 1982.

(11) E. Paul, Diplomarbeit TU Berlin 1984; R. Zocher and E. Paul,
     unpublished data.

(12) Ø. Frøyshov: Synthesis of Secondary Products During Sporulation.
     In: Regulation of Secondary Product and Plant Hormone Metabolism
     (M. Luckner and K. Schreiber, eds.) p. 189, Pergamon Elmsford
     1979.

(13) H. v. Döhren and Ø. Frøyshov, unpublished results.

(14) H. Brückner, G. Jung, M. Przybylski, Chromatographia 17, 679 (1983).

(15) H. Brückner, M. Prybylski, Chromatographia 19, 188 (1984).

(16) H. Brückner, H. Graf, M. Bokel, Experientia 40, 1189 (1984).

(17) M. Prybylski, I. Dietrich, I. Manz, H. Brückner, Biomed. Mass
     Spectrom. 11, 569 (1984).

(18) H. Kleinkauf and H. v. Döhren: Biosynthetic Aspects of Antitumor
     Peptides. In: Cellular Regulation and Malignant Growth. (S. Ebashi,
     ed.) p. 473, Japan Sci. Soc. Press, Tokyo and Springer Verlag
     Berlin 1985.

(19) D. Bothe, M. Simonis and H. v. Döhren, manuscript in preparation.

(20) H. Kleinkauf and H. v. Döhren: Enzymatic Production of Secondary Metabolites. In: Industrial Aspects of Biochemistry and Genetics (N. G. Alaeddinoglu, ed.) p. 107, Plenum Publ. Corp., New York 1985.

(21) H. Kleinkauf, H. v. Döhren, B. Tesche, R. Zocher, 14th FEBS Meeting Edinburgh 1981, Abstract Tue-S 14-22.

(22) W. Freist, H. Sternbach and F. Cramer, Hoppe Seyler's Z. Physiol. Chem. 302, 1247 (1981).

(23) H. v. Döhren and W. Freist, unpublished results.

(24) H. Kleinkauf and H. v. Döhren (eds.) Peptide Antibiotics - Biosynthesis and Functions, de Gruyter Berlin 1982.

(25) Y. Saito: Some Characteristics of Gramicidin S-Synthetase Obtained From Mutants of Bacillus brevis Which Could Not Form D-Phenylalanyl-L-prolyl-diketo-piperazine. In: Ref. 24, p. 195.

(26) M. A. Marahiel, W. Danders, M. Krause and H. Kleinkauf, Eur. J. Biochem. 99, 49 (1979).

(27) M. A. Marahiel, R. Lurz and H. Kleinkauf: Characterization of a Plasmid From Bacillus brevis ATCC 9999. In: Advances in Biotechnology, Vol. 3 (C. Vezina and K. Singh, eds.) p. 43, Pergamon Press 1981.

(28) M. A. Marahiel, R. Lurz and H. Kleinkauf, J. Antibiot. 34, 323 (1980).

(29) K. Stärko, Diplomarbeit TU Berlin 1982.

(30) L. Sankaran and B. M. Pogell, Nature New Biology 245, 257 (1973).

(31) M. Rogolsky, H. T. Nakamura, J. Bacteriol. 119, 57 (1974).

(32) W. F. Burke, Jr. and J. Spizizen, J. Bacteriol. 129, 1215 (1977).

(33) I. Takahashi and L. W. MacKenzie, Can. J. Microbiol. 28, 80 (1982).

(34) M. Krause, M. A. Marahiel, H. v. Döhren and H. Kleinkauf, J. Bacteriol., in press.

(35) M. Krause, Thesis, TU Berlin 1985.

(36) Y. Kawai, K. Nakahara, T. Gotoh, I. Uchida, H. Tanaka and H. Imanaka, J. Antibiot. 35, 1293 (1982).

(37) K. Murata and A. Kimura, Appl. Environm. Microbiol. 44, 1444 (1982).

(38)   H. Gushima, T. Miya, K. Murata and A. Kimura, Agric. Biol. Chem. 47, 1927 (1983).

(39)   A. Kimura, K. Murata, T. Miya, H. Gushima, Eur. Pat. 107, 400 (1984), Jap. Pat. 82/170, 727 (1982).

(40)   Y. Aharonowitz and A. L. Demain, Biotechnol. Bioeng. 22, Supl. 1,5 (1980).

(41)   R. Gross, F. Engelbrecht and V. Braun, Mol. Gen. Genet. 196, 74 (1984).

(42)   V. Braun, FEMS Microbiol. Lett. 11, 225 (1981).

(43)   A. Bindereif, J. B. Neilands, J. Bacteriol. 153, 1111 (1983).

(44)   R. Lewin, Science 225, 401 (1984).

(45)   K. T. Greenwood and R. K. J. Luke, Biochim. Biophys. Acta 660, 371 (1981).

(46)   D. G. Cooper, C. R. MacDonald, J. B. Duff and N. Kosaric, Appl. Environm. Microbiol. 42, 408 (1981).

(47)   E. J. Vandamme: Properties, Biosynthesis and Fermentation of the Cyclic Decapeptide, Gramicidin S. In: Topics in Enzyme and Fermentation Biotechnology (A. Wiseman, ed.) p. 187, Ellis Horwood, Chichester 1981.

(48)   J. V. Formica and M. J. Waring, Antimicrob. Agents Chemother. 24, 735 (1983)

(49)   H.-J. Aust, Thesis TU Berlin 1983.

(50)   C. W. Chiu, Thesis TU Berlin 1983.

(51)   T. Mitani, J. E. Heinze and E. Freese, Biochem. Biophys. Res. Comm. 77, 1118 (1977).

(52)   J. M. Lopez, C. L. Marks and E. Freese, Biochim. Biophys. Acta 587, 238 (1979).

(53)   N. Vasantha and E. Freese, J. Bacteriol. 144, 1119 (1980).

(54)   K. Ikehara, M. Okamoto and K. Sugae, J. Biochem. 91, 1089 (1982).

(55)   G. W. Hanlon and N. A. Hodges, J. Bacteriol. 147, 427 (1981).

(56)   Ø. Frøyshov, FEBS Lett. 81, 315 (1977).

(57)   A. L. Demain and C. C. Matteo, Antimicrob. Agents Chemother. 9, 1000 (1976).

(58)   V. Haring, Diplomarbeit TU Berlin 1983.

(59)   S. Ohuchi, A. Okuyama, K. Kawamura, T. Aoyasi and H. Umezawa, Agric. Biol. Chem. 48, 1661 (1984).

(60)   D. Gauvreau and M. J. Waring, Can. J. Microbiol. 30, 721 (1984).

(61)   D. Gauvreau and M. J. Waring, Can. J. Microbiol. 30, 439 (1984).

(62)   M. P. Williamson, D. Gauvreau and D. H. Williams, J. Antibiot. 35, 62 (1982).

(63)   D. Gauvreau and M. J. Waring, Can. J. Microbiol. 30, 730 (1984).

(64)   G. H. Jones and D. A. Hopwood, J. Biol. Chem. 259, 14151 (1984).

(65)   G. H. Jones and D. A. Hopwood, J. Biol. Chem. 259, 14158 (1984).

(66)   U. Keller, J. Biol. Chem. 259, 8226 (1984).

(67)   S. C. Pruitt and R. H. Reeder, Mol. Cell. Biol. 4, 2851 (1984).

Genetic and Physiological Control of Chloramphenicol Production

Leo C. Vining, Stuart Shapiro, Zia U. Ahmed, Sushma Vats, Janice Doull* and Colin Stuttard*

Dalhousie University, Departments of Biology and Microbiology*, Halifax, Nova Scotia, Canada B3H 4J1

Abstract

Formation of chloramphenicol in cultures of Streptomyces venezuelae is influenced by the form in which carbon and nitrogen are supplied and can be maximized by limiting either nutrient. Under such conditions, antibiotic production is associated with biomass accumulation. With glucose as a nonlimiting carbon source, ammonium supports rapid growth and low antibiotic titres. However, investigations in both batch and continuous cultures have shown that ammonium does not repress chloramphenicol biosynthesis. Earlier studies discounted the possibility of carbon catabolite repression by glucose or of phosphate regulation. Thus S. venezuelae appears to lack a general mechanism for regulating secondary metabolism. Antibiotic titres are probably determined by precursor availability and rates of enzyme synthesis, each inversely responsive to the growth rate, and to feedback effects.

Most chloramphenicol-producing organisms lack readily detectable extrachromosomal DNA and those in which a plasmid has been found retain antibiotic production after the plasmid has been eliminated. In nonproducing mutant strains of S. venezuelae ISP5230, genes associated with specific lesions in the pathway of chloramphenicol biosynthesis have been mapped by conjugation with a fertile variant. All of the cml genes are located in a single region of the chromosome. The availability of a transducing phage for S. venezuelae makes it possible to test for cotransduction of antibiotic production and auxotrophic marker genes. Such evidence, linking cml and pdx genes, has recently been obtained.

1 Introduction

Chloramphenicol is a relatively simple acylated phenylpropanoid antibiotic, related in structure to the phenylpropanoid amino acids. It is produced in some strains of <u>Streptomyces</u> <u>venezuelae</u> as the sole antibiotically active metabolite and the early stages of its formation make use of the shikimate pathway for aromatic biosynthesis. At the chorismate branch point, transfer of the amide nitrogen from glutamine generates 4-aminochorismate, which is then converted to <u>p</u>-aminophenylalanine in a sequence of reactions paralleling those by which tyrosine is usually made (1). Stepwise modification of <u>p</u>-aminophenylalanine (Fig. 1) eventually yields chloramphenicol (2).

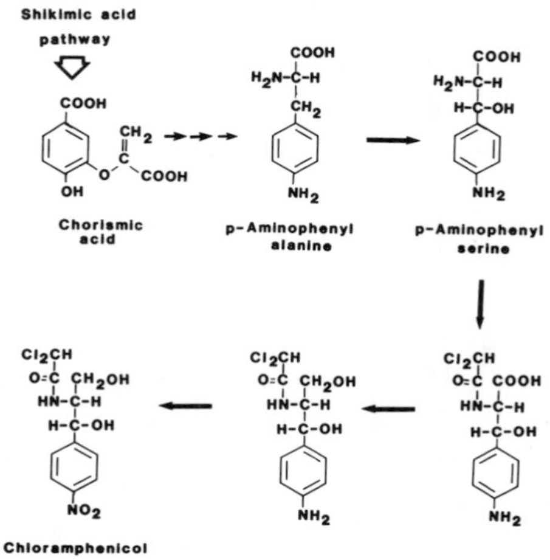

Fig. 1. Pathway for the biosynthesis of chloramphenicol from chorismate.

There is a large body of evidence suggesting that the production of antibiotics such as chloramphenicol, and secondary metabolites in general, is regulated at two levels. The first is manifest as an overall control of the onset and intensity of biosynthetic activity. The control mechanism responds primarily to environmental conditions experienced by the organism, including those related to nutrient availability. It enables secondary metabolic functions, ancillary to the primary growth processes, to be maintained in an active or inactive state according to the circumstances. Control at this level can be expected to operate on transcription or translation of a recognizably secondary metabolic gene system. Implicit is the organization of genes for the secondary metabolic pathway into a functional unit with regulatory elements able to sense changes in the growth status of the organism.

The second level of control is exerted on the activity of the biosynthetic enzymes and on the supply of precursors. The mechanisms expected here are activation and inhibition of enzyme function, as well as feedback repression of enzymes in the secondary pathway and in primary systems furnishing precursors. Operation of level-2 controls adjusts the intensity of secondary metabolism to the physiological circumstances of the organism and provides protection from overproduction of potentially toxic metabolites.

The work summarized below is concerned with control of chloramphenicol bio- synthesis in S. venezuelae. With this antibiotic, as with other secondary meta- bolites produced in concert with growth (i.e. in a uniphasic pattern) and not easily dissociated from it by nutritional manipulations, an important question is whether such control exists. We have addressed this issue by investigating both the physiological parameters associated with chloramphenicol production and the location and organization of genes responsible for the process in S. venezuelae.

2 Nutritional Control

Within broad limits, chloramphenicol production is insensitive to variations in phosphate concentration whereas it is markedly affected by the forms in which carbon and nitrogen are supplied in the medium (3). The pattern of response to different combinations of carbon and nitrogen reflects a situation commonly found with secondary metabolites -- high titres can be obtained with a good carbon source and a poor nitrogen source or vice versa, but not in a medium where both the carbon and nitrogen source support rapid growth (4).

2.1 Nitrogen Source
The inverse relationship between growth rate and optimum expression of anti- biotic producing potential is particularly strong when nitrogen availability is altered. With glucose as a nonrestrictive carbon source, media containing am- monium support rapid growth and low antibiotic titres. In contrast, slowly me- tabolized amino acids give high titres (5). Ammonium is well known for its re- pression of alternative nitrogen assimilation pathways and there is evidence that it is directly responsible for suppressing antibiotic production in other actino- mycetes (6). We therefore examined whether it is a repressive nitrogen source in S. venezuelae.

Mixtures of ammonium and a less readily assimilated amino acid such as pro- line are taken up from the medium and used concurrently (Fig. 2). With each ami- no acid that has been tested in this way, there is no evidence of catabolite repression by ammonium (7). In contrast, when a mixture of ammonium and nitrate is provided the two forms of nitrogen are used in succession, with nitrate being taken up from the medium only when ammonium is exhausted (Fig. 3). Athough the latter situation might appear to be due to catabolite repression of nitrate assimilation, intracellular nitrate reductase activity shows no response to the presence or depletion of ammonium. The enzyme is constitutive in S. venezuelae and is not sensitive to ammonium inhibition at the concentrations used (8).

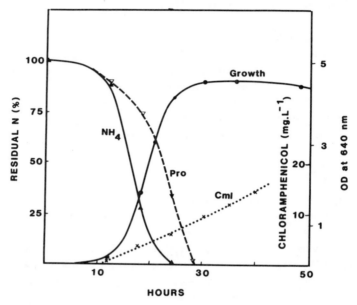

Fig. 2. Growth and chloramphenicol production in cultures of S. venezuelae in a medium containing glucose (50 g.L^{-1}), ammonium sulfate (15 mM) and proline (30 mM).

The mechanism by which ammonium suppresses the utilization of nitrate has not been explored further but apparently it does not involve a general repression of assimilative enzymes. The absence of such regulation for both amino acids and nitrate is consistent with the relatively constant level of glutamine synthetase found in cell extracts during growth on different nitrogen sources (5). Assuming a similarity to enteric bacteria where repression of assimilative pathways involves regulatory genes for glutamine synthetase, the cellular content of this enzyme should serve as a sensitive indicator of the state of repression or derepression of nitrogen utilization pathways.

Although ammonium does not appear to repress assimilation enzymes for alternative nitrogen sources, it does depress the formation of chloramphenicol (7).

In cultures supplied a mixture of ammonium and proline, production follows a
course intermediate between that with either source alone. Moreover, its onset
is not related to ammonium depletion. When ammonium is added to cultures already
growing on proline, chloramphenicol biosynthesis is temporarily halted but re-
sumes at close to the presupplement rate after several hours. Since the delay is
of similar length, regardless of the amount of ammonium added, resumption of
antibiotic synthesis does not depend upon depletion of the supplement. In short,
the response to ammonium does not have the characteristics expected for repression of enzyme synthesis.

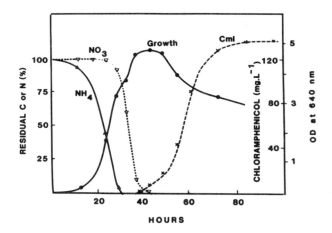

Fig. 3. Growth and chloramphenicol production in cultures of $\underline{S}$. $\underline{venezuelae}$
in a medium containing glucose (50 g.L^{-1}), ammonium nitrate (30 m$\underline{M}$)
and ammonium sulfate (15 m$\underline{M}$).

With mixtures of ammonium and nitrate, chloramphenicol is not produced until
both nitrogen sources have been depleted and then accumulates at a high rate (8).
The pattern of growth and secondary metabolism is classically biphasic, a situation not often achieved in chloramphenicol fermentations with defined media.
However, the onset of antibiotic production does not correlate with ammonium
depletion, nor is there any change in activity of arylamine synthetase until
nitrate has also been consumed. Thus the results again fail to provide evidence
of catabolite repression by ammonium.

To obtain more definitive information about the role of ammonium in
chloramphenicol production, cultures were grown in a chemostat with growth
limited by the concentration of nitrogen source in the medium (7). Varying the
dilution rate to bring about alternations in the specific growth rate did not

significantly affect the specific rate of chloramphenicol production (Table 1).
Such results indicate that the specific rate of antibiotic synthesis is not only
insensitive to nitrogen concentration under steady state conditions but also that
it does not respond to changes in the growth rate per se. It is apparent that
nutritional control of chloramphenicol producion differs from that exerted over
cephamycin C production in Streptomyces cattleya where the titre in continuous
cultures is affected by changes in growth rate regardless of whether carbon,
nitrogen or phosphate is the limiting nutrient (9).

Table 1. Effect of dilution rate on chloramphenicol production in nitrogen-
limited chemostat cultures.

Input (meq $NH_4^+.L^{-1}$)	Dilution rate (h^{-1})	Specific production (q_{cml}) ($\mu g.h^{-1}.mg\ DNA^{-1}$)
14	0.06	6.8
	0.10	5.7
	0.23	7.6
46	0.03	0.96
	0.12	0.71
	0.19	1.3

2.2 Carbon Source

In S. cattleya, thienamycin is produced only if phosphate is limiting. Under these conditions, changing the growth rate by altering the phosphate level
causes an inverse response in specific thienamycin output. Since chloramphenicol
production tolerates wide variations in phosphate concentration but is strongly
influenced by changes in the carbon/energy source, it is with the latter nutrient
that a parallel to the nutritional control of thienamycin biosynthesis is most
likely to be found. Indeed, preliminary evidence from chemostat cultures points
to an inverse relationship between chloramphenicol output and growth rate in
carbon-limited media (R. K. Bhatnagar, private communication). This is in agreement with results obtained by limiting glucose utilization through addition of
the nonmetabolizable inhibitor, methyl α-glucoside (10).

Incompatibility between active secondary metabolism and vigorous growth in
glucose-containing media is a common occurrence and is usually attributed to
carbon catabolite repression (4). In S. venezuelae, enzymes for the utilization
of less preferred carbon sources are inducible, and with some substrates are not

produced when glucose is present (11). Whether catabolite repression, inducer exclusion or some other mechanism is responsible for sequential assimilation of these substrates has not yet been established but changes in cytoplasmic cyclic AMP levels are not required (12).

Although glucose suppresses assimilation of less rapidly metabolized carbon sources, it does not directly suppress chloramphenicol biosynthesis (Fig. 4).

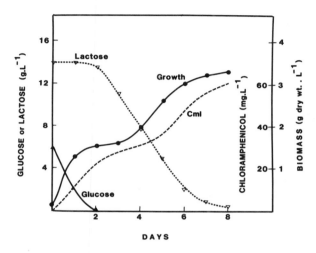

Fig. 4. Growth and chloramphenicol production in a medium containing glucose (6 g.L^{-1}), lactose (14 g.L^{-1}) and ammonium sulfate (15 m$\underline{M}$).

Not only can high rates of antibiotic production be attained in media containing glucose and a poor nitrogen source but, in media where glucose is mixed with a repressible second carbon source, the onset of antibiotic production precedes exhaustion of glucose (11). Thus carbon source limitation is not the sole and absolute requirement for chloramphenicol biosynthesis in the way that a deficiency of phosphate is necessary for thienamycin biosynthesis in <u>S</u>. <u>cattleya</u>.. In <u>S</u>. <u>venezuelae</u> there appears to be no linkage between catabolite regulation of carbon source assimilation and control of antibiotic production; moreover the effect of carbon sources on the latter activity does not have the characteristics associated with catabolite regulation of gene expression.

3 Metabolic Control

<u>Streptomyces</u> <u>venezuelae</u> resembles other actinomycetes in that the shikimate pathway, supplying the major primary intermediate for chloramphenicol biosynthesis, is unregulated at its entry point. No evidence for isozymes of DAHP synthe-

tase has been reported and primary end products of the pathway cause neither inhibition nor repression of the enzyme(13). This is also true of chorismate mutase but prephenate dehydratase and anthranilate synthetase are inhibited by
phenylalanine and tryptophan, respectively (14,15); anthranilate synthetase activity is also controlled through feedback repression by tryptophan. Thus regulation of the shikimate pathway by primary metabolites depends upon feedback
control of the branch sequences by their specific endproducts.

In vitro, chloramphenicol does not inhibit enzymes of the shikimate pathway,
nor any of those yet isolated in the specific sequence beginning with arylamine
synthetase (13,14). However, addition of excess antibiotic to cultures suppresses arylamine synthetase activity (16). Reduced enzyme activity is at least
partly due to a decrease in enzyme synthesis, presumably mediated by an intracellular effector. Since chloramphenicol does not penetrate the mycelium of producing cultures (17), the effector may be an intermediate that accumulates because export becomes rate limiting. Back up of intermediates could be responsible also for feedback effects on enzyme activity since p–aminophenylalanine and
other intermediates inhibit arylamine synthetase (16).

The general conclusion from these studies is that chloramphenicol biosynthesis is unregulated up to the limit tolerated by the producer, this limit being
determined by feedback mechanisms. The rate at which antibiotic is accumulated
in a culture will depend upon the concentration of specific pathway enzymes in
the cells and on the flow of precursors from primary metabolism. Whether there is
interaction between these two determinants has not been investigated, but the
presence of enzymes able to convert chorismate to chloramphenicol should draw
primary intermediates into the shikimate pathway. The possibility that accumulation of a precursor such as chorismate could induce the enzymes converting it
to chloramphenicol is more remote. Precursor induction of secondary pathway enzymes has only infrequently been observed (4), and the low permeability of S.
venezuelae mycelium to shikimate and chorismate makes a direct test difficult.

In the absence of specific control from environmental signals, transcription
of genes for the secondary metabolic pathway might be expected to depend on factors such as promoter strength, competition for RNA polymerase and the cellular
concentration of ppGpp or other nucleotide effectors. The overall result is
likely to produce a concentration of secondary pathway enzymes inversely related
to the growth rate of the culture.

Arylamine synthetase supplying intermediates for chloramphenicol biosynthesis competes directly for chorismate with enzymes making protein amino acids ;
this also should result in an inverse relationship between growth rate and
secondary metabolism. In general, the most efficient conversion of substrates

to biomass takes place during unrestricted growth of microorganisms on abundant
and easily assimilated nutrients. Nutrient-limited growth characteristically
exhibits energy-spilling and related metabolic balancing behaviour that leads to
accumulation and excretion of specific intermediates. The nature of the accumulated metabolites varies with the limiting nutrient and undoubtedly also with the
microorganism(18). Little is yet known about regulation of the central metabolic
pathways in S. venezuelae, but assuming that the general pattern of physiological
control is similar to that described above and that appropriate metabolic imbalance is needed to generate the precursors for chloramphenicol biosynthesis in
large amounts, there are several observations that appear to be significant. One
is that in S. venezuelae phosphofructokinase activity is inhibited by phosphoenolpyruvate rather than by Krebs cycle intermediates (unpublished results).
This may explain the early discovery (19) that supplementing cultures with lactate markedly stimulates chloramphenicol production; metabolism of lactate to pyruvate could result in elevated phosphoenolpyruvate levels and a consequent diversion of glucose-6-phosphate into the pentose phosphate pathway. On the other
hand, depletion of pyruvate (e.g. by excretion, see later) and lowering of the
phosphoenolpyruvate concentration would drain glucose-6-phosphate by allowing
increased flux through the glycolytic pathway and so reduce the availability of
erythrose-4-phosphate for aromatic biosynthesis.

Streptomyces venezuelae is prone to acid production (Fig. 5). As occasio-

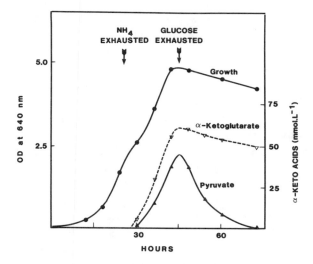

Fig. 5. Excretion of α-keto acids by S. venezuelae during growth in a glucose
(50 g.L^{-1}), potassium nitrate (30 mM), ammonium nitrate (30 mM) medium.

nally noted in other actinomycetes and as reported for <u>Klebsiella</u> <u>aerogenes</u> in nitrogen-limited media (18), cultures excrete large amounts of pyruvate and α-ketoglutarate into the broth under certain conditions (20). In lightly buffered media, the rising acidity halts further biomass production, but where pH control is maintained the output of keto acids is a severe drain on metabolism. The most plausible explanation for the accumulation of these intermediates lies in the known repression of α-keto acid dehydrogenase activity in <u>E</u>. <u>coli</u> by glucose (21). Cells of <u>S</u>. <u>venezuelae</u> are passively permeable to pyruvate and α-ketoglutarate, and if Krebs cycle activity were repressed in this way, the acids would accumulate and leak into the medium. Evidence for this comes from the discovery within the wild-type population of low-acidity variants. The principal difference between these and the wild-type majority is their higher content of α-keto acid dehydrogenase.

Since keto acid excretion is associated with nitrogen-limited growth on glucose, it might be predicted that the use of poorly metabolized amino acids as nitrogen sources would cause strong acidification of the culture during growth. However, this is true only for some amino acids. With others (e.g. proline) no acid is excreted. It seems likely that metabolites released during deamination of amino acid nitrogen sources have a significant role in regulating intermediary metabolism and it is worthy of note that non-acidifying amino acids support the best yields of chloramphenicol.

The high growth rates that develop in cultures supplied with easily assimilated nutrients can lead to partial oxygen insufficiency under normal conditions of cultivation (22). In <u>S</u>. <u>venezuelae</u>, anaerobiosis leads to a severe drain on central pathways, distorting pool concentrations probably involved in metabolic control. This has been observed (Fig. 6) during an investigation of [^{15}N]ammonium utilization using ^{15}N-nuclear magnetic resonance spectroscopy to analyze cellular contents (23). Glutamine and glutamate are the most rapidly labeled components in the cytoplasm of well aerated cultures undergoing rapid growth. When oxygen is withdrawn, the concentration of these amino acids falls and alanine builds up rapidly. The change is accompanied by excretion of pyruvate and α-ketoglutarate and is reversed by restoring aeration. The overall pattern is consistent with an accumulation of pyruvate due to reduced Krebs cycle activity, which in turn results from the shortage of NAD attendant upon diminished electron transport. With abundant ammonium and NADH available, the alanine dehydrogenase known to be present in <u>S</u>. <u>venezuelae</u> (5) acts upon the excess pyruvate, thereby regenerating sufficient NAD to sustain the organism. The distortion of metabolic flow entailed by such a sequence of events at growth rates creating high oxygen demand may well be a factor in limiting secondary metabolism.

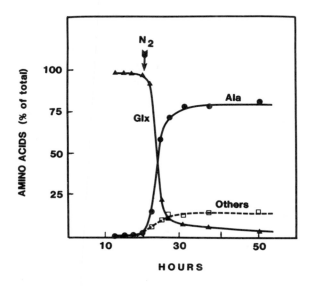

Fig. 6. Effect of oxygen deprivation on the composition of the amino acid
pool in S. venezuelae.

In summary, failure to demonstrate transcriptional control of the secondary
metabolic pathway responsible for chloramphenicol biosynthesis in S. venezuelae
could simply mean that no such control is present. The responses to nutritional
imbalance that have been observed may be due to alterations in biosynthetic enzyme levels due to normal adjustment of gene expression at different cell growth
rates, and to alterations in the supply of precursors. Changes in precursor flow
are plausibly related to responses of the primary metabolic network to nutrient
availability and to growth rate. An additional factor is the existence of feedback control by the antibiotic itself.

4 Location of Genes

Chloramphenicol production is lost at high frequency or reduced to trace
levels when wild-type cultures of S. venezuelae are treated with plasmid-curing
agents (24,25). Moreover, attempts to map the genetic locus associated with such
changes suggested an absence of linkage to chromosomal markers (26). This evidence initially pointed to one or more of the genes controlling production of
chloramphenicol being plasmid borne. However, subsequent work has not supported
such a conclusion and recent studies on variation in actinomycetes indicate that
the accentuation of spontaneous run down commonly observed when antibiotic producers are treated with plasmid-curing agents is caused by rearrangements in the
genome DNA (27).

Plasmids have been detected in only two of 11 strains of chloramphenicol producing species examined (28,29). In both of these, plasmid-free progeny obtained from regenerated protoplasts retain the ability to produce chloramphenicol, and Southern hybridizations of plasmid DNA with total DNA from the cured strains indicate that this is not due to integration. The results, together with the absence of a detectable plasmid in other producing strains, suggest strongly that none of the genes responsible for antibiotic biosynthesis are located on extrachromosomal DNA.

5 Blocked Mutants

By treating S. venezuelae ISP5230 with a variety of mutagenic agents, prototrophic strains that fail to produce antibiotic have been recovered at a frequency averaging 0.03% (30). These were accompanied by a higher proportion (0.3%) of strains producing very low levels of chloramphenicol. Of the 12 nonproducing mutants isolated, two (Cml-1 and Cml-12) will produce chloramphenicol when supplemented with p-aminophenylalanine and are crossfed when grown in mixed culture with mutants that accumulate this amino acid. These characteristics indicate that Cml-1 and Cml-12 are blocked in genes coding for enzyme(s) in the arylamine synthetase complex (Fig. 7). Three of the mutants (Cml-4, Cml-5 and Cml-8) ex-

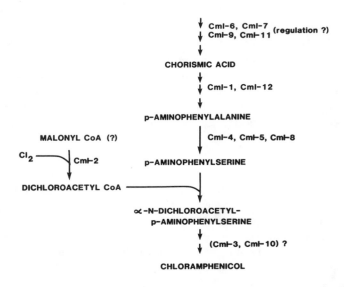

Fig. 7. Probable sites of mutations in the pathway of chloramphenicol
       biosynthesis.

crete p-aminophenylalanine and are probably blocked in the conversion of p-aminophenylalanine to p-aminophenylserine. Two other mutants (Cml-3 and Cml-10) accumulate small amounts of p-aminophenylalanine intracellularly and may be blocked
in a later reaction, the substrate for which either feedback inhibits arylamine
synthetase or is shunted to an undetected product. Mutant Cml-2 accumulates a
mixture of nonchlorinated acyl analogues of chloramphenicol. Similar compounds
are made by wild-type S. venezuelae when chlorination is prevented by eliminating
halogen ions from the medium (31); they are also produced by Corynebacterium
hydrocarboclastus which, like Cml-2, appears to lack an enzyme for introducing
chlorine into the dichloroacetyl precursor of chloramphenicol (32). The remaining four nonproducing strains do not accumulate any detectable intermediates or
shunt products and may be regulatory mutants. However, they differ from putative
regulatory strains obtained by plasmid-curing treatments in producing no trace of
the antibiotic.

6 Genetic Mapping

Initial attempts to generate a linkage map by conjugation of genetically
marked strains of S. venezuelae ISP5230 were frustrated by low fertility. In a
series of crosses the frequency with which recombinant progeny were recovered
ranged between 4×10^{-7} and 6×10^{-8} per c.f.u. This was not significantly higher
than the frequency of reversion for many of the auxotrophic markers used. A fertile strain was obtained by transforming S. venezuelae with pIJ701, a derivative
of the low copy number plasmid SLP1.2 from Streptomyces lividans 66 (33). However, the plasmid was not stably replicated in its new host. In crosses where a
pIJ701-containing strain was used, recombination frequencies varied widely, both
in different matings and in repetitions of the same mating. Attempts to obtain
fertile strains by transformation with pIJ303, a derivative of the high copy
number plasmid pIJ101 that mediates fertility in S. lividans ISP5434 (34), failed
when the plasmid could not be transferred into S. venezuelae.

Difficulties with fertility were resolved when approximately 2% of spores
from a doubly auxotrophic mutant, VS113 (his-6 ade-10), of S. venezuelae ISP5230
were found to exhibit a "lethal zygosis" (aerial mycelium inhibition, Ami) response (35) when they were patched on agar and partially overlaid with a suspension of bulk VS113 spores. Variants sensitive to aerial mycelium inhibition
(Ami-S) displayed markedly increased fertility and yielded recombinants at frequencies ranging from 1×10^{-4} to 1×10^{-3} per c.f.u. of the minority parent, when
mated with auxotrophic strains that were insensitive to aerial mycelium inhibition (Ami-I). No plasmids could be detected in strains with either the Ami-S or
Ami-I phenotype, nor was there any difference in their production of chloramphenicol.

Conjugational crosses were carried out using strain VS206 (<u>his-6 ade-10</u>), an
Ami-S derivative of VS113, and nonproducing mutants of <u>S. venezuelae</u> ISP5230 into
which single auxotrophic markers had been introduced by further mutagenic treatment. In each instance, a 20-fold excess of VS206 spores gave a balanced cross
with reciprocal transfer of markers. Relative locations of the auxotrophic and
resistance markers were first determined as described by Hopwood (36). The segregation of the Cml marker was then analysed by examining approximately 100 recombinants for antibiotic production. From the results of such crosses, the location of markers relative to those of the VS206 parent (<u>his-6 ade-10 strA6</u>) on a
circular linkage map were determined. The data do not allow ordering of markers
within the three segments defined by <u>his-6</u>, <u>ade-10</u> and <u>strA6</u>. However, assign-
ment of auxotrophic and resistance markers to locations where corresponding markers have been reported in the genetic map of <u>Streptomyces coelicolor</u> A3(2) (37)
yields a self-consistent interpretation of the results (Fig. 8). On this basis,

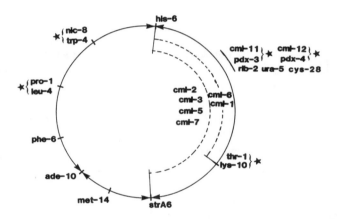

Fig. 8. Genetic map of <u>S. venezuelae</u> ISP5230. Pairs of cotransducible
genes are indicated with a star.

basis, a provisional genetic map of <u>S. venezuelae</u> ISP5230 has been prepared. The
eight Cml markers so far examined show linkage to chromosomal markers; no
infectious transfer of the Cml+ phenotype was observed. Thus all of the evidence
obtained in these studies is consistent with a chromosomal location for the genes
specifying chloramphenicol biosynthesis.

From the mapping data, all <u>cml</u> genes are located in the arc between <u>his-6</u>
and <u>strA6</u>, opposite to <u>ade-10</u>. While the position of <u>cml-3</u>, <u>cml-5</u> and <u>cml-7</u> has
not been more closely defined, <u>cml-1</u> can be positioned between <u>his-6</u> and <u>lys-10</u>.

In separate crosses, cml-2 has been shown to be near ura-5 and rib-2 in the arc
between strA6 and his-6. Similarly, the cml-6 gene has been mapped to the region
between lys-10 and his-6. In other crosses, recombination frequencies indicate
cml-6 is also close to ura-5 and rib-2. The cml-11 gene is located near pdx-3,
in the arc between strA6 and his-6; likewise, cml-12 has been mapped between
strA6 and his-6, and is close to cys-28.

7 Transduction of Cml Markers

Development of the phage SV1 for transduction in S. venezuelae (38) has made
it possible to test the conjugational mapping evidence of a close linkage between
certain auxotrophic and Cml markers. With strain VS263 carrying the cml-11 pdx-3
marker pair as recipient and phage grown on a wild type donor, 11% of the prototrophic progeny produced chloramphenicol. Similar results were obtained with
strain VS258 carrying mutations in cml-12 and pdx-4. In contrast, no cotrans-
ductants were obtained with VS227 (cml-2 ura-5) nor with VS242 (cml-6 rib-2).
Failure to obtain auxotrophic transductants when a ura-5 recipient was infected
with phage from donor strains carrying either cys-28, pdx-3 or rib-2 is consistent with ura-5 being some distance from these markers. The absence of cotransduction between cml-2 and ura-5 may mean that cml-2 lies close to the pdx markers. Thus at least some of the cml genes form a cluster in close proximity to
pdx-3 and pdx-4.

8 References

(1) C.-Y. P. Teng, B. Ganem, S. Z. Doktor, B. P. Nichols, R. K. Bhatnagar,
L. C. Vining, J. Am. Chem. Soc. in press.
(2) L. C. Vining, D. W. S. Westlake, in Biotechnology of Industrial Antibiotics
(ed. E. J. Vandamme), Marcel Dekker, New York, 1984, p. 387.
(3) S. Chatterjee, L. C. Vining, D. W. S. Westlake, Can. J. Microbiol., 29
(1983) 247.
(4) A. L. Demain, Y. Aharonowitz, J.-F. Martin, in Biochemistry and Genetic Regulation of Commercially Important Antibiotics (ed. L. C. Vining), Addison
Wesley, Reading, MA, 1983, p. 49.
(5) S. Shapiro, L. C. Vining, Can. J. Microbiol. 29 (1983) 1706.
(6) Y. Aharonowitz, Spec. Publ. Soc. Gen. Microbiol. Vol. 10, 1983, p. 33.
(7) S. Shapiro, L. C. Vining, Can. J. Microbiol. 31 (1985) 119.
(8) S. Shapiro, L. C. Vining, Can. J. Microbiol. 30 (1984) 798.
(9) G. Lilley, A. E. Clark, G. C. Lawrence, J. Chem. Technol. Biotechnol. 31
(1981) 127.
(10) L. C. Vining, S. Shapiro, J. Antibiot. 37 (1984) 74.

(11) S. Chatterjee, L. C. Vining, Can. J. Microbiol. 28 (1982) 311.

(12) L. C. Vining, S. Chatterjee, in Overproduction of Microbial Products. FEMS
     Symp. No. 13, 1982, p. 35.

(13) D. A. Lowe, D. W. S. Westlake, Can. J. Biochem. 49 (1971) 448.

(14) D. A. Lowe, D. W. S. Westlake, Can. J. Biochem. 50 (1972) 1064.

(15) M. M. Francis, L. C. Vining, D. W. S. Westlake, J. Bacteriol. 134 (1978)

(16) A. Jones, D. W. S. Westlake, Can. J. Microbiol. 20 (1974) 1599.

(17) V. S. Malik, L. C. Vining, Can. J. Microbiol. 18 (1972) 583.

(18) O. M. Neijssel, D. W. Tempest, in Microbial Technology (eds. A. T. Bull, D.
     C. Ellwood, C. Ratledge), Soc. Gen. Microbiol. Symp. No. 29,   1979, p. 53.

(19) D. Gottlieb, L. Diamond, Bull. Torrey Bot. Club 78 (1951) 56.

(20) Z. U. Ahmed, S. Shapiro, L. C. Vining, Can. J. Microbiol. 30 (1984) 1014.

(21) C. R. Amarasingham, B. D. Davis, J. Biol. Chem. 240 (1965) 3664.

(22) J. S. Schultz, Appl. Microbiol. 12 (1964) 305.

(23) S. Shapiro, L. C. Vining, M. Laycock, A. G. McInnes, J. A. Walter, Can. J.
     Microbiol. in press.

(24) M. Okanishi, H. Umezawa, in Genetics of Actinomycetales (eds. E. Freerksen,
     I. Tarnock, J. H. Thumin), Gustav Fischer, Stuttgart, 1978, p. 19.

(25) A. M. Michelson, L. C. Vining, Can. J. Microbiol. 24 (1978) 662.

(26) H. Akagawa, M. Okanishi, H. Umezawa, J. Antibiot. 32 (1979) 610.

(27) H. Schrempf, in Genetic Rearrangement, Fifth John Innes Symposium (eds. K.
     F. Chater, C. A. Cullis, D. A. Hopwood, A. W. B. Johnston, H. W. Woolhouse),
     1983, p.131.

(28) Z. U. Ahmed, L. C. Vining, J. Bacteriol. 154 (1983) 239.

(29) J. L. Doull, L. C. Vining, C. Stuttard, FEMS Microbiology Letters 16 (1983)
     349.

(30) J. Doull, Z. Ahmed, C. Stuttard, L. C. Vining, J. Gen. Microbiol. 131 (1985)
     97.

(31) C. G. Smith, J. Bacteriol. 75 (1958) 577.

(32) K. Shirahata, T. Hayashi, T. Deguchi, T. Suzuki, I. Matsubara, Agric. Biol.
     Chem. 36 (1972) 2229.

(33) E. Katz, C. J. Thompson, D. A. Hopwood, J. Gen. Microbiol. 129 (1983) 2703.

(34) T. Kieser, D. A. Hopwood, H. M. Wright, C. J. Thompson, Mol. Gen. Genet. 185
     (1982) 223.

(35) M. J. Bibb, R. F. Freeman, D. A. Hopwood, Mol. Gen. Genet. 154 (1977) 155.

(36) D. A. Hopwood, in Methods in Microbiology Vol. 7B (eds. J. R. Norris, D. W.
     Ribbons) Academic Press, London, 1972, p. 29.

(37) D. A. Hopwood, Bacteriol. Rev. 31 (1967) 373.

(38) C. Stuttard, J. Gen. Microbiol. 110 (1979) 479.

Factors Governing Polyketide and Glycopeptide Productions by Streptomycetes

Udo Gräfe, Inge Eritt, Frank Hänel, Walter Friedrich, Martin Roth, Bernd Röder
and Ernst J. Bormann

GDR Academy of Sciences, Central Institute of Microbiology and Experimental Therapy,
Box 73, DDR-6900 Jena, GDR

ABSTRACT

Interwoven regulatory networks play an important but poorly elucidated role in the expression of the complex phenotype and secondary
metabolism of streptomycetes. As a model, the role of the A-factor
[2-(6'-methylheptanoyl)-3-hydroxymethyl-4-butanolide] and its derivatives in the restoration of aerial mycelium formation and anthracycline production by blocked mutants of S. griseus has been investigated. The general variability of the genetic and metabolic organization of signal chains of the differentiation-associated metabolism
greatly hampers the directed screening for antibiotic-overproducing
strains. Examples have been given by our selection for mutants of
S. noursei JA 3890b insensitive to either inhibition by phosphate of
the nourseothricin production or toxic agents including the antibiotic produced.

1 INTRODUCTION

In contrast to animal or plant cells, whose differentiation occurs
in full coincidence with the functional requirements of the macroor-
ganism, cytodifferentiation of the microorganisms provides a tool of
adaptation to changing environmental conditions. In the latter, differentiation has to enable either, that a given cell can adapt properly
to various limitations of nutrients by expressing a suitable programme of development, or that few clones out of a population can
survive under adverse conditions. A high variability of these processes could be ascertained by the low selection pressure which crea-

tes an enlarged playground for evolutionary modifications of structures, pathways, and even features of control (1).

Variability of cytodifferentiation as a general feature

Obviously, every microorganism appears to follow its individual rules throughout the biosynthesis of antibiotics even more than in the
formation of the cellular constituents. That there is a non-uniform
pattern of biosynthesis even for a particular antibiotic structure
has been shown with the formation of the ß-lactam ring,which can be
generated by different genera,from quite different precursor molecules (2). Furthermore, investigations into the control by phosphate
and carbon catabolites of several antibiotic biosyntheses suggested
the absence of uniform regulatory mechanisms (3). Thus, catabolite
regulation of the ß-lactam productions by glucose occurs at the level
of different enzymes and mediated by various mechanisms (4).
Up to now,investigations into the role of known microbial 'alarmons'
as,for example ,cyclic AMP and guanosine tetraphosphate (ppGpp) have
not essentially aided understanding of the control of antibiotic productions. Apparently, the role of such molecules as mediators of the
cellular response to nutrient limitation may vary considerably from
one genus,or species,to another. Although cAMP has been shown to govern germination of spores in S. hygroscopicus (5), there have been
no other indications of an outstanding regulatory function either
in the catabolite repression of inducible enzymes (6,7), or in the
regulation of antibiotic syntheses by streptomycetes (8,9). In Bacillus sp.,in presence of glucose,the increased level of cAMP appears
to suppress formation of extracellular hydrolases (10) but no involvement in the sporulation has yet been established.
Similarly, confusion exists in the case of ppGpp which mediates the
stringent response to amino acid starvation in the Gram-negative bacteria by affecting the RNA polymerase. Though this endogenous signal
compound appears to be involved in the secretion of α-amylase by
Bacillus sp. (11), a role as a trigger of sporulation and antibiotic
biosynthesis still seems to be at variance. In the streptomycetes
the mechanism of the stringent response has been proved but the intramycelial level of ppGpp was much lower than in Klebsiella sp.
(12,13), and its participation in the control of antibiotic productions still remains obscure (14).

Variability of the genetic organization of cytodifferentiation in the actinomycetes and the involvement of pleiotropic effectors

An additional problem arises from the frequently noticeable location of the differentiation-associated genes on instable genetic ele-

ments such as plasmids and transposon-like structures (15), and their
encoding for particular biochemical and morphological alterations
(16). Due to the possible transposition of such genes, novel clones
could segregate permanently which are distinguishable from the parental genotype by their morphology, secondary metabolism, and type of
differentiation. These genetic changes seem to realise the long-term
adaptability and the resulting survival of the species, and should be
regarded therefore, as a constitutive part of the cytodifferentiation.
In some cases pleitropic regulatory genes are responsible for the
formation of particular endogenous effectors which are specific to a
given species of microorganism and which control exclusively the individual cellular development. Examples of such autoregulatory molecules have been reported but, conceivably, the majority of these peculiar endogenous factors still awaits elucidation (17). In order to
learn more about the complex cellular organization of the pleiotropic
regulatory systems involved in the cytodifferentiation of antibiotic-
producing streptomycetes, it may prove promising to explore the mode
of action of such autoregulatory effectors. The present communication
summarizes the results of our previous studies on the role of 2,3-di-
substituted γ-butyrolactones in the regulation of the production of
polyketide-derived anthracyclines by Streptomyces griseus strains.
These studies revealed the complexity of the regulatory levels and
their interactions. This situation complicates the elucidation of the
individual patterns of control of the morphogenesis as well as of the
production of antibiotics. Because of the limited insight into the
complex processes of development, the directed screening aimed at the
antibiotic-overproducing strains is still in search of more effective
strategies. This will be shown by the results of our recent efforts
towards isolation of nourseothricin-overproducing strains of Streptomyces noursei (18).

2 FACTORS GOVERNING POLYKETIDE FORMATION AND CYTODIFFERENTIATION OF ANTHRACYCLINE-PRODUCING STRAINS OF S. GRISEUS

An intriguing example of an autoregulatory signal compound of the
cytodifferentiation of streptomycetes has been provided by the pio-
neer work of KHOKHLOV et al. (17) who detected the so-called A-factor (2-(6'-methylheptanoyl)-3R-hydroxymethyl-4-butanolide; 1a; R=
C_7H_{15} ; Fig. 1) as the inducer of streptomycin biosynthesis and aerial
mycelium formation by S. griseus mutants blocked in the cytodifferentiation. The effect of 1a on streptomycin-non-producing strains, the
development of resistance to the produced antibiotic in the presence
of this effector and other concomitant biochemical and morphological
changes have been reported elsewhere (17,19) and will not be treated

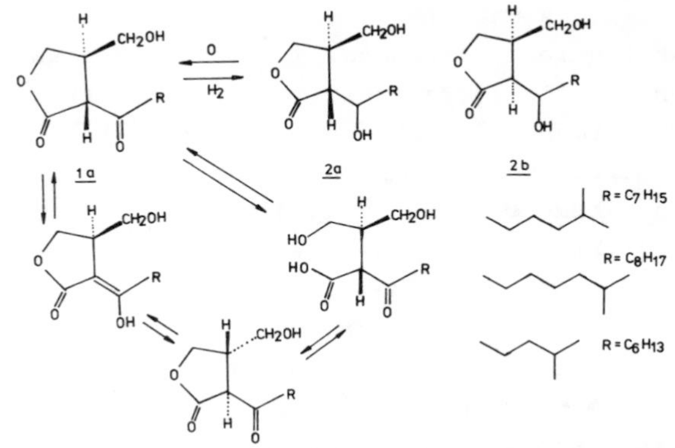

Fig. 1. Chemical constitutions of naturally occurring inducers and
their possible interconversions.

here. More recently, studies using the rDNA technique have uncovered
the genetic organization of A-factor formation (20,21,22). A pleiotropic regulatory gene triggering the onset of A-factor production
and the structure genes have been identified by cloning procedures
and transferred to other streptomycetes.

Occurrence of the A-factor and its derivatives

By means of A-factor⁻ strains it has been demonstrated that inducers of cytodifferentiation similar to A-factor can be produced by
many different Streptomyces species and strains, and even by members
of other genera (19,23,24). Such inducers were isolated from the fermentation broth of S. griseus (25,26), S. viridochromogenes (27),
S. bikiniensis, S. cyaneofuscatus (28) and other Streptomyces species. In contrast to S. griseus JA 5142, which produced a substance
related at least constitutionally to the A-factor 1a (R=C_7H_{15}), the
other strains generated the homologuous dihydro-derivatives (2a or
2b, Figs. 1 and 2, R=C_7H_{15}; C_8H_{17}; C_6H_{13}; absolute stereochemistry
undetermined) either as single component or as mixtures containing
compounds harbouring a relative cis or trans configuration at the C2
and C3 positions of the γ-butyrolactone ring. Many strains coproduced
both the 1'-keto (1a, 1b) and the 1'-OH structures (2a, 2b) (24).

Mode of action on blocked indicator strains of S. griseus

All these naturally occurring effectors had the same effect at
approximately the same concentration on some aerial-mycelium and an-
thracycline-negative mutants (Amy⁻Ant⁻) of the ancestral Amy⁺Ant⁺
strains of S. griseus JA 5142 and JA 3933 producing the daunomycin-
type antibiotic leukaemomycin (23). In the presence of these factors

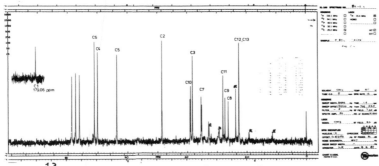

Fig. 2. 25 MHz ^{13}C NMR spectrum of $\underline{2b}$ (R=C_7H_{15}) from $\underline{S}$. $\underline{bikiniensis}$
JA 8031. The additional signals nearby C7 and C10 are due to
the presence of the homologue with R=C_6H_{13}. ($\mathbf{x}$ impurities)

(10-50 ng applied to an agar well, or filled into a cup plate positioned on the agar surface at zero time), blocked indicator mutants (Amy$^-$
Ant$^-$A-factor$^-$), reestablished both the wild-type morphology and the
production of the anthracyclines (Amy$^+$Ant$^+$)(Fig. 3). Cobalt (5-70 mg
Co(NO$_3$)$_2$/l agar) specifically enhanced synergistically the effect of
$\underline{1a}$, or its derivatives, on surface cultures of the blocked mutant 86
(28). This feature suggested that the initial effect of $\underline{1a}$ could be

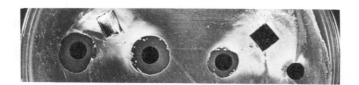

Fig. 3. Induction of the formation of aerial mycelium and anthracyclines by $\underline{1a}$ (0.1 µg adsorbed to silufol sheet and placed on
an agar culture of the blocked mutant 86 at zero time).
Co(NO$_3$)$_2$ (200,100,50,20 mg; left to right) in the agar wells
stimulated the inducing effect.

ascribed to the chelating properties of the enole form of the ß-keto-
lactone structure (Fig. 1), which could presumably scavenge small
amounts of this trace element from the medium and transport it
through the cytoplasmatic membrane as a specific lipophilic carrier
ionophore. As far as   cobalt is concerned it appears as a particularly important cofactor of some enzymes such as xylose isomerase,
alkaline phosphatase and methylmalonyl coenzyme A mutase. It might be
the latter enzyme which could provide the building blocks of the anthracyclines from succinyl coenzyme A, but further experiments are

in progress at our laboratory in order to check this point further. Some other examples from the literature witness the outstanding role of this trace metal (30) as well as of others, such as nickel (31), regarding the regulation of the secondary metabolism of <u>streptomyce-</u> <u>tes</u> (32). The fact that the dihydro derivatives <u>2a</u> and <u>2b</u> displayed about the same effect on indicator mutants, can be explained by the assumption that an oxidation at C-1'-OH and configurational changes at C2 and C3 positions, due to enolizations and transesterifications, although the chelating properties probably do not depend essentially on the presence of one single configuration (Fig. 1).

These contentions have received support due to the kinetics of A-factor production in submerged cultures of the parental strain <u>S</u>. <u>gri-</u> <u>seus</u> JA 3933 (24,29). The amount of <u>1a</u> grew after the decrease of the specific growth rate and attained its maximum many hours before the beginning of anthracycline biosynthesis (29). The addition of inorganic phosphate to the medium suppressed formation of leukaemomycin, but not the A-factor (<u>1a</u>) (25), and in later stages of fermentation the inducer level declined, this was probably due to the presence of inactivating enzymes (Fig. 4). These findings suggested the absence of a direct relationship between the biosynthesis of the antibiotic

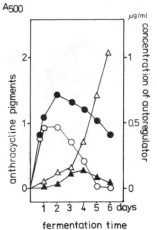

Fig. 4. Production of A-factor (1a) (-o-) and anthracyclines (-△-) by cultures of <u>S</u>. <u>griseus</u> JA 5142. Open symbols: complex medium; shaded symbols: complex medium + 0.1 % KH_2PO_4 (25).

and the production of the A-factor <u>1a</u>. The presence of <u>1a</u> in the medium at an early stage of cultivation of the blocked mutants (0 to 10 hours) is thus a prerequisite of the normal cytodifferentiation in which formation of

leukaemomycin appears to be embedded (33). Experiments with the purified trans-2-(6'-methylheptanol-1'-yl)-3-hydroxymethyl-4-butanolide
($\underline{2a}$; R=C$_7$H$_{15}$) indicated a membranotropic activity of this effector
molecule towards several in vitro cell systems and physicochemical
models as well (34). Hence it could be concluded, that due to their
polar structure the effectors such as $\underline{1a}$, $\underline{1b}$, $\underline{2a}$ and $\underline{2b}$ (R: varying
length of the side chain) could interfere with the function of the
cytoplasmic membrane, on the other hand, the effect of $\underline{2a}$ on $\underline{E}$. $\underline{coli}$
systems of replication, transcription, and translation was negligible
below a concentration of 25 μg/ml (34).

Integration of the A-factor into a pleitropic regulatory network

In order to elucidate the mode of action of $\underline{1a}$ and its derivatives on the A-factor⁻ mutants 86, 15, 16 and 6 (Amy⁻Ant⁻), the morphological and biochemical changes were studied during submerged growth on
Hickey-Tresner's medium (34,35): The presence of $\underline{1a}$ (0.1-0.5 μg/ml)
or $\underline{2a}$ (0.5-2 μg/ml) stimulated slightly biomass formation by the
blocked strains 86 and 15, concomitant with the restoration of antibiotic production, and the parental morphology of the mycelium, provided the effectors had been added at zero time of cultivation (35,36)
(Fig. 5). Under these conditions, the A-factor induced a transition
from either strongly fragmented or pellet-like structures of mycelia
to the filamentous hyphae which are characteristic of the parental
strains (33). In addition, biochemical changes were observed which
showed the integration of the A-factor into a system of interconnected levels of signal transformation (33,35,36).

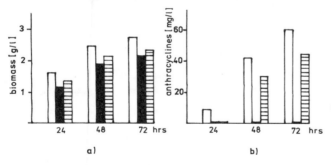

Fig. 5. Effect of $\underline{1a}$ on formation of biomass (a) and anthracyclines
(b) by submerged cultures of blocked mutant 86 (black co-
lumns: control, strain 86: half-shaded: strain 86 + $\underline{1a}$; fair:
parental strain JA 5142).

A first arbitrary level of this signal system could be represented by a pleiotropic regulatory gene in the anthracycline-producing

parental strains JA 5142 and JA 3933 which controls positively or
even negatively the expression of various groups of genes being
either needed or not for spore and antibiotic formation. A deletion
of this gene function in the mutants 86, 15, and others did cause not
only the loss of A-factor production but concomitantly also the absence of NAD(P)-glycohydrolase, a green sporulation pigment, as well
as the control over the proper composition of fatty acids (35,36).
This has been demonstrated also by the protein spectra of cell-free
mycelium extracts during SDS polyacrylamide gel electrophoresis. Mutant 86 was distinguished from the parental strain JA 5142 by both
the presence and the absence of respective proteins (Fig. 6). Though

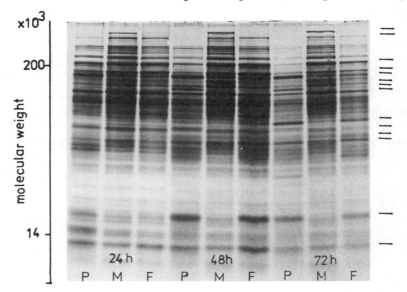

Fig. 6. Protein spectra of S. griseus JA 5142 (P), mutant 86 (M) and
        Mutant 86 grown in presence of 1a (F) (38) as shown by SDS
        polyacrylamide gel electrophoresis. The bars indicate diffe-
        rences.

administration of the A-factor 1a (or 2a) restored greatly the parental protein pattern in the mutant, several protein bands remained unaffected, irrespective of the reconstitution of the parental phenotype
(35). The control of A-factor production as well as its degradation
and interaction with cellular target sites might represent a further
regulatory level. Thus, mutant strain 39 neither produced anthracyclines nor aerial mycelium but still continued the secretion of both
the A-factor and NAD(P)-glycohydrolase into the medium (37). This
could indicate that a genetic change affected the interference of the

A-factor with the cellular machinery in this mutant strain.

On a further tentative level of regulation, at least three different kinds of protein syntheses were controlled by 1a: the biosynthesis of lipid material, the formation of neutral proteinases and the
biosynthetic pathway of the anthracyclines (35,36). Duplication
of the content of mycelial lipids was observed in mutants 86 and 15
concomitant with a decrease of the portion of the polar lipids (35,
36). However, this latter phenomenon might be ascribed to the strict
phosphate limitation of the medium which favoured the non-proportio-
nal increase of the neutral lipids. The synthesis of the neutral and
serine proteinases was stimulated although the parental level could
not be attained again. Conceivably this change could alter the acquisition of complex nutrients and the pattern of intramycelial proteolysis as well. Supporting evidence to this proposal has been provided by studies with the cell-free mycelium extracts of the parental
strain JA 5142, its Amy⁻Ant⁻ mutant 86 grown in the presence and absence of 1a: after they had been kept at ambient temperature for 24
hours, differences in protein digestion by the endogenous proteinases
became evident between the parental strain and the mutant 86 grown in
the presence of 1a, on the one hand, and the mutant strain 86 grown
without 1a, on the other (38). Moreover, the A-factor switched on the
biosynthetic pathway of the anthracyclines beginning with the formation of polyketide-derived aglycone precursors and closing with daunomycin (Fig. 7) and all the other components of the leukaemomycin
complex (23). Additional mutations in the A-factor⁻ indicator strains

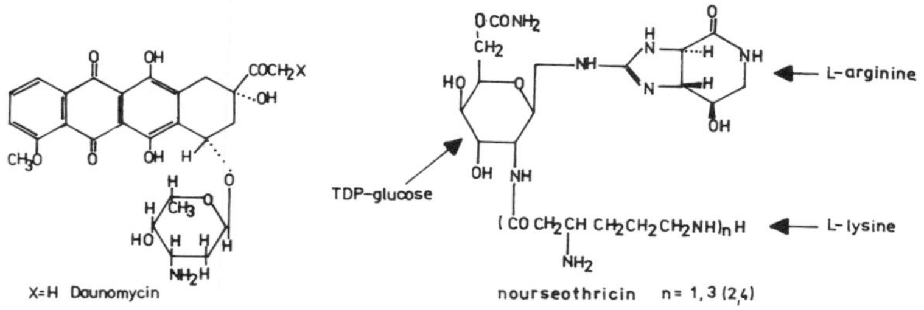

Fig. 7. Chemical structures of daunomycin (left) and nourseothricin
(right).

interfered with the inducing effect of 1a on the secondary metabolism. For instance, mutant 16 (A-factor⁻ Amy⁻Ant⁻) responded to 1a
solely with formation of aerial mycelium but did not form any anthracyclines (24). Another mutant strain, no. 6, (A-factor⁻Ant⁻Amy⁻),
though regaining formation of aerial mycelium in the presence of 1a,
failed to form the red daunomycin-type antibiotics and produced in-

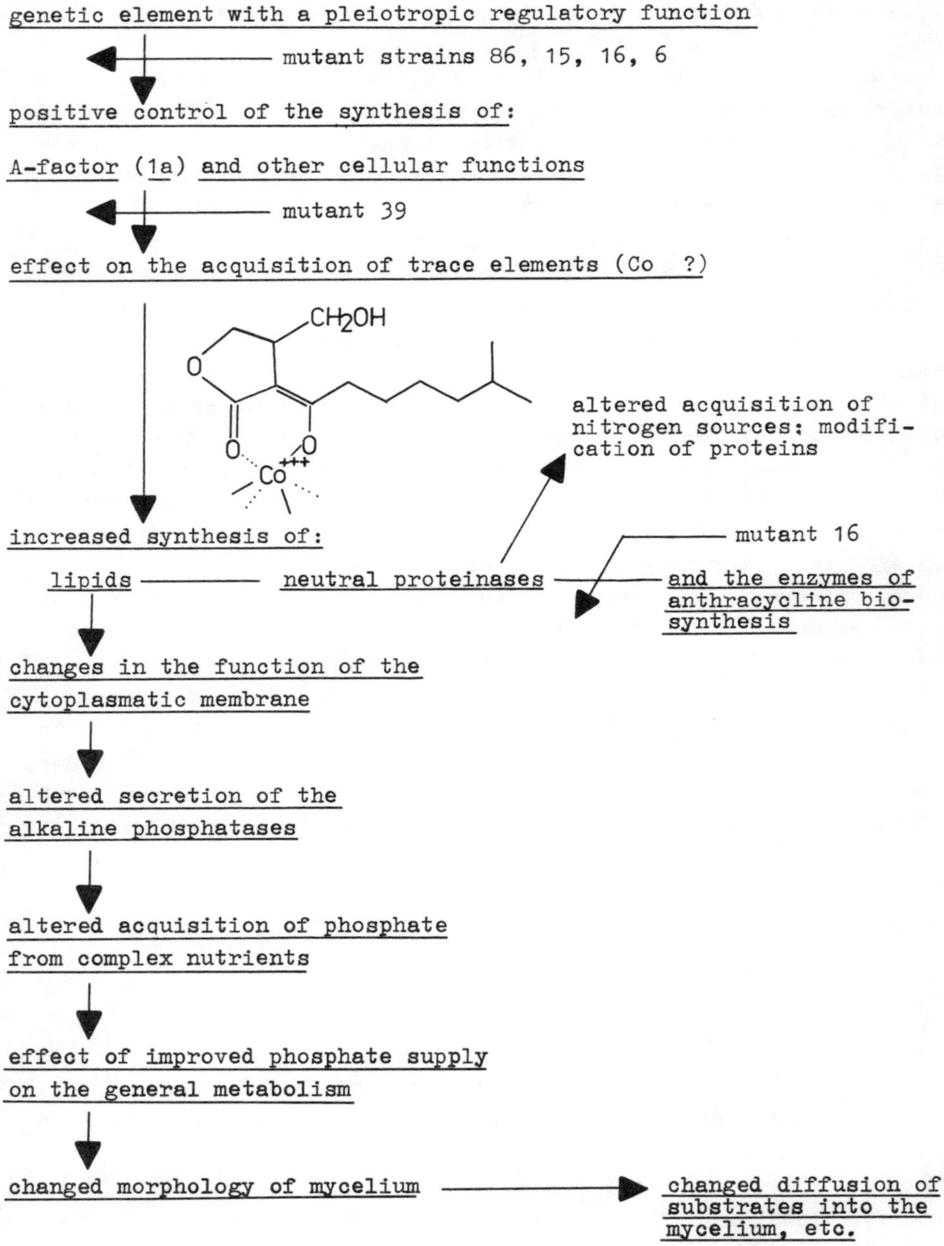

<u>genetic element with a pleiotropic regulatory function</u>

⟵———————— mutant strains 86, 15, 16, 6

<u>positive control of the synthesis of:</u>

<u>A-factor (1a) and other cellular functions</u>

⟵———— mutant 39

<u>effect on the acquisition of trace elements (Co ?)</u>

altered acquisition of
nitrogen sources; modifi-
cation of proteins

<u>increased synthesis of:</u>

<u>lipids</u> ————— <u>neutral proteinases</u> ——————— mutant 16

<u>and the enzymes of
anthracycline bio-
synthesis</u>

<u>changes in the function of the
cytoplasmatic membrane</u>

<u>altered secretion of the
alkaline phosphatases</u>

<u>altered acquisition of phosphate
from complex nutrients</u>

<u>effect of improved phosphate supply
on the general metabolism</u>

<u>changed morphology of mycelium</u> ——————▶ <u>changed diffusion of
substrates into the
mycelium, etc.</u>

Possible signal chain of the A-factor-mediated control of the cytodifferentiation of anthracycline-producing strains of <u>S</u>. <u>griseus</u>

stead, blue pigments (24).

Probably, the observed changes of the lipid metabolism induce on a further regulatory level alterations of the membrane function, which could affect the secretion of enzymes, the uptake of substrates, and the energy metabolism. At least one of these functions has been altered due to the presence of 1a in cultures of the blocked mutants 86 and 15. The parental strain JA 5142 thus displayed comparably low intracellular, but high extracellular activities, of the alkaline phosphatase during growth on the phosphate-limited Hickey-Tresner's medium. In contrast, mutant 86 produced a much higher intracellular activity but the comparable secretion of the enzyme into the medium (33) was missing. Most of the activity had been restrained to the sediment of the 22000 g centrifugation. This suggests that the enzyme remained attached to membrane particles. After administration of 1a to growing cultures of mutant 86, enzyme secretion was markedly enhanced, and concomitantly, filamentous non-fragmented hyphae were produced (33). Addition of phosphate ions (0.2 % KH_2PO_4) to the medium prevented fragmentation of mutant 86 in the absence of 1a but gave rise to formation of very dense mycelial aggregates. It might be concluded that the acquisition of complex nutrients and the effect of the A-factor thereon represents a further regulatory level (33). Recently, the profound effect of extreme nutrient depletion on the morphology of submerged mycelia of other strains of S. griseus was demonstrated (39).

It should be considered further that the structure of mycelium could affect the passive diffusion of substrates inside the mycelial aggregates. We have shown by pulse labelling with ^{14}C-(U)-leucine that the pellet-like mycelia of strain 15 (Amy⁻Ant⁻) absorbed much less radioactivity into proteins than the filamentous mycelia of the parental strain JA 3933. This indicates that alterations of the morphology interfered with the overall metabolic activity. These observations may have shown that the incidental effect of the A-factor 1a (or 2a) on the cytodifferentiation of blocked mutants of the anthracycline-producing strains of S. griseus, should be embedded into a chain of interwoven levels of signal transformation. This chain could be characterized by the broadening of the regulatory levels, the increasing complexity of the individual regulatory circuits and their integration into an interconnected regulatory network (33).

Variability of the control of the cytodifferentiation by A-factor
The model given above is subject to manifold variations depending

stead, blue pigments (24).

Probably, the observed changes of the lipid metabolism induce on a
further regulatory level alterations of the membrane function, which
could affect the secretion of enzymes, the uptake of substrates, and
the energy metabolism. At least one of these functions has been altered due to the presence of 1a in cultures of the blocked mutants 86
and 15. The parental strain JA 5142 thus displayed comparably low
intracellular, but high extracellular activities, of the alkaline phosphatase during growth on the phosphate-limited Hickey-Tresner's medium. In contrast, mutant 86 produced a much higher intracellular activity but the comparable secretion of the enzyme into the medium was
missing (33). Most of the activity had been restrained to the sediment of the 22000 g centrifugation. This suggests that the enzyme remained attached to membrane particles. After administration of 1a to
growing cultures of strain 86, enzyme secretion was markedly enhanced,
and concomitantly, filamentous non-fragmented hyphae were produced.
Addition of phosphate ions (0.2 % KH_2PO_4) to the medium prevented
fragmentation of mutant 86 in the absence of 1a but gave rise to formation of very dense mycelial aggregates. It might be concluded that
the acquisition of complex nutrients and the effect of the A-factor
thereon represents a further regulatory level (33). Recently,
the profound effect of extreme nutrient depletion on the morphology of submerged mycelia of other strains of S. griseus was demonstrated (39).

It should be considered further that the structure of mycelium
could affect the passive diffusion of substrates inside the mycelial
aggregates. We have shown by pulse labelling with ^{14}C-(U)-leucine
that the pellet-like mycelia of strain 15 (Amy⁻Ant⁻) incorporated
much less of radioactivity into proteins than the filamentous mycelia
of the parental strain JA 3933. This indicates that alterations of
the morphology interfered with the overall metabolic activity. These
observations may have shown that the incidental effect of the A-factor 1a (or 2a) on the cytodifferentiation of blocked mutants of the
anthracycline-producing strains of S. griseus, should be embedded into
a chain of interwoven levels of signal transformation. This chain
could be characterized by the broadening of the regulatory levels,
the increasing complexity of the individual regulatory circuits and
their integration into an interconnected regulatory network (33).

Variablity of the control of the cytodifferentiation by A-factor

The model given above is subject to manifold variations depending

on the strain and its taxonomic position. Although the formation of
A-factor <u>1a</u> (R=C$_7$H$_{15}$) and similar **butyrolactone-type** autoregulators
appears widely distributed among actinomycetes and other microorganisms (19,24) the significance of these compounds for the formation
of aerial mycelium and secondary metabolites has been demonstrated
in only a few cases. In most of these strains these molecules seem to
be present without having a comparable function. Furthermore, the
structure of the inducer molecule 2-(6'-methyl-heptanoyl)-3-hydroxy-
methyl-4-butanolide (<u>1a</u>; R=C$_7$H$_{15}$) has been subject to wide variation
in the course of the evolution thus giving rise to the appearance of
a plethora of homologues, stereoisomers, and derivatives, which can
exert about the same activity. In other cases similar, but inactive
γ **-butyrolactones, have been produced as congenors (26).**

It should be taken into account that the cellular response of the
A-factor-negative strains to this effector can be highly variable in
dependence on the species or additional genetic changes. Quite
different kinds of antibiotic productions, either the formation of
aminoglycosides or polyketides, can be switched on by <u>1a</u> in the different strains of <u>S</u>. <u>griseus</u> which are unable to yield this endogenous signal. While <u>1a</u> stimulated, for instance, the biosynthesis of
lipids by the Amy⁻Ant⁻ indicator mutants 86 and 15 of <u>S</u>. <u>griseus</u>, no
adequate effect has been observed in the same range of concentration
with the A-factor-negative strain <u>S</u>. <u>hygroscopicus</u> JA 6599. This suggested that the cellular response to A-factor is highly specific with
respect to a given microorganism. It was shown further with our mutant
strains 6 and 16 (Amy⁻Ant⁻A-factor⁻) that the cellular answer to the
A-factor of the blocked indicator strains can be altered by genetic
changes as well as by the medium composition (36). In the presence of
high concentrations of phosphate in cultures of the indicator strain
86, the biosynthesis of the anthracyclines was negligible although the
A-factor had been administered. Previously, high variability had been
demonstrated in the genetic control of A-factor production (20,21,22).
The involvement of both stable chromosomal, and instable plasmid-borne
genes, was observed with different species of streptomycetes. It
appears that the A-factor provides an instructive example demonstra-
ting the variable organization of the cytodifferentiation of streptomycetes, both on the genetical and the physiological level. Furthermore
this model shows that exploration of the proper sequence of the A-
factor-mediated chain of signal transformation represents a rather
difficult or even impossible enterprise. Many similar effector compounds might be formed by the actinomycetes and other producers of
secondary metabolites which could trigger particular stages of their

cytodifferentiation such as the germination of spores, the retainment
of their dormancy, the regulation of morphological changes, and also
the formation of secondary metabolites. As a corollary, we
should mention here our recent results with polyether-producing
Streptomyces strains. Spores of S. griseus HP, S. cinnamonensis IMET
33358, and S. lasaliensis IMET 33359 contained up to 2 % griseochelin
(40), 1.5 % monensins A and B, and 0.8 % of the lasalocid complex
suggesting that these cation-selective ionophores have some importance
for their producer organisms. Griseochelin was found particularly to
transport heavy metals such as zinc, and cadmium, through layers of
organic solvents.

3 DIRECTED SEARCHING FOR STRAINS OF S. NOURSEI JA 3890b OVERPRODUCING
   THE GLYCOPEPTIDE ANTIBIOTIC NOURSEOTHRICIN (FIG. 7)

As far as the development of directed methods of strain improvement
is concerned we have to consider   the complex organization of programs of cytodifferentiation starting with the excessive length of
the secondary pathways (41) and ending with the need for those particular morphological changes throughout the cell cycle which are
correlated with an optimal expression of the secondary metabolism.
Because of the control of the secondary pathways by very many genetic
functions, the variability of the regulatory systems, and the non-
availability of a directed selection pressure which could support the
vegetative development of antibiotic-overproducing clones, elaboration of biochemical criteria of selection can only aid the detection
of the desired mutants but success should not be taken for granted (41).
Apparently, directed screening methods have given the best results as
far as the secondary pathways themselves had been subjected to genetical and biochemical manipulations. Thus, new procedures of the directed biosynthesis, mutational biosynthesis, and hybrid biosynthesis
enlarged the scale of available antibiotics. Other directed methods
were aimed at manipulations of the production of precursor molecules.
Pertinent changes could afford both alterations of the composition
and the quantity of the produced mixture of secondary metabolites.
Frequently, overproductions of precursors installed either occasio-
nally during randomized screening or during selection of strains resistant to antimetabolites corresponded to an increased antibiotic
production (41). The isolation of mutants displaying an altered life
cycle should be regarded as a third way of isolating strains deregulated in the control of antibiotic production. In this context it
could be claimed that mutants particularly well adapting to extreme
environmental conditions (environmental stress) preferentially might
display an altered regulation of the secondary metabolism. Irrespec-

tive of the frequently noticeable genetic instability of such mutants, the main problem with this type of rational selection might be
the variability of the cellular response to a given situation.
Different genetic changes could so contribute to the same degree of
adaptation in the presence of toxic agents. Due to alterations at the
level of overlapping pleiotropic gene functions many different phenotypic characteristics could be altered concomitantly.

Mutants of S. noursei JA 3890b resistant to benzyl alcohol

Recently we isolated a collection of mutants resistant to benzyl
alcohol (Bal) as an inhibitor of the synthesis of fatty acids (34)
from natural colony populations of the nourseothricin-producing
strain UV 12 of S. noursei JA 3890b. The aim was to search for
strains altered in their lipid metabolism which possess differing
properties of the cytoplasmatic membrane corresponding to an increased production of the glycopeptide antibiotic nourseothricin (Fig. 7).
Only a few of the respective derivatives were found. They still produced the identical amount of antibiotic as their parental strains
whilst the formation of spores and aerial mycelium were missing. Although both the Bal^R strains and their ancestors responded to the
presence of benzyl alcohol in the medium with a reduction of their
lipid content, the former grew almost normal up to a concentration of
0.1 % in the medium. In the absence of benzyl alcohol the Bal^R strain
2/8 was distinguishable from its parent strain, UV 12, by an almost
duplicated content of lipids. When 0.1 % of the toxic agent had been
administered, it amounted to about the same as found in the parental
strain when grown in the absence of the inhibitor (Fig. 8). This re-

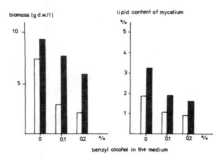

Fig. 8. Effect of benzyl alcohol on biomass production and mycelial
lipid content (48 hrs cultures). Fair columns: parental
strain BF 32; black columns: Bal^R strain 2/8.

vealed that Bal^R strains are deregulated concerning the metabolism
of the fatty acids but it seems unclear whether the lack of forma-

tion of aerial mycelium should be ascribed to this particular change.
More likely, a pleiotropic gene may control concomitantly the
rate of fatty acid synthesis and any an important step in spore formation (16). As another consequence of the presence of several pleiotropic genes and their overlapping functions, a series of phenotypi-
cally similar mutant strains could be obtained by quite different methods of directed screening.

Phosphate-deregulated strains of Streptomyces noursei

Thus, by the use of two different methods, i. e. by searching for
arsenate-resistant strains and by chemostat cultivation, we succeeded
in isolating mutants of S. noursei which displayed reduced sensitivity of the nourseothricin production to inhibition by inorganic phosphate (43,44,45). The majority of the As^R strains, obtained from natural colony populations by the paper strip method, produced the same
amount of antibiotic when the phosphate concentration in the medium
was low (43), but was exceeded by a comparably higher yield in the presence of this inhibitor. It is interesting that the higher producing
strains UV 12 and NG 13, found by conventional screening techniques
were distinguishable from the wild-type strain JA 3890b by both the
decreased sensitivity to phosphate inhibition of the antibiotic production, and by improved resistance to the toxic arsenate, as an analogue of the phosphate. Measurements of the intracellular ATP level revealed that this observation could be explained by an altered regulation of the energy metabolism rather than by changes at the level of
phosphate influx (44). During short-time incubation of mycelia with
AsO_4^{3-}, the level of ATP declined moderately in the As^R strains while
a drastic reduction has been observed in their As^S ancestors. Since
many streptomycetes seem to display an inversed correlation between
the ATP content of the mycelium and the expression of the secondary
metabolism, it can be supposed that ATP production was altered in the
As^R strains in presence of phosphate. Corroborating evidence to this
contention has been provided by the higher ATP level found in the
wild-type strain (44).

Quite another type of a phosphate-deregulated, nourseothricin-producing strain, RG 2, was isolated recently from the wild-type strain
JA 3890b after mutagenesis of mycelia and subsequent chemostat cultivation of the surviving cells under ammonia limitation in the presence of 0.1 mol/l inorganic phosphate (45). Apparently, these conditions supported the survival of those clones producing decreased
amounts of phospholipids. They would be able to prevent the wasteful
use of nitrogen for the enlarged formation of aminophospholipids

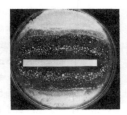
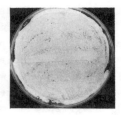

Fig. 9. Selection for As^R strains by the use of the paper strip method (paper strip soaked with 1.5 mol/l AsO_4^{3-}) left: parental strain JA 3890b; right: strain RG2.

which occurs usually in the presence of excessive phosphate. During
growth under phosphate limitation the mutant RG 2 displayed the same
level of both total and phosphorus-containing lipids as the parental
strain and the same production of nourseothricin as well (Fig.10)(45).

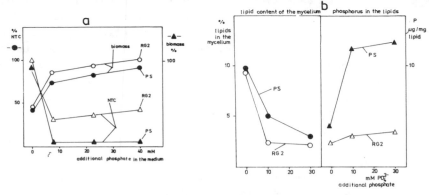

Fig. 10. Effect of increasing phosphate concentration on a) production of biomass (-o-), biosynthesis of nourseothricin (-△-),
b) mycelial lipid content (-o-), and phosphorus content of
lipids (-△-) from 48 hour cultures. PS: parental strain
JA 3890b, black symbols; strain RG 2: fair symbols.

However, increasing concentrations of phosphate in the medium failed
to raise the synthesis of phospholipids. This suggests that strain
RG 2 could adapt particularly well to a nutritional imbalance.
     Surprisingly, deregulation of phospholipid synthesis (phosphati-
dylethanolamine and cardiolipin) corresponds to insensitivity of the
nourseothricin production to phosphate inhibition, to higher resistance of growth to arsenate ions (Fig. 9), and to an increased secretion of the alkaline phosphatase into the medium (45). An explanation
for these seemingly divergent features could be given by assuming a

pleiotropic genetic change which deranged the energy metabolism in a similar manner as it has been found with the As^R derivatives. Contrarily, respective alterations were produced in case of strain RG 2 by changes at the level of the cytoplasmatic membrane and the regulation of lipid composition. The results with the phosphate-deregulated mutants of S. noursei JA 3890b are reminiscent of those obtained by Martin et al. (46). They isolated mutants of the candicidin-producing S. griseus which were not only discernible from their ancestors by reduced sensitivity to phosphate but showed also differences in their developmental behaviour.

As a generalization it could be proposed that under stressing environmental conditions particularly those mutants get an advantage over the parental genotype which are altered in their cytodifferentiation. Due to the highly variable organization of development in the streptomycetes, the same type of adaptation to peculiar conditions could be achieved by various genetic changes affecting different biochemical levels. As far as the control of antibiotic formation is concerned it appears to be altered in many of these strains, but insensitivity to phosphate inhibition is only one prerequisite for an increased antibiotic production. This has been demonstrated by the finding that none of the phosphate-deregulated strains of S. noursei obtained so far by directed methods excelled the parent by higher antibiotic production during phosphate limitation.

Nourseothricin-resistant strains of S. noursei

Though higher tolerance to the toxicity of produced secondary metabolites may be typical for the higher-yielding strains of streptomycetes, as a rule, additional genetic changes are required for overproduction such as improved generation of precursors and intermediates, alterations of the spectrum of metabolites and others. For the producers of macrolide, lincosamine, and streptogramine antibiotics a mechanism of inducible resistance has been demonstrated involving 23S RNA methylation (47). By virtue of an autoregulatory effect of these antibiotics, resistance develops concomitantly to the increase of productivity.

In the case of the nourseothricin-producing S. noursei JA 3890b the vegetative mycelia were resistant up to 3 g antibiotic/l in the medium though the nourseothricin inhibited the ribosomal protein synthesis (48). In contrast, the germination of spores was inhibited severely by 0.1 g/l. Since the resistance increased when the spores were pregerminated, we suppose that S. noursei JA 3890b also posses-

sed an inducible mechanism of detoxification. As in the other strep-
tothricin-producing strains of streptomycetes (49) inactivation of
the antibiotic could occur by the aid of an acetylating enzyme present in the cell-free mycelium extracts. Due to the increased intracellular titre of the antibiotic in the high—producing mutants they
might maintain a higher activity of the protecting enzyme than the
wild-type strains. This could explain why a nearly linear correlation
was found   between the level of productivity of the mutants and the
degree of their resistance to exogenous nourseothricin when the number of the surviving colonies had been taken as a measure which originated from spores in the presence of the antibiotic (Fig. 11) (47).

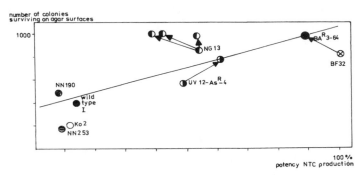

Fig. 11. Correlation of the maximum potency of nourseothricin-produ-
         cing strains and the degree of resistance of spore out-
         growth to the presence of 0.1 mg/ml antibiotic in the agar.

All attempts aimed at the isolation of higher producing
strains by searching for the antibiotic-resistant colonies failed to
yield a success. We thus have to observe that the higher producing mutants UV 12, NG13, and BF 32, which were obtained by conventional
screening techniques, possessed some common properties such as resistance to arsenate, to the antibiotic produced, and insensitivity of
the nourseothricin production to inhibition by phosphate. Since directed searching for these properties did not afford overproducing
strains it could be concluded that many other additional changes
would be needed as to improve productivity. For example, it has been
shown previously that the high producing strain BF 32 could be distinguished from the wild-type strain JA 3890b by the absence of
concerted feedback inhibition of the aspartokinase by both lysine
and threonine. This enzyme seems to be involved in formation of the
lysine precursor of nourseothricin (33). Similarly, Mendelovitz and
Aharonowitz (50) obtained cephamycin-overproducing strains of S. clavuligerus by searching for AEC[R] mutants displaying a deregulated ly-

sine formation. But accordingly with the high variability of the cellular adaptation to stressing environmental conditions, the same
authors isolated by their method a collection of mutants distinguishable from each other by additional biochemical properties.

That predictions concerning a more rational manipulation of the
secondary pathways suffer greatly from the incomplete knowledge about
the interwoven metabolic features could be shown further by our expe-
riences with S. noursei. As published recently, the wild-type strain
alkalizes strongly when grown on an alanine-starch medium concomitant
with repression of both the formation of glutamate dehydrogenase and
nourseothricin (51). Hence, abolition of the nitrogen regulation has
been proposed as a major goal of the directed search for the overproducing strains. None of the higher yielding strains isolated by conventional techniques of screening displayed an altered pattern of fermentation and glutamate dehydrogenase formation under the above conditions. This finding can be rationalized when we consider that those
complex media have been used for the selection which did not support
excessive production of ammonia. Instead of the excessive formation
of nitrogen catabolites throughout the fermentation, proper administration of inorganic phosphate represents a critical factor controlling antibiotic formation by S. noursei JA 3890b on complex
media (52).

4 CONCLUDING REMARKS

Since the secondary metabolism of the streptomycetes and other
microorganisms forms an integral part of their differentiation behaviour, we should not expect to find uniform structures here of metabolites or generally distributed regulatory mechanisms, but in the
search for more rational methods of strain improvement, including
the 'metabolic engineering' of the antibiotic-producing pathways
we should take into account the high variability of the genetic and
metabolic organization of the secondary metabolism and its embedding
in pleiotropic regulatory chains of the cytodifferentiation. The variability of the cellular development provides a major obstacle when
directed methods of screening aimed at the antibiotic-overproducing
strains are envisaged. In any case the individual features of control
have to be explored for a given strain before a biochemically motiva-
ted strategy of selection may be installed as to detect the overproducing mutants. Irrespective of the difficulties portrayed above,
this survey should be understood as far from drawing a pessimistic
picture. On the contrary, if we are continuing to learn more about
the principles of organization of the cytodifferentiation and their

variability we would be enabled to manipulate more and more successfully the expression of the secondary metabolism.

5 REFERENCES

(1) H. Zähner, H. Drautz, W. Weber, in: Bioactive microbial pro-
    ducts: search and discovery (eds. D. Winstanley et al.) (1983)
    p. 51, Academic Press.
(2) A. L. Demain, in: Antibiotics containing the ß-lactam structure
    Vol. 1 (eds. A. L. Demain, N. A. Solomon) (1983) p. 189, Sprin-
    ger Verlag.
(3) J. F. Martin, Adv. Biochem. Engin. 6 (1977) 105.
(4) J. F. Martin, Y. Aharonowitz, in: Antibiotics containing the
    ß-lactame structure (eds. A. L. Demain and N. A. Solomon) (1983)
    p. 229, Springer Verlag.
(5) D. Gersch, C. Strunk, Curr. Microbiol. 4 (1980) 272.
(6) S. Chatterjee, L. C. Vining, Can. J. Microbiol. 28 (1982) 311.
(7) Z. Dobrava, J. Naprstek, M. Jerešova, J. Janeček, FEMS Microbiol.
    Lett. 22 (1984) 197.
(8) C. M. Ragan, L. C. Vining, Can. J. Microbiol. 24 (1978) 1012.
(9) J. Terry, P. G. Springham, Can. J. Microbiol. 27 (1981) 1044.
(10) R. Esteban, A. R. Negreda, J. R. Villanueava, T. G. Villa, FEMS
    Microbiol. Lett. 23 (1984) 91.
(11) R. Wambutt, D. Riesenberg, M. Krüger, M. Schultze, Z. Allg.
    Mikrobiol. 24 (1984) 575.
(12) D. Riesenberg, F. Bergter, C. Kari, J. Gen. Microbiol. 130
    (1984) 2549.
(13) D. Riesenberg, C. Kari, Molec. Gen. Genet. 181 (1981) 467.
(14) G. An, L. C. Vining, Can. J. Microbiol. 24 (1978) 502.
(15) D. A. Hopwood, in: Biochemistry and Genetic Regulation of Com-
    mercially Important Antibiotics. (ed. L. C. Vining) (1983) p. 1,
    Addison Wesley Publ. Compl.
(16) M. Okanishi, Trends Antib. Res. (ed. Jap. Antib. Res. Assoc.)
    (1982) p. 32, Kodansha Tokyo.
(17) A. S. Khokhlov, in: Overproduction of Microbial Products (eds.
    V. Krumphanzl et al.) (1982) p. 96, Academic Press London.
(18) H. Thrum, in Biotechnol. Ind. Antibiotics (ed. E. J. Vandamme)
    (1984) p. 367, Marcel Dekker Inc.
(19) O. Hara, T. Beppu, J. Antibiot. 35 (1982) 349 and 1208.
(20) O. Hara, S. Horinouchi, T. Uozumi, T. Beppu, J. Gen. Microbiol.
    129 (1983) 2933.
(21) S. Horinouchi, O. Hara, T. Beppu, J. Bacteriol. 155 (1983) 1238.
(22) S. Horinouchi, Y. Kumada, T. Beppu, J. Bacteriol. 158 (1984) 481.

(23) I. Eritt, U. Gräfe, W. F. Fleck, Z. Allg. Mikrobiol. 22 (1982) 91.

(24) I. Eritt, U. Gräfe, W. F. Fleck, Z. Allg. Mikrobiol. 24 (1984) 3.

(25) U. Gräfe, I. Eritt, J. Antibiot. 36 (1983) 1592.

(26) U. Gräfe, G. Reinhardt, W. Schade, D. Krebs, I. Eritt, W. F. Fleck, E. Heinrich, L. Radics, J. Antibiot. 35 (1982) 609.

(27) U. Gräfe, W. Schade, I. Eritt, W. F. Fleck, L. Radics, J. Antibiot. 35 (1982) 1722.

(28) U. Gräfe, G. Reinhardt, W. Schade, I. Eritt, W. F. Fleck, L. Radics, Biotechnol. Lett. 5 (1983) 591.

(29) U. Gräfe, I. Eritt, D. Riesenberg, J. Basic Microbiol. 25 (1985), in the press.

(30) C. A. Claridge, R. P. Elander, K. E. Rice, in: Biotechnology of industrial antibiotics (ed. E. J. Vandamme) (1984) p. 413, Marcel Dekker Inc.

(31) A. M. Biot, in: Biotechnology of industrial antibiotics (ed. E. J. Vandamme) (1984) p. 695, Marcel Dekker Inc.

(32) E. D. Weinberg, Folia microbiol. 23 (1978) 496.

(33) U. Gräfe, I. Eritt, W. F. Fleck, The Actinomycetes 18 (1983 - 1984) 220.

(34) unpublished results.

(35) U. Gräfe, G. Reinhardt, D. Krebs, I. Eritt, W. F. Fleck, J. Gen. Microbiol. 130 (1984) 1237.

(36) U. Gräfe, G. Reinhardt, D. Krebs, I. Eritt, W. F. Fleck, Z. Allg. Mikrobiol. 24 (1984) 515.

(37) U. Gräfe, I. Eritt, W. F. Fleck, J. Antibiot. 34 (1981) 1385.

(38) U. Gräfe, E. Sarfert (to be published).

(39) K. K. Kendrick, J. C. Ensign, J. Bacteriol. 155 (1983) 357.

(40) U. Gräfe, W. Schade, M. Roth, L. Radics, M. Incze, K. Ujszaszy, J. Antibiot. 37 (1984) 836.

(41) Z. Vaněk, J. Cudlin, M. Blumauerová, Z. Hošťálek, Folia microbiol. 16 (1971) 225.

(42) R. P. Elander, L. T. Chang, in: Microbiology Technology 2nd ed. (eds. H. Peppler, D. Perlman) Vol. 2 (1979) p. 243, Academic Press.

(43) W. Friedrich, E. J. Bormann, U. Gräfe, Z. Allg. Mikrobiol. 24 (1984) 13.

(44) F. Hänel, U. Gräfe, W. Friedrich, E. J. Bormann, Z. Allg. Mikrobiol. 24 (1984) 239.

(45) F. Hänel, U. Gräfe, M. Roth, E. J. Bormann, D. Krebs, J. Basic Microbiol. 25 (1985) in the press.

(46) J. F. Martin, G. Naharro, P. Liras, J. R. Villanueva, J. Antibiot. 6 (1979) 600.

(47) B. Weisblum, Y. Fujisawa, S. Horinouchi, Trends Antib. Res.
     (1982) p. 73 (ed. Japan Antib. Res. Assoc.) Kodanska Tokyo.
(48) B. Röder, U. Gräfe, J. Basic Microbiol. 25 (1985), in the press.
(49) S. Keeratipul, M. Sugiyama, R. Nomi, Biotechnol. Lett. 5 (1983)
     441.
(50) S. Mendelovitz, Y. Aharonowitz, J. Gen. Microbiol. 129 (1983)
     2063.
(51) U. Gräfe, H. Bocker, H. Thrum, Adv. Biotechn. Vol. III, Fermen-
     tation products (eds. M. Moo-Young et al.) (1981) p. 193, Per-
     gamon Press Canada Ltd.
(52) P. J. Müller, G. Haubold, M. Menner, H. H. Grosse, J. M. Oze-
     gowski, H. Bocker, Z. Allg. Mikrobiol. 24 (1984) 555.

6 ACKNOWLEDGEMENT

We wish to thank Dr. Lajos Radics (Central Research Institute of Chemistry, Budapest, Hungary) for recording and assigning the ^{13}C NMR spectrum of 2b from S. bikiniensis.

Regulation of Tetracycline Biosynthesis

Vladislav Běhal

Czechoslovak Academy of Sciences, Institute of Microbiology, Vídeňská 1083, 14220 Prague 4, Czechoslovakia

Summary

With the onset of tetracycline biosynthesis the amount of enzymes of primary metabolism in the producer cell decreases. The building units for the biosynthesis of tetracyclines are synthesized in altern- ative biosynthetic pathways. The magnitude of tetracycline production depends on the amount of tetracycline synthetase in the cell; the activity of anhydrotetracycline oxygenase can be taken as a marker determining the activity of the whole synthetase. We elaborated a math- ematical model simulating the behaviour of a Streptomyces aureofaciens culture during overproduction of the antibiotic. Benzylthiocyanate increases the amount of secondary metabolism enzymes in the cell and affects their cellular localization.

1 Introduction

Tetracyclines belong among the oldest clinically applied antibiot- ics. Their biosynthesis and its regulation are relatively well known. Their production makes use of two microorganisms, Streptomyces aureo- faciens which synthesizes a mixture of chlortetracycline (CTC) and tetracycline (TC) and Streptomyces rimosus synthesizing oxytetracycline (OTC). The production magnitudes attained' in industrial fermentations are in the range of tens of grammes per L.

There high productions are naturally achieved by strains obtained
by prolonged improvement. Industrial strains used for production of
antibiotics differ from their parent strains isolated from the nature
in the activity of their enzyme systems. During the improvement they
have lost the ability to synthesize some other secondary metabolites
(SM). The activity of basic metabolic processes crucial for growth at
sporulation, however, has to be retained for the most part; variants,
however high-producing, which exhibit serious disturbances of fundamental metabolic pathways are unsuitable for production as well as for
further improvement. Regulation of biosynthesis of SM in these high
producing strains is different from that found in wild strains. Some
control mechanisms which in wild strains stop the biosynthesis of SM
at low concentration are removed and replaced by others which make
possible a large-scale synthesis of SM. The regulation of biosynthesis
of SM is thus studied under conditions of SM overproduction.

2 Primary metabolism

Primary metabolism of microorganisms synthesizing tetracyclines
is controlled so as to ensure the synthesis of a sufficient amount of
mycelium with a high activity of enzymes of secondary metabolism (ESM)
and enzymes of primary metabolism synthesizing precursors of the tetracycline molecule (TCs). Producers of TCs are cultivated in complex
containing, in addition to sucrose in S. aureofaciens and starch in
S. rimosus, also soybean or peanut flour as a source of carbon and
nitrogen nutrients and phosphate. Growth substances are supplied in
corn-steep and molasses. The activity of primary metabolism is regulated by phosphate nutritive limitation. Exhaustion of phosphates from
the medium causes a substantial slowing-down of protein synthesis (1).
However, protein synthesis proceeds even during the synthesis of TCs,
albeit in a limited extent (2,3). RNA synthesis reaches a maximum
around the middle of the growth phase and then drops fairly sharply
(3,4).

The amount of enzymes of primary metabolism declines in the produ-
uction phase, as shown in acetyl-CoA carboxylase (5), malate dehydrogenase (6) and also glucose 6-phosphate dehydrogenase (7). The amount
of the last enzyme in the production and the wild strain in the growth
phase is the same; in production phase its amount in the production
strain decreases while in the wild strain it rises 2 - 3 times. The
activity of enzymes of the tricarboxylic acid cycle is markedly lower
in the production strain of S. aureofaciens (8).

Polysaccharides in nutrient media have to be degraded prior to
uptake into the cells. The media containing starch, which are used
for cultivating S. rimosus, are supplied with technical grade amylase
(9) at the beginning of cultivation. Sucrose is degraded by sucrase
bound to the mycelium of S. aureofaciens (7). This enzyme is obviously
constitutive.

2.1 Phosphorylation of monosaccharides

Phosphorylation of monosaccharides in the cell of S. aureofaciens
is catalyzed by hexokinases (7) relying on ATP as phosphate source.
Utilization of polyphosphates for phosphorylation of sugars, which
has been proved in a number of microorganisms (10) has not yet been
unambiguously proved in producers of TCs.

Glucose 6-phosphate, the product of glucose phosphorylation, is
utilized in two important metabolic pathways. In the glycolytic pathway it is degraded and serves for the synthesis of building units for
TCs. In addition, it is used for production of energy in the form of
NADH and ATP. In the pentose phosphate pathway it yields during its
metabolism NADPH necessary for some enzymatic reactions during TCs
biosynthesis. The relation between the glycolytic and the pentose
phosphate pathway was studied by Hošťálek (19) who assumed that the
ensuing TCs inhibit the pentose phosphate pathway in favour of the
glycolytic dissimilation and thus also block the formation of NADPH
necessary for the biosynthesis of TCs. Glucose 6-phosphate dehydrogenase in S. aureofaciens uses not only NADP but also NAD as a substrate

(Neužil et al. in press).

In the presence of medium phosphate concentrations 2-5-fold higher than optimal for production the cells of both the wild and the production strain of S. aureofaciens were found to accumulate glucose 6-phosphate, obviously owing to the inhibition of glucose 6-phosphate dehydrogenase (11). Higher accumulations were found in a mycelium growing on glucose relative to mycelium growing on sucrose. Madry et al. (12) have also found a higher content of glucose 6--phosphate in a mycelium of the tylosin producer Streptomyces T59235

2.2 ATP, polyphosphates and phosphatases

The amount of ATP in the mycelium of a wild strain of S. aureofaciens markedly differs from that in production strain in which it is much lower. After a maximum ATP level has been reached in the growth phase, its content decreases prior to the onset of TCs synthesis (13, 14). The amount of enzymes splitting ATP and other nucleoside triphosphates and nucleoside diphosphates was the highest in production phase (15,16). Synthesis of ATP-diphosphohydrolase stopped when inorganic phosphate was added to the medium. ATP-diphosphohydrolase and inorganic pyrophosphatase were found both in the cytoplasm and in membranes. Ultra-cytochemical localization showed that the activity was present in the capsular slime coat surrounding the hyphal surface and also in cytoplasmic metachromatic granules (17).

The amount of polyphosphates in the cells of S. aureofaciens during cultivation on media with increased phosphate levels was also increased. Cytochemical staining demonstrated in the wild strain polyphosphates in exocellular irregular granules of different size (18).

2.3 Formation of building units

Even in the period of decreased activity of enzymes of primary metabolism sufficient amount of malonyl-CoA for the biosynthesis of TCs has to be synthesized, in the glycolytic pathway from monosaccharides by carboxylation of acetyl-CoA. Another source of acetyl-CoA for biosynthesis of TCs includes fatty acids (Běhal, unpublished results).

Another reaction of malonyl-CoA formation is decarboxylation of oxaloacetate. This metabolic pathway was also found in S. aureofaciens
(20). Oxaloacetate may arise by carboxylation of phosphoenolpyruvate.
Phosphoenolpyruvate carboxylase in the production strain of S. aureofaciens was found to be most active in the production phase. In addition, oxaloacetate may also arise from amino acids entering the tricarboxylic acid cycle during their degradation.

Biosynthesis of TCs includes a considerable utilization of acetate
units from degradation products by alternative metabolic pathways.
Experiments with incorporation of $2\text{-}^{14}C$ acetate (and also $3\text{-}^{14}C$ pyruvate and $2\text{-}^{14}C$ malonate) into Tc showed 28 % radioactivity to be present
in carbons derived from the acetate carboxyl (20). This result implies
that at least 53 % of the acetate units from which the TC was synthesized had already been utilized for the synthesis of other compounds.
Likewise the carbons of OTC originating biogenetically from the acetate
carboxyl were found to contain considerable radioactivity after incorporation of $2\text{-}^{14}C$ acetate. The data published by Catlin et al. (21)
point out that about 30 % OTC is synthesized from acetate units formed
by alternative metabolic pathways. These proportions may differ depending on experimental conditions, particularly on the length of presence
of radioactive substrate in the culture medium.

Malonylsemiamide, which is the terminal group in the biosynthesis
of TCs, is also formed from diverse compounds. $3\text{-}^{14}C$ propionate and
$5\text{-}^{14}C$ glutamate were incorporated only after the loss of specificity
of labelling (22). However, carbon atoms originating in asparagine
were preferentially incorporated into the terminal group (23).

3 Secondary metabolism

Synthesis of skeleton of TCs begins with the condensation of one
molecule of malonylsemiamide-CoA with eight molecules of malonyl-CoA.
The polymerization apparently takes place analogously as described by
Lynen and Tada (24) in fatty acids and by Dimroth et al. (25) in
6-methylsalicyl acid. In contrast to the biosynthesis of fatty acids

no reduction of keto groups takes place which promotes the formation
of aromatic rings. The sequence of reactions giving rise to TCs has
been elucidated by the McCormick group. With the aid of blocked
mutants they isolated individual intermediates and proposed a bio-
genetic scheme (26). Newer reviews of the metabolic pathways have been
published by Hošťálek et al. (27) and Běhal et al. (28).

3.1 Enzymes of Secondary Metabolism

The first intermediate to be isolated was 6-methylpretetramide.
This compound was first hydrolyzed on C-4 and the hydroxygroup was
then oxidized to ketone. The next reaction is the hydroxylation in
position 12a. Substitution of the keto group on C-4 with amino group
gives rise to 4-dedimethylamino-4-aminoanhydrotetracycline. This is
followed by a two-step methylation of the amino group to form anhydrotetracycline (ATC) (Fig.1). The enzyme catalyzing this reaction was
designated S-adenosylmethionine: dedimethylamino-4-aminoATC-N-methyl-
transferase (29). ATC is hydrated to 5a,11a-dehydrotetracycline by
ATC oxygenase (41) in the presence of NADPH and atmospheric oxygen.
The last step of TC biosynthesis is the reduction of the double bond
between C-5a and C-11a. This reaction is catalyzed by TC(5a-11a)
dehydrogenase (30). The activity of this enzyme is regulated by a
cosynthetic factor I (42).

The sequence of reactions which give rise to OTC was arrayed
into a consistent scheme by P.A. Miller et al. (43). The scheme pres-
umes the reaction sequence ATC   dehydro TC   dehydro OTC   OTC. Since
the hydroxylation of anhydro OTC to dehydro OTC was proved even in vitro, we may asume also a reverse sequence of the first and the second
reaction (28).

4 Regulation of biosynthesis

When optimum bioengineering parameters are maintained, the biosynthesis of TCs is regulated by the amount of nutrients and the regime of their dosage. The dependence of production of TCs on the type
of nitrogen nutrition has not yet been studied in detail. In industr-

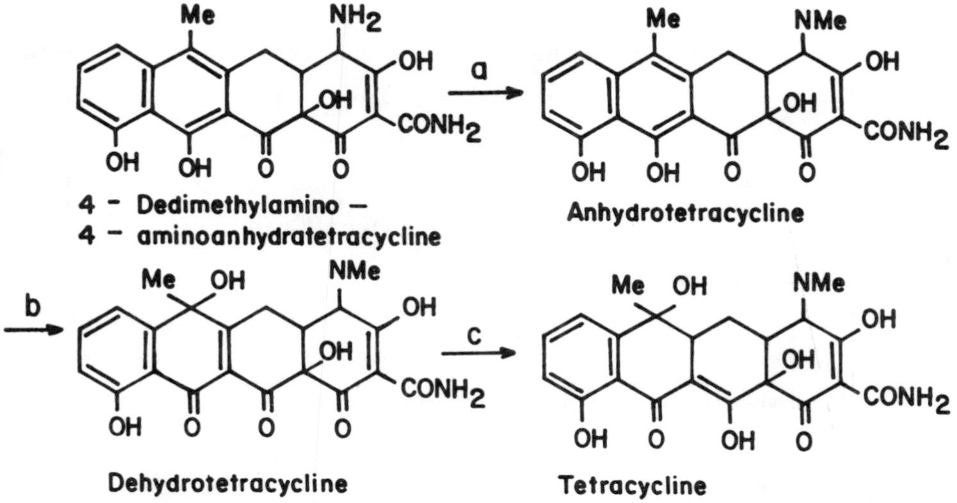

Fig. 1 The enzymes synthesizing tetracycline

a - S-adenosylmethionine: dedimethylamino-4-aminoATC-
    -N-methyltransferase

b - anhydrotetracycline oxygenase

c - tetracycline(5a-11a)dehydrogenase

ial cultivations the amount of ammonia nitrogen decreases from the
initial 1.3 % to about 0.4 % which is maintained nearly till the end
of cultivation (28). Additions of ammonia help to maintain the required pH of 5.6 - 6.2 suitable for S. aureofaciens.

4.2 Regulation by phosphate

Producers of TCs are cultivated on media with phosphate concentrations suboptimal for growth. Exhaustion of phosphate from the medium
serves as a signal for S. aureofaciens to commence the synthesis of
ESM synthesizing TCs (31). A marker for measuring the amount of enzymes cf the tetracycline synthesizing complex may be the amount of ATC
oxygenase; production of TCs is essentially proportional to its activity (41). As the amount of TC dehydrogenase throughout the cultivation

followed the curve of amount of TC oxygenase it may be assumed that
the amount of the latter enzyme determines the activity of the whole
complex (37). Higher concentrations of phosphate in the medium at the
beginning of cultivation repress the synthesis of ATC oxygenase while
addition of phosphate in the production phase has no effect on the
synthesis of the enzyme and on TCs production (42,31).

4.2 Regulation by sugars

The biosynthesis of CTC and TC is subject to catabolite repression (32). The mechanism of action of glucose, fructose and sucrose
on the biosynthesis of TCs in S. aureofaciens was studied by Erban
et al. (33) who found a repression of synthesis of ATC oxygenase in
the presence of glucose. In industrial cultivations the amount of
sucrose must not drop below a certain concentration. Even a short-
-term exhaustion of the sugar causes an irreversible cessation of
biosynthesis of TCs.

5 Mathematical model

The way in which the biosynthesis of TCs in S. aureofaciens is
affected by sugars and phosphate ions has been described a mathematical
model (34,35). Experimental data were evaluated by means of a set of
programmes BIOKIN (36). The initial phase included the setup of a
verbal model encompassing the consumption of substrate, biomass growth,
the amount of ESM (ATC oxygenase), forming TC and its negative feedback effect on the transport of the sugar into the cell and synthesis
of ATC oxygenase. The model included also the effect of benzylthiocyanate (BT) on the biosynthesis of TCs.

The mathematical model pointed to several important data and
confirmed the validity of experimental data in wider context. It
demonstrated the dependence of expression of genes encoding the ESM
on the level of phosphates in the medium and repression of ESM by the
product. Characteristics of the course of sugar consumption showed
that sugars are transported into the cells by both passive and active
transport mechanisms. In passive transport the rate obeys a first-

-order kinetics relative to the concentration of the substrate and
process is inhibited by high concentrations of TC. Active transport
also depends on substrate concentration. The relationship between the
rate of consumption of glucose, fructose and sucrose and the amount
of the sugars in the medium is shown in Fig.2. Whereas the passive
transport was not affected by the type of the sugar, the active transport was affected in both wild and production strain.

The rate of growth was proportional to the rate of sugar consumption. Production of TC in the given range was then inversely proportional to the consumption of sugars and was characteristic for each
strain.

The kinetics of production of TCs and ATC oxygenase has an analogous character for all three sugars. The lowest kinetic values were
found for glucose; the rate of degradation of ATC oxygenase was also
the lowest with this sugar. The model showed that the rate of degradation of ATC oxygenase was 5-8-fold higher in the wild strain than in
the production one, with all sugars tested.

6 Effect of benzylthiocyanate

The pronounced increase in the production of CTC and TC which
takes place in the presence of BT in the culture medium of S. aureofaciens, poses the question of what is the mechanism of action of this
low molecular compound. BT has so far been observed to affect the rate
of sugar consumption (19), with a concomitant inhibition of the growth
of the culture (33). The amount of glucose 6-P-dehydrogenase was also
markedly lowered in a mycelium growing in the presence of BT but the
activity of the enzyme in vitro was not affected by the agent (7).

The most important effect with regard to production of TCs is
on the amount of ATC oxygenase in the mycelium. The level of this
enzyme in the presence of BT conspicuously increased and the production of TCs was enhanced in proportion (1). However, BT was practically
without effect when added in the production phase. The effectivity of
BT towards the wild strain was many times higher than on the product-

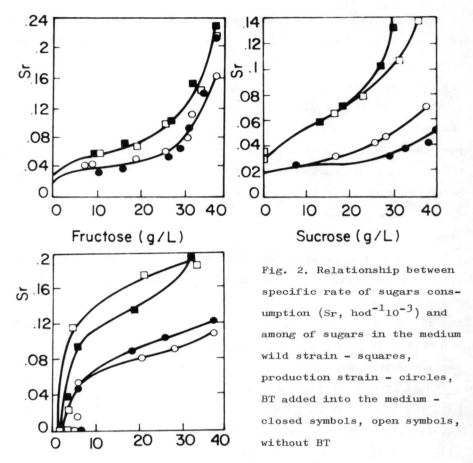

Fig. 2. Relationship between specific rate of sugars consumption (Sr, hod^{-1}10^{-3}) and among of sugars in the medium wild strain - squares, production strain - circles, BT added into the medium - closed symbols, open symbols, without BT

ion strain.

The increased synthesis of ATC oxygenase commenced 2 h after the addition of BT during the synthesis of the enzyme, Fig.3. The agent eliminated for the most part the effect of higher concentrations of phosphate but had no effect on protein synthesis.

The site of effect of BT on the biosynthesis of TCs is probably the plasma membrane. This can be inferred from the way in which it affects the localization of the last two enzymes of TCs synthesis. Apart from an overall increase in the level of these enzymes their localization was clearly shifted from membranes to the cytoplasm and

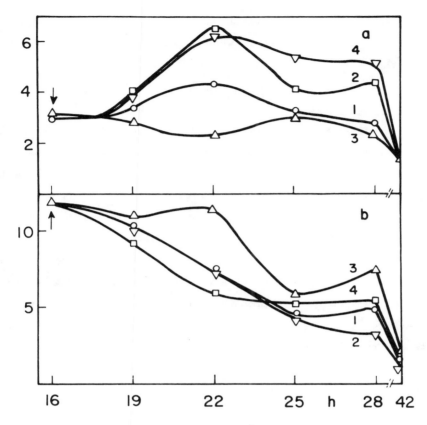

Fig. 3. Effect of phosphate (1 μmol ml^{-1} medium) and benzylthiocyanate (2 μmol ml^{-1} medium) on the activity of ATC oxygenase and proteosynthesis: a, activity of ATC oxygenase (pkat mg^{-1} protein); b, activity of proteosynthesis (dpm x 10^{-4} mg^{-1} dry wt); 1, control; 2, benzylthiocyanate added at 16 h; 3, phosphate added at 16 g; 4, benzylthiocyanate and phosphate added at 16 h. Arrows indicate the time of addition of phosphate or benzylthiocyanate.

periplasm (37) (cf. Tables 3 and 4 in Běhal: Enzymes of secondary metabolism, this volume).

The appearance of the S. aureofaciens culture growing on the solid medium was also affected by BT. In the presence of the agent the pigmentation of both the medium and the surface of the culture

was changed. The amount of spores was lower, the spores appared as
a later stage and were thicker: whereas in the control the length/
width ratio of the spores was 1.64, in a culture growing on a medium
with BT it was 1.26 (38).

7 Continuous cultivation

The conditions for a continuous cultivation of S. aureofaciens
in a two-stage fermentation equipment were described by Sikyta et
al. (39). At a dilution rate $D = 0,092$ h^{-1} they reached a constant
rate of CTC biosynthesis while at dilution rate $D = 0.049$ h^{-1} the
content of CTC during the first 30 h of cultivation was more than
twice as high but dropped sharply at later stages. The drop in CTC
level was stopped by lowering the level of phosphate in the medium
feed to a minimum. The effect of growth rate and different nutrient
limitation on specific CTC production rate was investigated in a
single-stage chemostat culture (40). Under conditions of phosphate
limitation the rate of OTC formation increased up to the dilution
rate $D = 0.02$ h^{-1}, then remained constant up to the value of $D = 0.03$
h^{-1} and then dropped sharply. The cause of this drop was the accumulation of rapidly growing mutants which prevented the attainment of an
actual steady state. Studies dealing with the continuous cultivation
of TCs lack the data on the amount of ESM and the activity of primary
metabolism. Without these data it is very difficult to assess the
physiological state of the culture and the role of dilution rate in
TCs production. Change in dilution rate alters a number of factors
affecting the physiology of the culture. The physiological state
characteritic for production of SM is then attained at a certain
dilution rate which in turn depends on the history of the culture.

8 Conclusion

In conclusion we may say that tetracyclines belong to models in
which the regulation of biosynthesis is relatively well understood.
Even so, further knowledge is necessary for their production to be
regulated and governed according to our requirements.

9 References

(1) V.Běhal, Overproduction of Microbial Products, Academic Press, London, 1982.

(2) V.Běhal, Z.Vaněk, Z.Hošťálek, A.Ramadan, Folia Microbiol. 24 (1979) 211.

(3) J.Šimúth, J.Hudec, H.T.Chan, O.Dányi, J.Zelinka, J.Antibiot. 32 (1979) 53.

(4) K.Mikulík, Z.Vaněk, Regulation of Secondary Product and Plant hormone metabolism, Pergamon Press, Oxford, 1979.

(5) V.Běhal, Z.Vaněk, Folia Microbiol. 15 (1970) 354.

(6) V.Jechová, Z.Hošťálek, Z.Vaněk, Folia Microbiol. 14 (1969) 128.

(7) J.Novotná, PhD thesis, Inst. of Microbiology, Prague 1981.

(8) Z.Hošťálek, M.Tintěrová, V.Jechová, M.Blumauerová, J.Suchý, Z.Vaněk, Biotechnol.Bioeng. 11 (1969) 539.

(9) M.Podojil, M.Blumauerová, K.Čulík, Z.Vaněk, Marcel Dekker, New York, 1984.

(10) I.S.Kulayev, Biochemistry of Inorganic Polyphosphates, John Willey and Sons, Chickester, 1979.

(11) E.Čurdová, V.Jechová, Z.Hošťálek, Symposium of Socialist Countries in Biotechnology, Bratislava, 1983.

(12) N.Madry, R.Sprinkmeyer, H.Pape, Eur.J.Appl.Microbiol.Biotechnol. 7 (1979) 365.

(13) Z.Janglová, J.Suchý, Z.Vaněk, Folia Microbiol. 14 (1969) 208.

(14) E.Čurdová, A.Křemen, Z.Vaněk, Folia Microbiol. 21,(1976) 481.

(15) V.Jechová, E.Čurdová, Z.Hošťálek, Folia Microbiol. 27,(1982) 153.

(16) E.Čurdová, V.Jechová, Z.Hošťálek, Folia Microbiol. 27 (1982) 159.

(17) Z.Hošťálek, V.Jechová, E.Čurdová, J.Voříšek, Actinomycetes, G.Fischer, Verlag, Stuttgart, 1981.

(18) J.Voříšek, E.Čurdová, V.Jechová, B.Lenc, Z.Hošťálek, Current Microbiology 8 (1983) 31.

(19) Z.Hošťálek, Folia Microbiol. 9 (1964) 96.

(20) V.Běhal, V.Jechová, Z.Vaněk, Z.Hošťálek, Phytochemistry, 16 (1977)

347.

(21) E.R.Catlin, C.A.Hassall, D.R.Parry, J.Chem.Soc. (1969) 1963.

(22) V.Běhal, M.Podojil, Z.Hošťálek, Z.Vaněk, F.Lynen, Folia Microbiol.
19 (1974) 146.

(23) M.Podojil, Z.Vaněk, V.Běhal, M.Blumauerová, Folia Microbiol. 18
((1973) 415.

(24) F.Lynen, M.Toda, Angen.Chem. 73 (1961) 513.

(25) P.Dimroth, H.Walker, F.Lynen, Eur.J.Biochem. 13 (1970) 98.

(26) J.R.D.McCormick, Academia, Prague, 1965.

(27) Z.Hošťálek, M.Blumauerová, Z.Vaněk, Academic Press, New York,
1979.

(28) V.Běhal, M.Bučko, Z.Hošťálek, Addison-Westley Pub.Comp. London,
1983.

(29) P.A.Miller, J.H.Hash, Meth.Enzymol. 43 (1975) 603.

(30) P.A.Miller, J.H.Hash, Meth.Enzymol. 43 (1975) 606.

(31) V.Běhal, J.Prušáková-Grégrová, Z.Hošťálek, Folia Microbiol. 27
(1982) 102.

(32) Z.Hošťálek, Folia Microbiol. 25 (1980) 445.

(33) V.Erban, J.Novotná, V.Běhal, Z.Hošťálek, Folia Microbiol. 28
(1983) 262.

(34) J.Votruba, V.Běhal, Appl.Microbiol.Biotechnol. 19,(1984) 153.

(35) V.Erban, PhD thesis, Inst. of Microbiology, Prague, 1984.

(36) J.Votruba, Acta Biotechnol. 2 (1982) 119.

(37) V.Erban, V.Běhal, L.Trilisenko, Z.Hošťálek, Symp.Physiology of
Microbial Growth and Differentiation Reinhardsbrunn (GDR), May,
1984.

(38) J.Novotná, V.Erban, V.Pokorný, Z.Hošťálek, Symp.Genetics and
Differentiation of Actinomycetes, Weimar, GRD, 1983.

(39) B.Sikyta, J.Slezák, M.Herold, Symp.Continuous Cultiv. of Microorg.
Prague, 1962.

(40) M.D.Rhodes, Biotechnol.Bioeng. 26 (1984) 382.

(41) V.Běhal, Z.Hošťálek, Z.Vaněk, Biotechnol.Lett. 1 (1979) 177.

(42) J.R.D. McCormick, G.O.Morton, J.Am.Chem.Soc. <u>104</u> (1982) 4014.

(43) P.A.Miller, J.H.Hash, M.Linchs, N.Bohonos, Biochem.Biophys.Res. Commun. <u>18</u> (1965) 325.

Enzymes of Secondary Metabolism: Regulation of Their Expression and Activity

Vladislav Běhal

Czechoslovak Academy of Sciences, Institute of Microbiology, Vídeňská 1083, 142 20 Prague 4, Czechoslovakia

Summary

Enzymes that participate directly in the biosynthesis of the molecule of a secondary metabolite (SM) are termed enzymes of secondary metabolism (ESM). They are usually organized in enzyme complexes. The amount of ESM in the cell is often a decisive factor in production of SM. The synthesis of ESM commences after exhaustion of rapidly utilizable sources of carbon, nitrogen and phosphorus. Cessation of biosynthesis of ESM is in some cases caused by the product of the biosynthesis itself.

1. Introduction

The term enzymes of secondary metabolism (ESM) denotes enzymes that participate directly in joining building units into more complex structures and transforming these structures to final products. They do not include enzymes synthesizing the basic building units of secondary metabolites (SM). A number of ESM have been found to be combined in vivo in complexes or multienzyme systems. The joining of enzymes into complexes that carry out multistage synthesis of metabolites without the appropriate intermediates being dissociated from the complex offers considerable advantages with regard to the rate of synthesis. The enzyme reaction may attain maximum rate at a complete saturation of the active centres of the enzyme by substrate. Intermediates that leave the enzyme and migrate, e.g., to the cytoplasm, have to approach the active centre by diffusion which implies a slow-

ing down of the reaction. We may hardly assume that all intermediates
in the cell will attain such concentration that the reaction rate will
become independent of their concentration. The statement that intermediates do not leave the enzyme complex naturally cannot be taken
absolutely. For instance, intermediates in the biosynthesis of patulin,
beginning with 6-methylsalicylic acid, are excreted into the fermentation medium.

Some of these complexes have been relatively thoroughly examined
as to their composition and organization of subunits or enzymes
catalyzing individual reaction steps in the biosynthesis. These
include in particular polypeptide synthetases (1); 6-methylsalicylic
acid synthetase along with fatty acid synthetases have been thoroughly
studied by the group of Lynen. Fatty acid synthetase can to a certain
extent be also considered an ESM.

2. Genetic regulation

Structural genes encoding ESM have in most cases been found on
chromosomes, some regulatory genes being found on extrachromosomal
particels. Plasmids have often been found to carry genes determining
the degree of resistance against the producer´s own product, and
they apparently also carry other genes related to the production of
ESM, which, however, have not been so frequently searched for.

The amount of an enzyme which can be synthesized by a given strain
is probably genetically governed. In Streptomyces aureofaciens, mutants
differing in tetracycline production differ also in the amount of
synthesized anhydrotetracycline oxygenase (ATC oxygenase), the penultimate enzyme of the pathway synthesizing chlortetracycline (CTC),
tetracycline (TC) and oxytetracycline (OTC). The amount of this enzyme
in the cells corresponds essentially to the magnitude of tetracycline
production (2). Since the amount of the last enzyme of tetracycline
dehydrogenase (TC-dehydrogenase) is identical with the amount of ATC-
-oxygenase throughout the cultivation (3), the amount of ATC oxygenase
can be taken as a marker determining the amount of TC synthetase
(CTC synthetase), fig.1.

It is not yet clear what part in the increased synthesis of
ESM during SM overproduction is played by increased number of genes
encoding them and what part is due to increased enzyme synthesis.
The studies of regulation of ESM synthesis are performed on strains
with known genetic equipment. In order to achieve the synthesis of
the highest possible amount of ESM it is necessary to adjust the
external medium and cultivation conditions accordingly. The amount
of ESM in the cell is one of the crucial factors in the production of
SM. In many cases a direct proportionality can be found between the

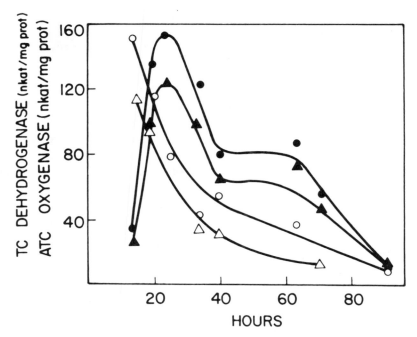

Fig.1 Activity of ATC oxygenase (circles) and TC dehydrogenase
        (triangles) in wild strain (open symbols) and production
        strain (closed symbols)

amount of ESM and the of metabolite production.

3. Onset of synthesis

During a batch fermentation the ESM are usually synthesized with
the highest intensity during the transition from the phase of intens-
ive growth to the stationary phase. In this phase the intensity of
protein synthesis declines. This state of decrease of growth of dry
matter and of protein synthesis is artificially induced by limiting
the nutrition of the microorganism by basic nutrients.

In principle we may say that synthesis of ESM does not occur if
the medium contains rapidly utilizable sources of carbon, nitrogen and
phosphorus. Among carbon sources we use mostly glucose which causes
catabolite repression, among nitrogen sources ammonium salts, nitra-
tes, and, for some metabolites, certain amino acids. Among phosphorus
compounds this holds for phosphate ions which are not bound to organic
compounds. A sufficient supply of carbon or nitrogen sources necessary
for biosynthesis of SM is ensured by slowly utilizable substances
such as lactose, starch or fatty acids. The same effect as with slowly
utilizable carbon sources may be achieved by dosage of glucose during

the cultivation which keeps low glucose level in the medium.

Slowly utilizable nitrogen sources are mostly proteins which the·
microorganisms producing SM are capable of degrading by exoproteina-
ses (4).

3.1   Phosphate limitation

A somewhat more complex situation is found with regard to phosphate limitation. As shown for biosynthesis of tetracyclines (2,5,6,7),
candicidin, tylosine and gramicidin S concentrations of phosphate
supraoptimal with respect to SM production inhibit the synthesis of
ESM. Hence the inhibitory effect of higher concentrations of phosphates on the production of antibiotics and other SM can be explained as
being due to this mechanism. Addition of phosphate into the medium of
a culture in which ESM have already been partially synthesized brings
about the cessation of their synthesis. This is followed by a sharp
drop in their activity, faster than would correspond to the dilution
by newly synthesized proteins (7,8,9). The ESM synthesis is restored
only after the level of phosphates in the medium has dropped to a
limiting concentration. Addition of phosphates to S. aureofaciens re-
stores protein synthesis (9) and apparently causes degradation or inactivation of ESM. The increase in protein synthesis has not been observed after addition of phosphates during candicidin biosynthesis
(10) obviously because in this case the protein synthesis does not
decrease before the onset of SM biosynthesis but proceeds intensively
even after that.

Phosphate added to a growing culture is exhausted from the medium
at a very high rate (11,12,7,8), higher that can be considered to correspond to its utilization in primary metabolism.. The excess phosphate
is probably polymerized in the cells to polyphosphates (13,14,15).
Polyphosphates have been found also in the S. aureofaciens glycocalyx
(16). The polymerized phosphate no longer inhibits the synthesis of
ESM.

The cause of the lower sensitivity to higher concentrations
of phosphate in mutants obtained by Martin et al. (17) in the candicidin producer S. griseus IMRU 3570, by Haenel et al. (18) in S. noursei
JA 38906 producing streptothricin and by Novotná et al. (19) in
S. aureofaciens is unclear. The mutants of S. griseus and S. noursei
have been found to differ from permeability mutants. The S.aureofa-
ciens mutant was found to exhibit no decrease in the amount of ATC-
-oxygenase at higher phosphate concentrations, or, the decrease was
much less than that found in the parent strain(Tab.1 and 2). Some of
the mutants contained ATC-oxygenase; the amount of the enzyme did not

Table 1   Phosphate tolerant mutants of productive strain 8425

Strain code	Phosphate added (mmol/L)	CTC production (g/L)	CTC %	ATC oxygenase pkat/mg prot. Hours of cultivation	
				24	42
Control	0	1000		111	98
(8425)	1	741	74	52	69
	5	161	16	30	33
70/132	0	947		122	97
	1	1059	111	85	89
	5	231	24	65	31
70/93	0	675		77	101
	1	1045	155	88	51
30/19	0	95		89	34
	5	157	166	126	47

decrease at higher phosphate concentrations but the production of CTC was 10-fold lower than in the parent strain.

Table 2   Phosphate tolerant mutants of low-productive strain Bg

Strain	Phosphate added (mmol/L)	CTC production (g/L)	CTC %	ATC oxgenase pkat/mg prot. Hours of cultivation	
				24	42
Control	0	165		7.2	8.1
(Bg)	5	29	17.4	1.4	1.8
S/60/109	0	90		15.9	10.5
	5	92	103	12.6	5.6
S/40/44	0	212		36.4	22.1
	5	71	33.5	12,3	23.8
Pl 60/86	0	109		30.1	18.5
	5	89	81.6	23.4	23

3.2 Transition from the growth phase to the production phase

The commencement of ESM synthesis can also be taken as a transition from the growth phase to the production phase, or a transition from the phase characterized by the predominance of primary metabolism to the phase of secondary metabolism. The cell dry weight, especially in filamentous microorganisms, is not always suitable criterion for judging whether the culture still grows or whether its growth stagnates. A sharp drop in intensity of protein synthesis can be observed much earlier than the cessation of increase in dry weight (20,8,9).

In cases when no marked decrease in the dry weight increment takes place in the production phase, e.g. in the biosynthesis of candicidin, no conspicuous decrease in protein synthesis occur (21). Production of SM during the growth phase can be induced by using medium poor in nutrients, such as has been used in chloramphenicol biosynthesis. However, the production of chloramphenicol on poor media is low. On rich media, when high yields are attained, the synthesis of chloramphenicol takes place only towards the end of the growth phase. This quantitative aspect should not be dismissed in our considerations; there is a great difference between the physiology of wild or only slightly improved strains producing SM on the one hand, and the physiology of high-production strains under conditions of overproduction.

The drop in the rate of protein synthesis is preceded by a drop in the rate of RNA and DNA biosynthesis (20,21,53,22).

The decrease in the rate of protein synthesis corresponds in time also to a drop in the specific activities of enzymes of primary metabolism (23,24,25) and deceleration of fatty acid biosynthesis (30).

3.3 Production and the cellular level of ATP

The decrease in the activity of primary metabolism is associated with a drop in the cellular level of ATP. In most of cases under study (26,27,28,29) the biosynthesis of SM is preceded by a sharp drop in the level of ATP; ATP is thus considered as an effector causing the transition from primary to secondary metabolism. Even though this role" is not excluded in some cases, the intracellular content of ATP should rather be taken as a marker of activity of primary metabolism. Even in metabolites whose synthesis is accompanied by synthesis of ESM during the culture growth, such as tylosin, the exhaustion of rapidly utilizable nutrient sources is accompanied by a drop in the level of ATP which is in turn followed by synthesis of ESM or SM. During biosynthesis of tylosin (Fig.2) the depletion of glucose is followed by

a decline in ATP level to a certain limit, which coincides with
the synthesis of enzymes of tylosin synthetase. Addition of glucose
causes first a drop in ATP level relative to control, probably owing
to ATP utilization in glucose phosphorylation. Even in this period,

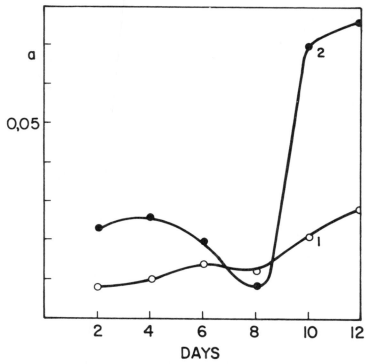

Fig.2 Specific activity of chorismatmutase of Oudemansiella mucida
       cultivated in the medium with glucose (open symbols) and
       glucose with tryptophan (closed symbols)

when the ATP level is lowered, the biosynthesis of tylosin stagnates.
After several hours the level of ATP rises transiently and tylosin
synthesis starts again until the ATP level drops again, apparently due
to exhaustion of added glucose (29).

    A similar lack of specificity is found in the action of substan-
ces such as ppG$_{pp}$ and cAMP.

3.4 The signal molecules

    ESM synthesis can also be induced by compounds such as tryptophan
which increases the amount of chorismate mutase (Fig.3) and phenylala-
nine-ammonia lyase in the mucidin producer, the basidiomycete
Oudemansiella mucida (31,32). Phenylalanine transaminase, which does
not take part in mucidin synthesis, is not affected by tryptophan.

Tryptophan also induces alkaloid synthesis (33). The fact that tryptophan is effective only when added in the growth phase indicates that the compound also induces the synthesis of ESM. Under the same

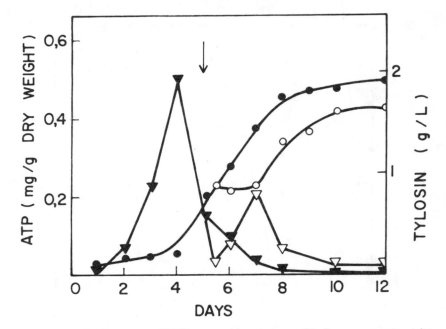

Fig.3 Effect of glucose addition on the intracellular concentration
       of ATP (triangles) and tylosin production (circles).
       Closed symbols-control, open symbols - glucose added.
       (Redrew from Vu-Trong et al., Antimicrob.Agents and Chemother.
       17 (1980) p.519.

conditions methionine stimulates the biosynthesis of cephalosporin C (34).

4. Cessation of synthesis

    The magnitude of metabolite production is crucially affected by the type of regulation of cessation of ESM biosynthesis. We should distinguish in this respect between the cultivation of high-production or low-production or wild strains. In high-production strains we must assume that a number of factors inhibiting the biosynthesis of ESM, and other factors inhibiting the synthesis of SM are eliminated by mutation treatments of the strain genome.

    One of the important inhibitors of ESM biosynthesis is the meta-bolite produced by the enzymes. This has been unequivocally proved with chloramphenicol which inhibits the synthesis of arylamine synthetase (35).

4.1 Resistance towards the product

Inhibition of its own biosynthesis by an antibiotic is a frequently encountered phenomenon. However, high-production mutants possess at
least a partial resistance towards the product. Several types of resistance have been described. Increased resistance may result, e.g.,
from a modification of the producer´s chromosomes, synthesis of proteins binding the product, or other mechanisms of protection of ribosomes, altered permeability of the plasma membrane, etc. In principle,
resistance to higher concentrations of the products was observed in
strains with higher production.

Inhibition of ESM synthesis can be prevented by localizing the
SM synthesis outside the plasma membrane or by separating this synthesis from ribosomes by intracellular membranes.

4.2 ESM in industrial fermentations

Cessation of ESM biosynthesis occurs in most cases towards the
end of the growth phase. In the production phase their amount in the
culture decreases, sometimes at a considerable rate. If the same holds
in industrial fermentation is difficult to say since the available literature data refer to laboratory experiments in which relatively low
productions were achieved even in putative production strains. During
an industrial cultivation of S. aureofaciens (Fig.4) we recorded
a drop in ATC-oxygenase from a maximum around the 50th hour to 45 %
in the 80th hour. Further decrease was gradual (36).

During laboratory fermentations of a production strain of
S.aureofaciens the biosynthesis of ATC oxygenase begins on exhaustion
of inorganic phosphate from the medium and ceases due to synthesized
tetracyclines. Under normal conditions the biosynthesis of tetracyclines proceeds even though a partial decrease of the amount of ESM
takes place. Restoration of synthesis of the enzymes apparently does
not take place. A different situation may be found in other strains
resistant to CTC and TC.

The blocking of ESM synthesis by OTC apparently does not occur
in S. rimosus. Bosnjak (37) reported on the results of a repeated
fed batch cultivation. Both the culture growth and the level
of ESM increased even at high concentrations of OTC in the fermentation medium. In S.aureofaciens this type of production was unsuccessful.

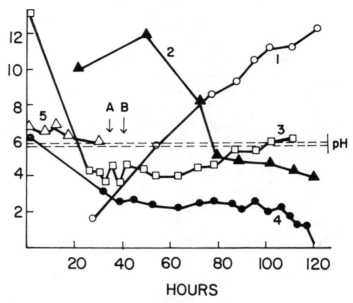

Fig.4   Parameters of an industrial fermentation of S.aureofaciens:
1=CTC production (mg.mL^{-1}); 2=ATC oxygenase (pkat.mg^{-1} protein
x 2); 3=NH$_3$-nitrogen (mg.mL^{-1} x 0.1); 4=sucrose (mg.mL^{-1} x 10);
5=pH. Aqueous ammonia was added after 27 h to maintain the pH
at 5.7-5.9; sucrose was added from 33 h to 115 h to hold the
concentration at 22-25 mg.mL^{-1}. Ammonium sulfate supplements
were added at points A and B.

5. Mathematical modelling

We may thus assume that in a number of SM the magnitude of production will be determined in a relatively short period in which ESM
are synthesized. The search for optimum regime of culture fermentation, including all the factors affecting the expression of genes
encoding ESM, should be performed with the aid of a computer. This
requires a mathematical model which would simulate the behaviour of
the culture and its response to change in conditions. Data obtained
in the study of tetracycline biosynthesis in S. aureofaciens served
us for setting up a mathematical model simulating the behaviour of
the culture (38) which is being further improved (39). The model will
require further elaboration and verification under cultivation conditions identical with those of industrial fermentations. The model
pointed to analogous relationships pertaining to the biosynthesis of
ergot alkaloids (40) and tylosine; the relevant data were obtained
both from industrial fermentatiorns and from the literature.

The behaviour of SM producers could thus be probably simulated by a few models. Mathematical models can also be used to verify certain rules governing both the growth of a microbial culture and the production of SM.

6. Regulation of activity

The study of regulation of activities of ESM is very difficult. The isolation of an enzyme and measurement of the effect of a substance on its activity poses no problems. However, it is problematic whether the enzyme behaves identically when in complex with other enzymes and in vivo. In principle we may say that ESM are regulated by the same mechanisms as enzymes of primary metabolism. The biosynthesis of an antibiotic was in many cases found to be inhibited by the producer´s own antibiotic (41,42). Often it is difficult to decide if the inhibition concerns the synthesis of enzymes participating in the biosynthesis of the metabolite or if it concerns their activity. When the inhibition of production occurs after addition of the antibiotic in the growth phase while a much lower inhibition is found in the production phase a repression of ESM may be assumed to take place.

Regulation of the last enzyme of streptomycin biosynthesis, streptomycin-6P-phosphohydrolase, by phosphate was observed by Miller and Walker (43). A higher concentration of phosphate inhibited the splitting of phosphate from streptomycin-6-phosphate. Inhibition of activity of candicidin synthase by phosphate was also presumed by Martin et al. (11).

6.1 Regulation by the products and metal ions

We studied the effect of CTC, TC, OTC and some metal ions on ATC-oxygenase in vitro (44). The activity of the enzyme decreased with increasing concentration of tetracyclines. We may assume that under in vivo conditions the synthesized tetracyclines are transported away from the site of formation. As to the effect of Ca and Mg ions, a slight stimulation was observed at increasing concentration, to be replaced by a sharp drop in activity. The inhibitory effect of tetracyclines and Ca or Mg ions are additive. In the presence of other metal ions the activity of ATC-oxygenase also attains a maximum at a certain concentration and then decreases rapidly. Interestingly, the dependence of the concentration at which the maximum stimulation of activity takes place on the atomic number is linear.

The effect of metal ions on bacitracin-synthetase was studied by Froyshov et al. (45). They assumed that the activity of the enzymes was affected by substrate-metal ion complexes and product-

-metabolite complexes. Enzymes of Streptomyces sp. 3022, a chloramphenicol producer, were also found to be inhibited by metal ions. Magnesium, potassium and sodium ions stimulated the activity of anthranilic acid synthetase as well as arylamine synthetase while Ca^{2+}, Co^{2+},
Mn^{2+} and Zn^{2+} inhibited the activity, especially of the latter enzyme. Since SM producers require the presence of some metal ions in the
medium, we may assume that some ESM need for their function metal ions
and may be regulated by them.

The activity of ESM may be regulated by pH. The pH optima of the
last two enzymes of TC biosynthesis differ (Fig.5), whereas the pH
optimum of ATC oxygenase is 7.4 (2) the optimum of TC dehydrogenase

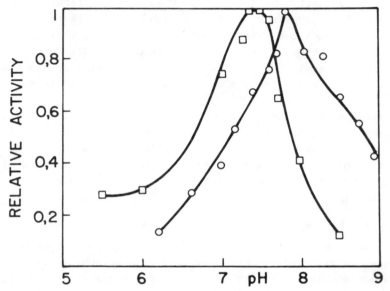

Fig.5   Relative activity of ATC oxygenase (squares) and TC dehydrogenase (circles) at different pH

is 7.8 (3).

7. Localization in the cell

ESM were found in different cellular fractions. The localization
of the ESM complex in the cell is important for production of SM. Production of gramicidin S and bacitracin (46) does not take place if the
appropriate synthetases are localized in the cytoplasm and is practically proportional to the amount of synthetases found at later stages
on pellets. Individual enzymes of the complexes, or probably complex

subunits or the whole complex are obviously synthesized in the cytoplasm and then transported to the part of the cell in which the
actual synthesis of SM takes place. We may assume that the whole enzyme complex is not synthesized at once since, for instance, the genes
coding for OTC have been found on two opposite loci of the chromosome (47).

7.1 Enzymes producing the building units

Localization of ESM is connected with the localization of enzymes of primary metabolism which produce the building units of SM.
In my opinion the notion of a pool of intermediates in the cell which
are freely accessible for various syntheses is not entirely correct.
More probable is the notion that enzymes producing the direct precursors of SM synthesis which are polymerized to form the SM skeleton
are localized in the close vicinity of ESM or are even their integral
part, albeit loosely bound.

The notion is supported by the behaviour of enzymes participating in the biosynthesis of propionate units. Methylmalonyl-CoA mutase
during the biosynthesis of eryhtromycin (48) and propionyl-CoA carboxylase and methylmalonyl-CoA carboxytransferase in the biosynthesis of
tylosine (29,49,50) follow the curve of biosynthesis of SM and the
curve of macrocin 3⁻-O-methyltransferase which is the ultimate enzyme
of tylosine biosynthesis. At any rate the decarboxylation of methylmalonyl-CoA to active propionyl-CoA and, analogously, decarboxylation
of malonyl-CoA to active acetyl-CoA has to proceed in the close vicinity of the polymerizing enzyme complex. If this is so, then, for
instance, the malonyl-CoA for the tricarboxylic acid cycle is synthesized by enzymes localized in the cell at a different place than the
malonyl-CoA for tetracycline biosynthesis.

7.2 Enzymes of tetracycline synthetase

Localization of ESM in S. aureofaciens was the subject of
Erban´s PhD thesis (39). The study of localization of ESM in the
cell has to be carried out by gentle methods; fine cell structures
on which the enzymes are localized may be disrupted or the enzymes
may be washed away by extraction buffers. The most suitable method
seems to be the preparation of protoplasts and their disintegration
by osmotic shock.

To prepare from Streptomycetes protoplasts containing ESM presents a problem. The cultivation medium for Streptomycetes described
by Okanishi et al. (51), which can be used for preparing protoplasts,
is unsuitable since it contains glycine and phosphate and ESM are
not synthesized. A suitable medium in which the synthesis of enzymes

of the tetracycline synthetase complex takes place has been described by Erban et al. (52); it contains fructose as the source
of carbon. As shown in Tables 3 and 4 both ATC-oxygenase and TC-
-dehydrogenase were localized in various cell fractions in dependence

Table 3   Localisation of ATC-oxygenase in cell fractions

Cell structure	ATC oxygenase (pkat/mg prot.)			
	Production strain		Wild strain	
	+ BT	– BT	+ BT	– BT
Cell-free extract	52.2	30	15.5	2.24
Periplasm	79.7	3.7	2.6	0
Periplasmatic vesicles	18.8	10	4.8	4
Membranes	30.2	15	12.8	43.8
Cytoplasm	130	21.2	17.9	15.5

Table 4   Localisation of TC-dehydrogenase in cell fractions

Cell structure	TC-dehydrogenase (pkat/mg prot.)	
	Production strain	Wild strain
	+ BT	+ BT
Periplasm	21.3	20
Periplasmatic vesicles	5.8	5.8
Membranes	9.5	86
Cytoplasm	31	18

on the strain and on the presence of benzylthiocyanate, a stimulator
of production of CTC and TC (3,39). When the cells were disintegrated
on X-press the ATC-oxygenase was found solely in the soluble fraction (2).

     The tables indicate that at higher production rates, whether
attained by using a mutant strain or by adding benzylthiocyanate, ATC-
-oxygenase and TC-dehydrogenase is transferred from the membranes to
the cytoplasm and periplasm. The localization of TC-dehydrogenase in
the periplasm facilitates the transfer of the product out of the cell
and the lowering of its concentration at the cell periphery, which

reduces the interference of the product with the metabolic processes inside the cell.

8. Conclusion

In conclusion it may be said that the amount of ESM plays a decisive role in the determination of the magnitude of production of many SM. Even though the conditions under which the synthesis of ESM takes place are known in rough outline, further study is necessary to elucidate the mechanisms causing the derepression of genes encoding them. Another aspect requiring elucidation is the processes that take place in the cell when rapidly utilizable sources are replaced by slowly utilizable ones. The dosage of basic nutrients can presumably be optimized so that the most suitable expression of ESM takes place, both with regard to their amount and to the time of their formation. Attention should also be given to the stability of the ESM, especially under conditions of overproduction under industrial or other comparable conditions. Closely associated is also the problem of effect of product on the synthesis and activity of ESM.

The mere listing of the above problems indicates how inadequate is our knowledge of the ESM. Without learning the rules which govern the regulation of their synthesis and activity we cannot expect to be able to regulate the formation of secondary metabolites.

9. References

(1)   H.Kleinkauf and H.von Döhren, Biochemistry and Genetic Regulation of Commercially Important Antibiotics, Addison-Westley Publishing Company, London, 1983.

(2)   V.Běhal, Z.Hošťálek, Z.Vaněk, Biotechnol.Lett 1 (1979) 177.

(3)   V.Erban, V.Běhal, L.Trilisenko, Z.Hošťálek, Symp.Physiology of Microbial Growth and Differentiation, Reinhardsbrun (GDR), May, 1984.

(4)   M.Pokorny, L.Vitole, V.Turk, M.Renko, J.Žuvanic, Eur.J.Appl. Microbiol.Biotechnol., 8 (1979) 81.

(5)   N.Madry and H.Pape, Actinomycetes, G.Fischer, Sttutgart, 1981.

(6)   J.F.Martin, M.T.Alegre, J.A.Gil, G.Naharro, Advances in Biotechnology: Fermentation Products Pergamon Press, Toronto, 1981.

(7)   C.W.Chin, T.Bernhard, G.Dellweg, Peptide Antibiotics - Biosynthesis and Functions, Gruyter, Berlin, 1982.

(8)   V.Běhal, J.Prušáková-Grégrová, Z.Hošťálek, Folia Microbiol. 27 (1982) 102.

(9)   V.Běhal, Overproduction of Microbial Products, Academic Press, London, 1982.

(10) J.F.Martin, A.L.Demain, Biochem.Biophys.Res.Commun. 71 (1976) 1103.

(11) J.F.Martin, Adv.Biochem.Eng. 6 (1977) 105.

(12) A.L.Colombo, N.Crespiperellino, A.Grein, A.Minghetti, C.Spalla, Biotechnol.Lett. 3 (1981) 71.

(13) A.M.Umnov, A.G.Steislyk, N.S.Umnova, S.E.Mansurova, I.S.Kulayev, Microbiology 44 (1975) 414.

(14) I.S.Kulayev, A.N.Belozerskii, D.N.Ostrovskii, Biokhimiya 26 (1961) 188.

(15) I.S.Kulayev, V.M.Vagebov, A.B.Isiomenko, Dokl.Akad.Nauk 204 (1972) 734.

(16) J.Voříšek, E.Čurdová, V.Jechová, B.Lenc, Z.Hošťálek, Current Microbiol. 8 (1983) 31.

(17) J.F.Martin, G.N.Naharro, P.Liras, J.R.Villanueva, J.Antibiot. 32 (1979) 600.

(18) F.Haenel, U.Graefe, W.Fridrich, E.J.Bovman, Ztsch.allgem.Mikrobiol. 24 (1984) 239.

(19) J.Novotná, O.A.Kadir, M.Blumauerová, V.Běhal, Z.Hošťálek, Folia Microbiol. 29 (1984) 399.

(20) J.Šimúth, J.Hudec, H.T.Chan, O.Dányi, J.Zelinka, J.Antibiot. 32 (1979) 53.

(21) P.Liras, J.R.Villanueva, J.F.Martin, J.Gen.Microbiol. 102 (1977) 269.

(22) N.Madry and H.Pape, Arch.Mikrobiol. 131 (1982) 170.

(23) V.Běhal and Z.Vaněk, Folia Microbiol. 15 (1970) 354.

(24) V.Jechová, Z.Hošťálek, Z.Vaněk, Folia Microbiol. 14 (1969) 128.

(25) J.Novotná, PhD thesis, Inst.of Microbiol., Praha,1981.

(26) Z.Janglová, J.Suchý, Z.Vaněk, Folia Microbiol. 14 (1969) 208.

(27) E.Čurdová, A.Křemen, Z.Vaněk, Folia Microbiol. 21 (1976) 481.

(28) N.Madry, R.Sprinkmeyer, H.Pape, Europ.J.Appl.Microbiol.Biotechnol. 7 (1979) 365.

(29) K.Vu-Trong, S.Bhuwapathanapuns, P.P.Gray, Antimicrob.Agents and Chemother. (1980) 519.

(30) V.Běhal, J.Cudlín, Z.Vaněk, Folia Microbiol. 14 (1969) 117.

(31) Z.Zouchová, PhD thesis, Inst.of Microbiol., Praha, 1980.

(32) F.Nerud, Z.Zouchová, V.Musílek, Folia Microbiol. 29 (1984) 389.

(33) J.E.Robbers, L.W.Robertson, K.M.Hornemann, A.Jindra, H.G.Floss, J.Bacteriol. 112 (1972) 791.

(34) J.Nuesch, H.J.Treichler, M.Liersch, Genetics of Industrial Microorganisms, Academia, Prague, 1973.

(35) A.Jones, D.W.S.Westlake, Can.J.Microbiol. 20 (1974) 599.

(36) V.Běhal, M.Bučko, Z.Hošťálek, Biochemistry and Genetic Regulation of Commercially Important Antibiotics, Addison-Westley Publishing

Company, London 1983.

(37) Z.Bosnjak, Symp.Physiology of Microbial Growth and Differentiation, Reinhardsbrunn (GDR) May, 1984.

(38) J.Votruba and V.Běhal, Appl.Microbiol.Biotechnol.19 (1984) 153.

(39) V.Erban, PhD thesis, Inst.of Microbiol., Praha 1984.

(40) S.Pažoutová, J.Votruba, Z.Řeháček, Biotechnol.Bioeng. 23 (1981) 2837.

(41) S.W.Drew, A.L.Demain, Ann.Rev.Microbiol. 31 (1977) 342.

(42) J.F.Martin, A.L.Demain, Microbiol.Rev. 44 (1980) 230.

(43) A.L.Miller, J.B.Walker, J.Bacteriol. 104 (1970) 8.

(44) V.Běhal, J.Neužil, Z.Hošťálek, Biotechnol.Lett. 5 (1983) 537.

(45) O.Froyshov, A.Mathiesen, H.I.Haavik, J.Gen.Microbiol. 117 (1980) 163.

(46) O.Froyshov, FEBS Lett. 81 (1977) 315.

(47) P.M.Rhodes, N.Winskil, E.J.Friend, M.W.Warren, J.Gen.Microbiol. 124 (1981) 329.

(48) A.A.Hunaiti and P.E.Kolattukudy, Antimicrob.Agents Chemother. 25 (1984) 173.

(49) K.Vu-Trong and P.P.Gray, Biotechnol.Bioeng. 24 (1982) 1093.

(50) N.Madry, H.Pape, Arch.Mikrobiol. 131 (1982) 170.

(51) M.Okanishi, K.Suzuki, H.Umezawa, J.Gen.Microbiol. 80 (1974) 389.

(52) V.Erban, V.Běhal, Z.Hošťálek, Folia Microbiol. 29 (1984) 402.

(53) V.Běhal, Z.VAněk, Z.Hošťálek, A.Ramadan, Folia Microbiol. 24 (1979) 211.

Biosynthesis of Polyketide Antibiotics

Heinz G. Floss, Sheri P. Cole, Xian-Guo He, Brian A. M. Rudd, Janice Duncan, Isao Fujii, Ching-jer Chang and Paul J. Keller

The Ohio State University, Department of Chemistry, 140 West 18th Avenue, Columbus, Ohio 43210, U.S.A.

SUMMARY

The biosynthesis of several members of the benzoisochromane quinone class of antibiotics has been studied in Streptomyces species. Their polyketide biosynthetic origin was established by stable isotope labeling in conjunction with NMR spectroscopy. Mechanistic aspects of their biosynthesis were unravelled by multiple and stereospecific isotopic labeling experiments. Biosynthetic interrelationships were revealed by observing interconversions of various compounds and by chemical analysis of blocked mutants using a bioassay-guided fractionation to isolate biosynthetic intermediates. Transformants of S. violaceoruber, a granaticin producer, containing plasmids carrying genes from S. coelicolor coding for the biosynthesis of actinorhodin were analyzed and found to produce a new compound, dihydrogranatirhodin, exhibiting structural features of both parent compounds.

INTRODUCTION

Work in our laboratory over the past decade has dealt with the biosynthesis of a number of antibiotics of polyketide origin. These include chlorothricin (1), aplasmomycin (2) and boromycin (3), naphthomycin and ansatrienine (4) and, most

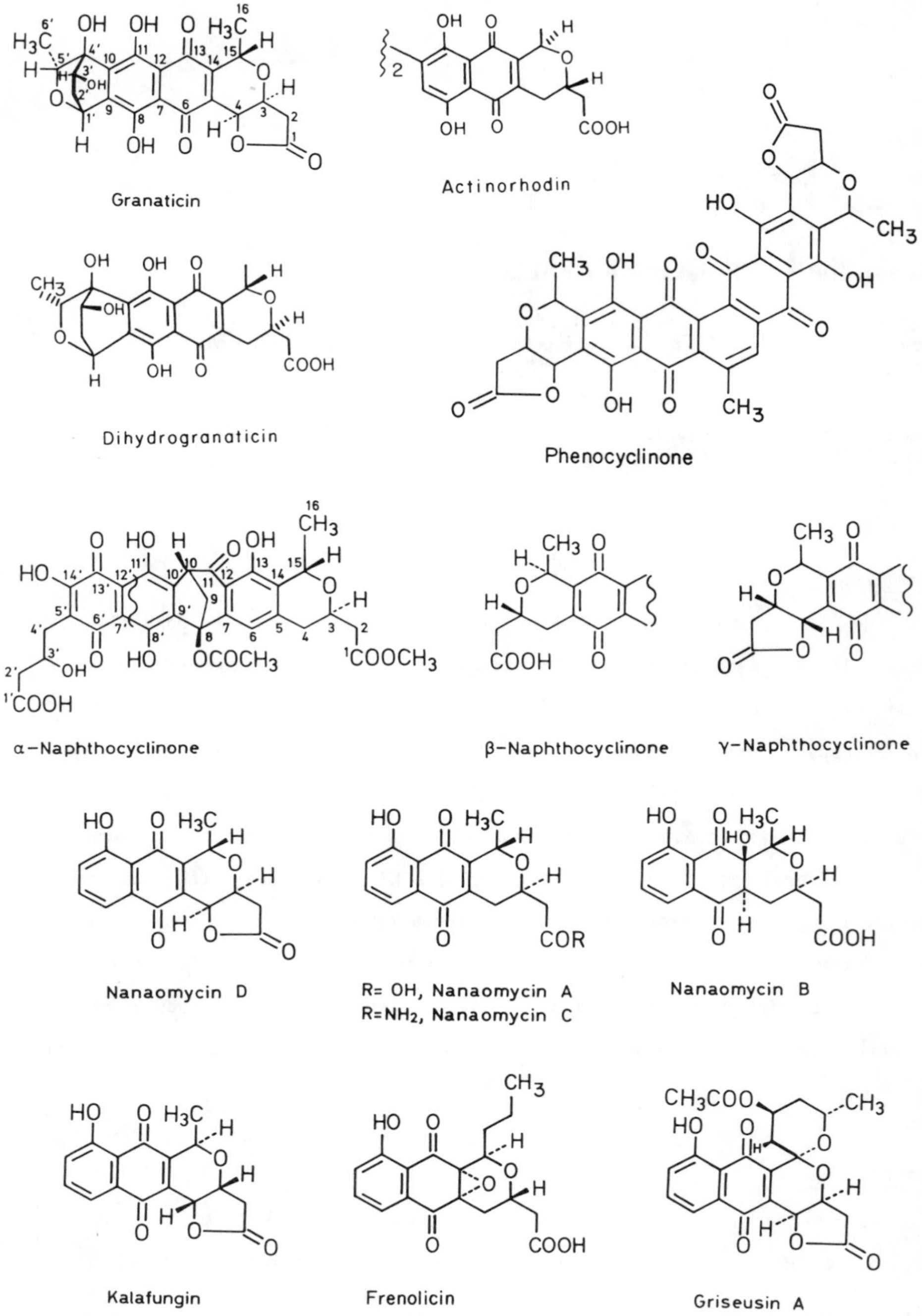

Fig. 1   Structures of benzoisochrome quinones

recently, asukamycin (5). In addition we have studied the formation of granaticin
(6), actinorhodin (7) and the naphthocyclinones (8,9), members of the class of
polyketides referred as to benzoisochromane quinones. This class also includes
kalafungin (10), the frenolicins (11,12), the nanaomycins (13-17), the griseusins
(18) and phenocyclinone (19). All these compounds are Streptomycete metabolites,
and they represent both the 15S and the enantiomeric 15R series. Actinorhodin,
the first member of this group (20-22) and the related γ-actinorhodin (23) were
isolated from S. coelicolor; they have little antibiotic activity, but their mode
of formation has been the subject of extensive genetic investigations (24-26).
α-Naphthocyclinone and several analogs were obtained from S. arenae (27,28); their
stereochemistry at C-8 and C-10 has recently been revised based on an X-ray
structure (29). Granaticin and other related compounds were isolated from S.
violaceoruber, but also from other species (30-35), and the structure is based on
chemical evidence and an X-ray analysis (36,37). Granaticin has modest antitumor
activity (T/C 166 in P-388) (33); it inhibits aminoacylation of leucyl-t-RNA in
bacteria (38) and maturation of ribosomal RNA in KB cells (39).

BIOSYNTHETIC ORIGIN

The polyketide origin of the benzoisochromane quinone skeleton was first
demonstrated for the nanaomycins by Ōmura and coworkers (13). Feeding of $[1-^{13}C]$-
acetate to S. rosa var. notoensis produced nanaomycin A, which upon ^{13}C-NMR
analysis displayed the typical alternating labeling pattern of an octaketide (Fig.
2). The same biosynthetic origin of the parent skeleton was demonstrated for
granaticin (6,40) and for actinorhodin (7). In the latter case, the biosynthetic
feeding experiment also established, in agreement with chemical evidence (22),
that the two monomeric units in actinorhodin are connected through carbon atoms 10

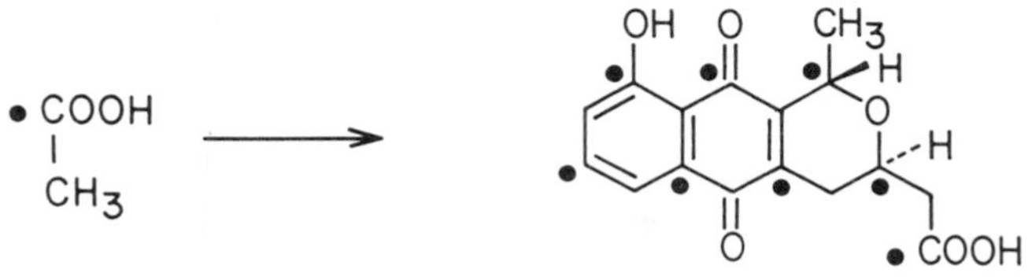

Fig. 2   Origin of nanaomycin A from $[1-^{13}C]$acetate

and 10' rather than 9 and 9' (41). In the naphthocyclinones all the carbon atoms, except the ester methyl group, are derived from either C-1 or C-2 of acetate (8). This includes the acetoxy group. The labeling pattern supports the proposal by Zeeck et al. (27) that the naphthocyclinones arise from two monomeric octaketide precursors. A rather peculiar result is the finding that [2-^{13}C]malonate, fed as the diethyl ester, labels all the polyketide carbons derived from C-2 of acetate, including the starter unit, but not the acetoxy group (8). Both the acetoxy group and the starter unit should come from acetyl-CoA; the labeling of the starter unit indicates rapid equilibration between acetyl-CoA and malonyl-CoA. One might argue that the actoxy group is added to the backbone at a late stage, when the labeled precursor has been used up. However, this does not account for the labeling of the acetoxy group in the acetate feeding experiments. An alternative, albeit entirely speculative, explanation would be that the starter unit is also malonyl-CoA, not acetyl-CoA, and that malonyl-CoA is not readily converted to acetyl-CoA. This would invoke a symmetrical, enzyme-bound intermediate, as shown in Fig. 3, which must selectively lose the carboxyl group of the starter unit.

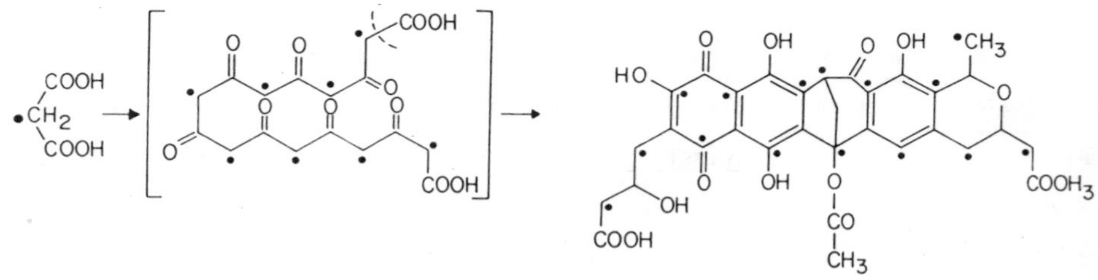

Fig. 3   Labeling of α-naphthocyclinone from [2-^{13}C]-malonate

The additional six carbon atoms found in granaticin represent a 2,6-dideoxy-hexose moiety derived from D-glucose. This was demonstrated in feeding experiments with [3,4-^{14}C]- and [6-^{14}C]glucose (6). Tracing of the fate of the individual hydrogen atoms of glucose in the conversion into the dideoxyhexose moiety of grana-ticin indicated (6) that the hydrogens at C-1 and C-2 are completely retained, whereas H-3 and H-5 are largely lost (less than 10% tritium retention). A large percentage of the tritium from positions 4 and 6 of glucose is washed out, but the remaining tritium incorporated into granaticin is located almost entirely in one or both of the C-methyl groups recovered by Kuhn-Roth oxidation to acetic acid, most likely at C-6', the methyl group of the dideoxyhexose moiety. The biosynthetic origin of granaticin is summarized in Fig. 4.

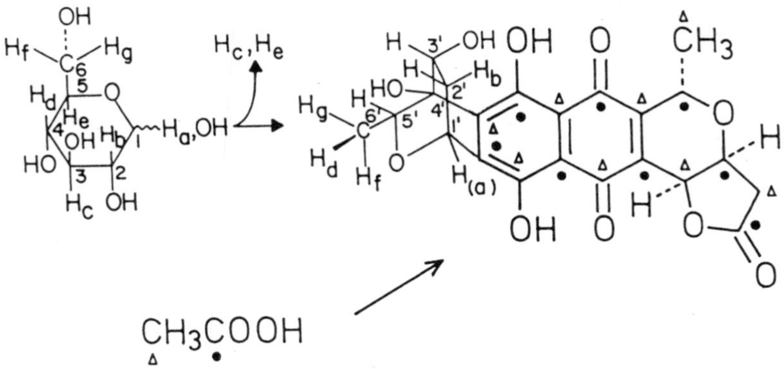

Fig. 4   Biosynthetic origin of granaticin

MECHANISTIC STUDIES

The above results on the fate of the glucose hydrogens in the biosynthesis of granaticin suggest the involvement of the TDP-glucose oxidoreductase reaction in the formation of the dideoxyhexose moiety. In this reaction (42) a tightly enzyme-bound pyridine nucleotide mediates a hydride transfer from C-4 to C-6 of the sugar moiety in the conversion of TDP-glucose to TDP-4-keto-6-deoxyglucose. This key enzyme connects normal hexose metabolism to the more specialized branch of deoxyhexose metabolism. The mechanism of this reaction was further probed by determining the steric course of the hydride migration. To this end we synthesized samples of glucose tritiated stereospecifically at C-6 and deuterated at C-4, such that each tritiated molecule also contained deuterium (43). Feeding of these glucose samples to S. violaceoruber gave granaticin which upon Kuhn-Roth oxidation produced acetic acid. Chirality analysis by the method of Arigoni and Cornforth (cf. 44) indicated that (6R)-[4-D,6-T]glucose had produced a methyl group of 45% ee S configuration, whereas the methyl group generated from (6S)-[4-D,6-T]glucose was 95% ee R. Consequently, the reaction is intramolecular

(45) and stereospecific; the replacement of the 6-hydroxy group by the migrating hydrogen from C-4 occurs with inversion configuration, as shown in Fig 5 (6).

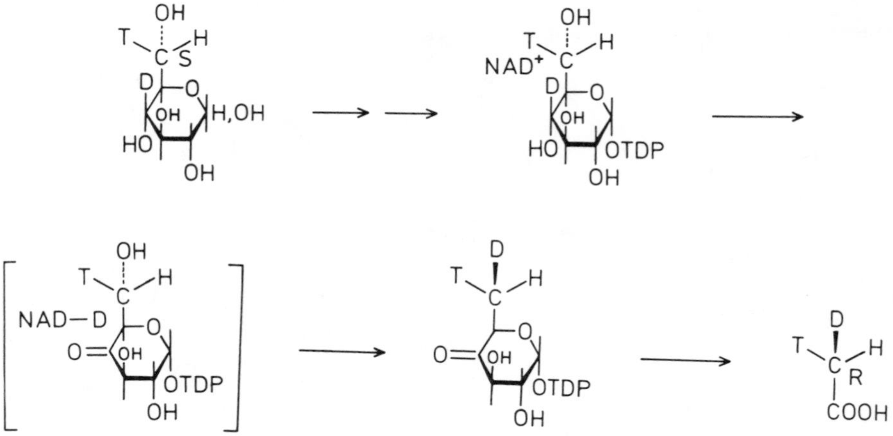

Fig. 5   Steric course of the TDP-glucose oxidoreductase reaction

This stereochemistry agrees with that deduced for the TDP-glucose oxidoreductase isolated from E. coli (43); it suggests a plausible arrangement of the reactants in the enzyme active site (Fig. 6) and a likely mechanism (6). We also determined the steric course of the replacement of the 2-hydroxy group of glucose by hydrogen in the formation of the 2-deoxy function. Feeding of [2-D]glucose gave granaticin

Fig. 6   Active site orientation of

reactants in TDP-glucose

oxidoreductase

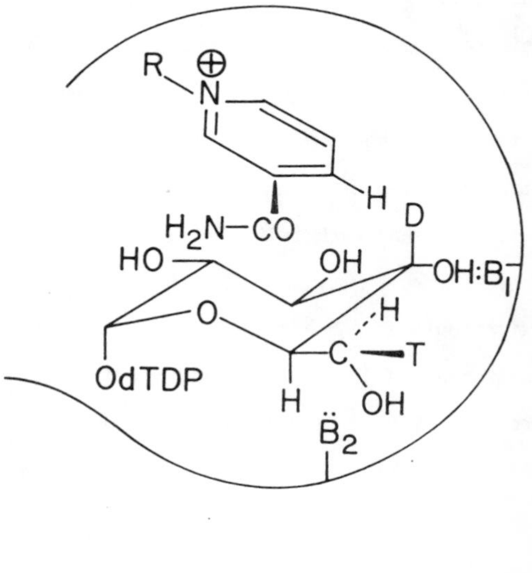

(75% D) which, as shown by proton NMR, carried the deuterium in the 2'-pro-S
position. Hence, replacement of the 2-OH group by hydrogen has occurred in a
retention mode (6). The mechanistic significance of this result, if there is any,
is not obvious at this time.

Pyrek et al. (34) had noted that in the fermentation producing granaticin
appearance of the latter was preceded by the appearance of dihydrogranaticin.
In accordance with the presumed biosynthetic sequence dihydrogranaticin → granaticin we observed that a cell-free extract of S. violaceoruber Tü22 catalyzed the
conversion of dihydrogranaticin to granaticin (6). When the incubation was carried
out in an $^{18}O_2$ atmosphere, no ^{18}O was incorporated into the granaticin formed.
This result suggests that the conversion does not proceed via a classical sequence
of hydroxylation followed by dehydration to the lactone. Rather, it suggests the
operation of a direct cyclization mechanism (Fig. 7) as has been invoked (18) in

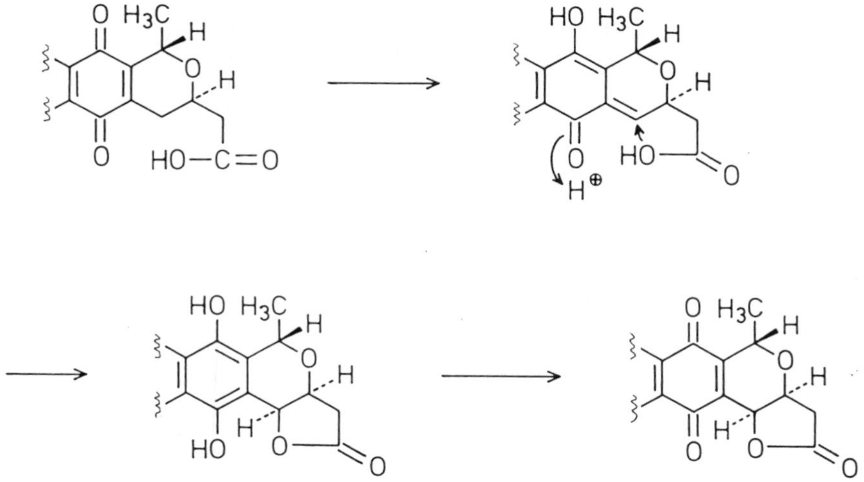

Fig. 7   Oxidative cyclization mechanism for lactone ring formation

the chemical interconversions of the lactone and the corresponding dihydro compound
first observed in the nanaomycin (15) and griseusin (18) series.

The origin of the oxygen in the pyran ring of granaticin was examined in a
feeding experiment with $CH_3{}^{13}C^{18}O_2Na$ (46). Analysis of the product by ^{13}C-NMR, in

collaboration with Prof. John Vederas (47) indicated that the signal for C-3, but not that for C-15 showed an ^{18}O shift. Therefore, the pyran ring oxygen originates from the acetate unit giving rise to C-3 and C-4, not from the starter unit (C-15 and C-16). Other carbons showing retention of the attached ^{18}O are C-11, C-13 and, to a smaller extent, C-1 (46,47) (Fig. 8). In a similar manner the fate of

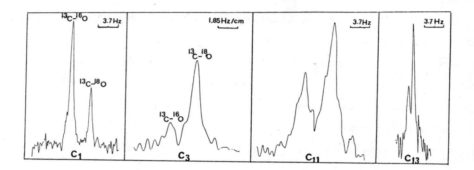

The $CH_3{}^{13}C^{18}O^{18}ONa$ Feeding (97.9% atom ^{13}C, 91.5% atom ^{18}O)

Carbon	Chemical Shift* (ppm)	Isotopic Shift (Hz)	% ^{18}O
1	170.8	3.7	32
3	63.1	2.2	75
6	174.9	none	0
8	162.5	none	0
11	168.5	6.0	70
13	174.8	0.9	65
15	67.4	not well resolved	

*as in dihydrogranaticin.in $CDCl_3$.

Fig. 8   Origin of oxygens in granaticin from acetate

the methyl hydrogens of acetate during the polyketide biosynthetis was probed by feeding $^{13}CD_3COONa$ (48). Analysis of the resulting granaticin and a derivative, dihydrogranaticin methyl ester, by triple-resonance ^{13}C-NMR spectroscopy (observe ^{13}C, broad-band decouple H and D), in collaboration with Dr. Gavin McInnes, showed the presence one atom of deuterium each at C-2 and C-4 (Fig. 9). The starter methyl group contained H_2D and CHD_2, but little if any CD_3 species (max. 2%). This latter finding would be consistent with the hypothesis of a malonyl-CoA

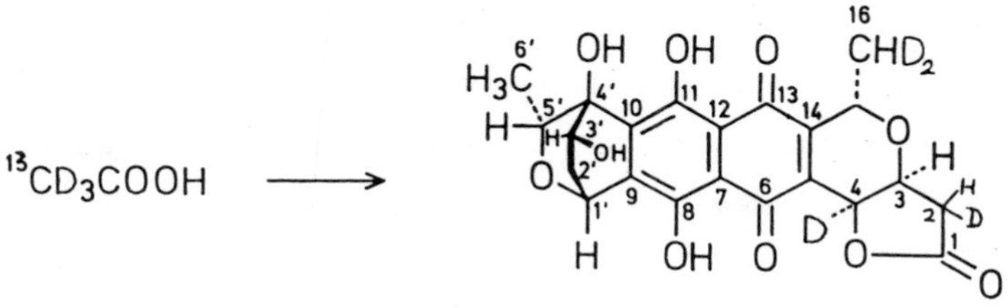

Fig. 9   Fate of acetate methyl hydrogens in granaticin biosynthesis

Carbon No.	δC^*		$\Delta\delta C^*$	$\%F_D$
		Granaticin		
2	38.9	CH_2	0	87
		CHD	0.27	13
		CD_2	?	
4	73.6	CH	0	89
		CD	0.30	11
16	18.5	CH_3	0	82
		CH_2D	0.23	10
		CHD_2	0.49	8
		CD_3	?	0

starter unit, as discussed above, but might also merely be due to exchange. The presence of only one atom of deuterium at C-2 suggests the possibilitiy of a 2,3-double bond at some intermediate stage.

BIOSYNTHETIC INTERRELATIONSHIPS

The biosynthetic relationships among the nanaomycins were studied by Ōmura and coworkers, making use of the inhibition of de novo polyketide synthesis by cerulenin (49). Addition of pure individual compounds to such inhibited cultures allows the observation of occurring biotransformations unobscured by internal production. In this way it was established that in S. rosa var. notoensis the lactone nanaomycin D is reduced to the open-chain nanaomycin A, which is then epoxidized to nanaomycin E, followed by reduction of the epoxide to nanaomycin B (50). The latter reaction as well as the reduction of D to A have been studied in a cell-free system (51). Nanaomycin D reductase has been purified and characterized (52). The reaction it catalyzes is unidirectional and seems to proceed by a reversal of the mechanism shown in Fig. 7 (53). In view of these results we reexamined the relationship between dihydrogranaticin and granaticin in <u>S. violaceoruber</u> by the cerulenin inhibition technique. Clearly, dihydrogranaticin was converted to granaticin by not vice versa (54). Thus, there is a definite difference between the nanaomycin and granaticin pathways in the direction of metabolic conversions. On the other hand, no significant interconversion between actinorhodin and γ-actinorhodin, the corresponding lactone, was observed in either direction in early blocked <u>act</u> mutants of <u>S. coelicolor</u> A3(2) (55), but this may be due to the poor solubility of both compounds and/or poor uptake into the cells.

A conversion sequence more resembling that observed in the nanaomycin series was seen among the naphthocyclinones. In this case the individual compounds were labeled biosynthetically from [1-^{14}C]acetate, purified, and refed to cultures of <u>S. arenae</u> (9). Biosynthetic conversions were indicated by the appearance of significant label in specific naphthocyclinones after feeding a particular precursor. The results indicate that the main biosynthetic sequence proceeds from the lactone γ-naphthocyclinone to the open-chain β-naphthocyclinone which is then oxidized to β-naphthocyclinone epoxide. The latter is converted to α-naphthocyclinone and α-naphthocyclinone acid (Fig. 10). This confirms that α-naphthocyclinone is formed by extrusion of two carbon atoms from a β-naphthocyclinone-type precursor and supports a mechanism for this conversion which is similar to that postulated for the corresponding photochemical process (9,28). It was also found that a monomer corresponding to the "eastern" half of the naphthocyclinones, but not the corresponding symmetrical dimer, was efficiently incorporated into all the naphthocyclinones (Fig. 10) (9). It seems likely that this compound labels only one half of the naphthocyclinone molecule and that the biosynthesis proceeds via an unsymmetrical dimer.

MUTANT STUDIES

As part of the extensive genetic studies on <u>S. coelicolor</u> A3(2) in Hopwood's laboratory, Rudd and Hopwood (25) prepared a large number of mutants of <u>S. coelicolor</u> blocked in the biosynthesis of actinorhodin. These were selected based on the pronounced pH indicator properties of actinorhodin, which results in a dark blue, diffusible pigmentation upon brief exposure of producing colonies to ammonia

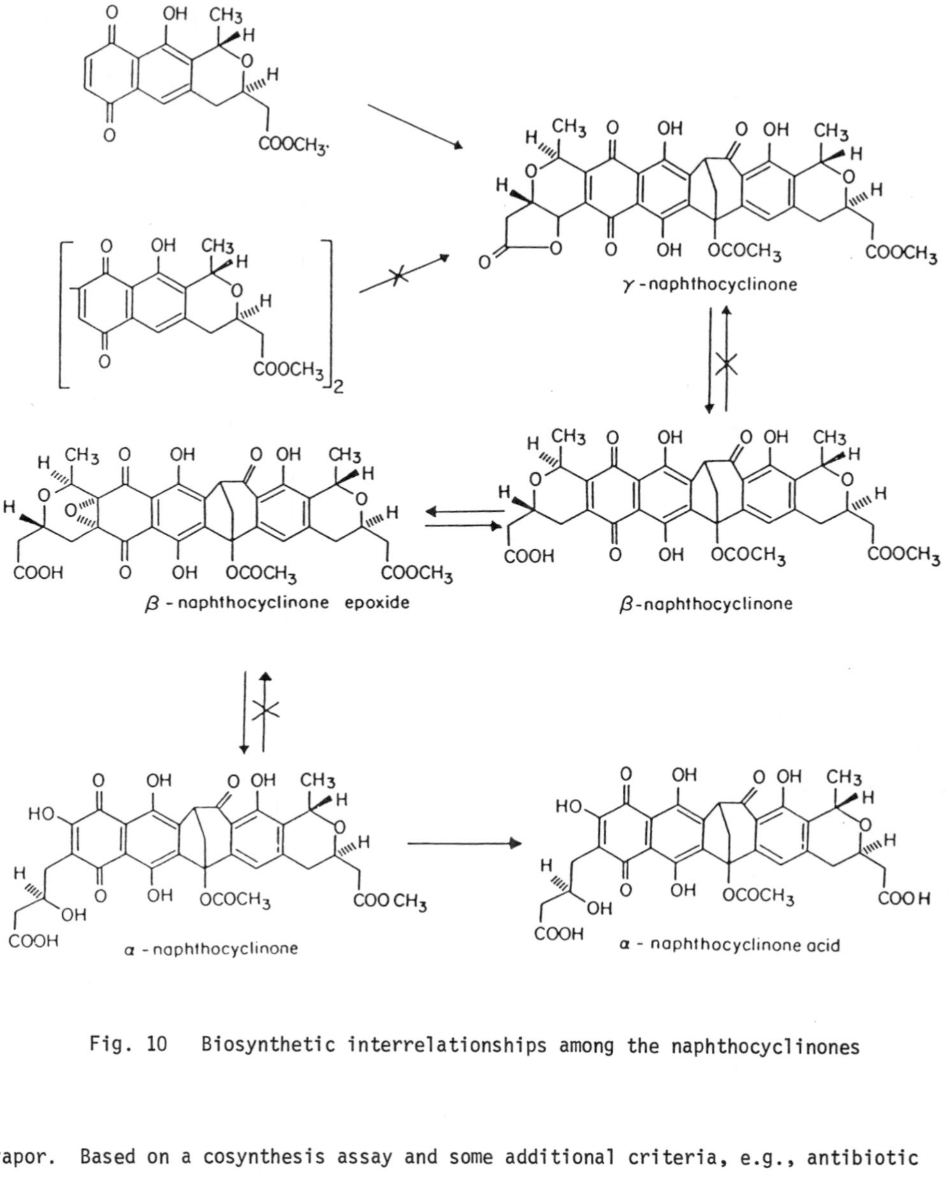

Fig. 10   Biosynthetic interrelationships among the naphthocyclinones

vapor. Based on a cosynthesis assay and some additional criteria, e.g., antibiotic activity, pigment formation, these were grouped into seven classes (Fig. 11) which constitute a series according to the position of the block in the biosynthetic sequence. All these classes mapped in a narrow region of the S. coelicolor chromosome. Mutant classes IV, V, VI and VII, by virtue of their ability to serve as secretors to other mutants, must produce diffusible intermediates of actino-

Classes of <u>act</u> mutants and their phenotype

Mutant class	Type strain	No. of mutants in class	Diffusible pigment	Antibiotic activity against S. aureus	Cosynthesis as convertor	as secretor
I	B78	13	-	-	IV,V,VI,VII	-
II	2377	26	-	-	-	-
III	B41	7	Red	-	IV,V,VI,VII	-
*VII	B40	2	Light golden brown	(+)	?,IV,V,VI	I,III
IV	B17	5	Reddish brown	-	V,VI	I,III
VI	B22	2	Light brown	-	V	I,III,IV
V	B1	21	Brown	+	-	I,III,IV,VI

*Mutants of class VII produced small quantities of actinorhodin which is presumed to be responsible for the limited inhibition of <u>Staph. aureus</u>. This also made it difficult to be sure of cosynthesis reactions, but it is probably that class VII mutants are cross-fed by mutants of IV, V and VI.

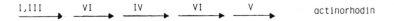

I,III ——→ VI ——→ IV ——→ VI ——→ V ——→   actinorhodin

Fig. 11   <u>Act</u> mutant classes, their characteristics and their position in the biosynthetic sequence

rhodin biosynthesis. We therefore set out to isolate these intermediates from the appropriate mutants (56).

The fractionation of mutant extracts was guided by a bioassay modified from the cosynthesis assay of Rudd and Hopwood (25). Filter paper discs impregnated with an aliquot of the extract or fraction to be tested were placed on a lawn of a converter strain in a Petri dish. After incubation, the dish was briefly exposed to ammonia vapor and inspected for blue zones surrounding the filter discs. Most of the intermediates proved to be extremely unstable and great care had to taken to avoid decomposition by solvents and air, as well as unfavorable pH. Nevertheless, some compounds could so far not be isolated and one was obtained only in a partially pure form. Problems were also encountered with decomposition during the acquisition of spectra.

Fractionation of extracts of mutant B1, a member of the "latest" mutant class, V, yielded as the biologically active material a compound $C_{16}H_{14}O_5$. Extensive proton NMR analysis at 500 MHz, including decoupling and NOE experiments, established the structure of this compound as shown in Fig. 12. Particularly diagnostic were a doublet-triplet-doublet pattern in the aromatic region with one doublet connected to a vinyl proton at 6.27 ppm by a 13.3% NOE, a methyl singlet at 2.65 ppm, and two ABX patterns involving the same methine group as X. The role of this compound as a biosynthetic intermediate was confirmed by labeling the material biosynthetically by feeding [1-^{14}C]acetate to a liquid culture of mutant B1. The purified compound was then refed to a wild-type culture of S. coelicolor and gave 3.9% incorporation into actinorhodin.

The conversion of the B1 compound to actinorhodin evidently still requires a substantial number of enzymatic steps which should involve additional inter-mediates. Class V is a rather large class of mutants, and we suspected that it might be inhomogeneous. We therefore examined the extracts of all class V mutants by tlc to compare their product patterns. Three mutants, B65, B135 and B185, produced a compound which was similar but not identical to the B1 compound. In agreement with this, Hopwood found that mutant B135 mapped in a slightly different region of the chromosome than B1 and the other class V mutants. Attempted isolation of this compound from the mutant B135 showed the presence of a yellow, high R_f spot on the tlc plates, which upon elution was spontaneously converted to a yellow, lower R_f material. The latter was isolated and found to be biologically active in the cosynthesis assay. By comparison with authentic reference material it was identified as kalafungin ($C_{16}H_{12}O_6$, m/z 300.067, calc. 300.063, $[\alpha]_D^{25}$ + 153°, c = 0.008, CHCl$_3$; lit. (10) $[\alpha]_D^{25}$ + 159°, c = 1.0, CHCl$_3$). Labeled

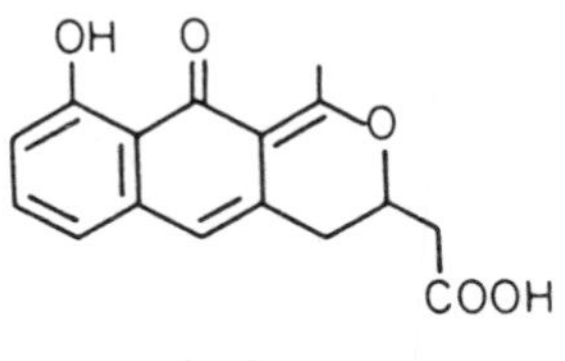

Compound from mutant
B1 (Class V)
(Biologically active)

Fig. 12

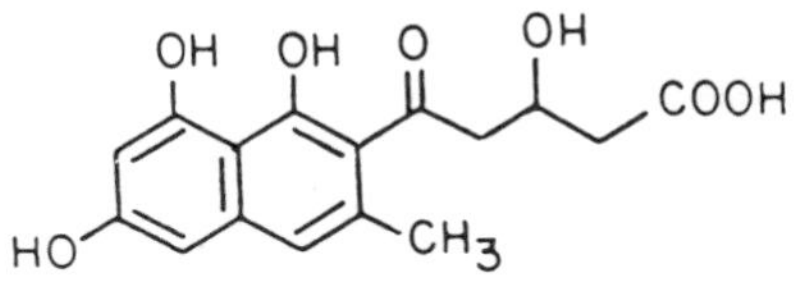

Compound from mutant
B40 (class VII)
(not biologically active)

Fig. 14

kalafungin, biosynthesized from [1-^{14}C]acetate, was efficiently incorporated (17.7%) into actinorhodin. The higher R_f compound originally present in the B135 extract was, by R_f, different from nanaomycin A, the enantiomer of dihydrokalafungin, and from kalafunginic acid, the lactone ring-open analog of kalafungin. Since the original extract was biologically active in the cosynthesis assay, it is assumed that the high R_f compound is an intermediate in actinorhodin biosynthesis. An attempt to interpret these relationships is given in Figure 13. It is

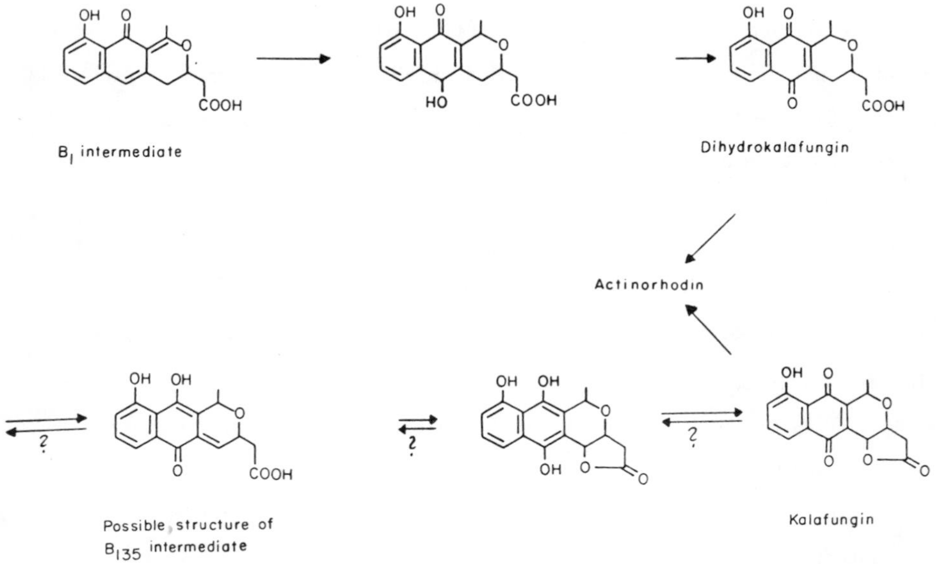

Fig. 13   Proposed relationship between the intermediates in mutants B1 and B135, kalafungin and actinorhodin

suggested that the B1 intermediate, either by 1,4-addition of water or by 1,4-reduction of the diene and hydroxylation, is converted into a 6-oxygenated compound, which is then further oxidized to dihydrokalafungin. Conversion of the latter to kalafungin by the direct oxidative cyclization mechanism discussed earlier could occur both enzymatically and nonenzymatically. Whether actinorhodin is formed from dihydrokalafungin via kalafungin or directly, with kalafungin only in equilibrium with dihydrokalafungin, can not be decided on the basis of the available data. Candidate structures for the high R_f intermediate accumulated in mutant B135 would be the enol of dihydrokalafungin or the 6-oxygenated compound formed from the B1 intermediate.

Analysis of extracts of mutant B40, a member of class VII, the earliest class of secretor mutants, revealed biological activity in the cosynthesis assay. However, the accumulated intermediate was extremely unstable and we were unable to isolate it. Instead, another, colorless compound was isolated which showed no biological activity. Since the mass spectrum showed it to be a C_{16} compound, we assumed that the compound was related to the actinorhodin pathway, possibly representing a shunt product. Proton- and ^{13}C-NMR analysis revealed the presence of a 1,3-dihydroxybenzene system connected to another, trisubstituted aromatic ring, a methyl group attached to a quaternary carbon and two connected ABX systems characteristic of the methylene-methine-methylene pattern of the side chain of compounds like dihydrokalafungin or the B1 intermediate. These and additional long-range ^{13}C-^{1}H coupling and NOE data lead us to propose the structure shown in Figure 14 for the shunt product from mutant B40. However, some alternatives, e.g., the corresponding dihydro-γ-pyrone structure (dehydration between C-3 and C-7) or attachment of the side chain para (rather than ortho) to the hydroxyl group, cannot be excluded with certainty. It seems likely that the shunt product is formed by a different mode of cyclization of the polyketide chain than that leading to actinorhodin, possibly primed by reduction of a different carbonyl group in the polyketide chain as shown in Fig. 15. Work by Harris et al. (57,58)

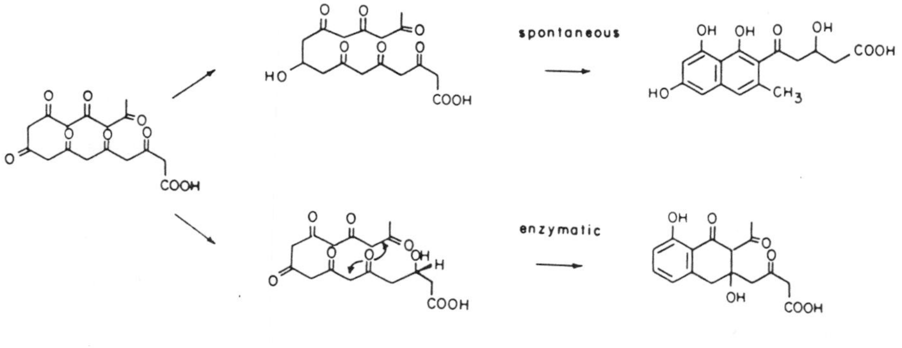

Fig. 15   Proposed relationship between the shunt product and the accummulated intermediate in mutant B40

suggests that chain folding leading to the kalafungin-type cyclization is favored by sp^3 hybridization at C-9 as would result from reduction of the 9-ketone to the alcohol.

Extracts of mutant B22, a member of class VI, contained a biologically active material which was colorless and extremely unstable. Efforts to isolate this material have so far proved futile. The intermediate accummulated by mutant B17 (class IV) is also colorless and rather unstable. However, careful workup under argon allowed us to purify the compound and to obtain structural information, despite problems with decomposition during spectral analysis. The mass spectrum indicates a molecular formula $C_{16}H_{14}O_6$ and ready loss of H_2O and CO_2 from the molecular ion. Proton NMR shows a singlet methyl group and a monosubstituted benzene ring, as in the B1 intermediate, but two isolated AB methylene patterns and a vinyl proton instead of the two ABX patterns seen in the B1 compound. Based on these data and detailed coupling analysis we propose the tentative structure shown in Figure 16 for the intermediate from mutant B17. The $\Delta 2,3$ isomer (rather

Fig. 16

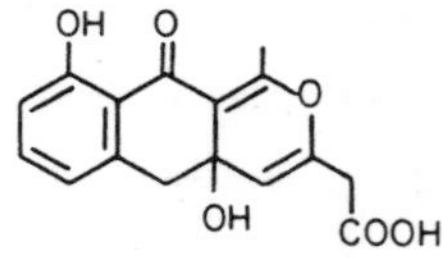

Tentative structure of
compound from mutant
B17 (class IV)
(Biologically active)

than $\Delta 3,4$) may be an alternative possibility. The compound, when labeled biosynthetically with ^{14}C and fed to a wild-type strain, showed excellent incorporation into actinorhodin (28.4%).

Based on the structures of the compounds isolated so far and the additional information available on can propose a reasonable pathway to actinorhodin which is shown in Figure 17. Clearly this biosynthetic pathway is still highly speculative in many respects. Initial assembly of 8 acetate/malonate units gives a polyketide which upon reduction of the 9-keto group and cyclization produces the structure

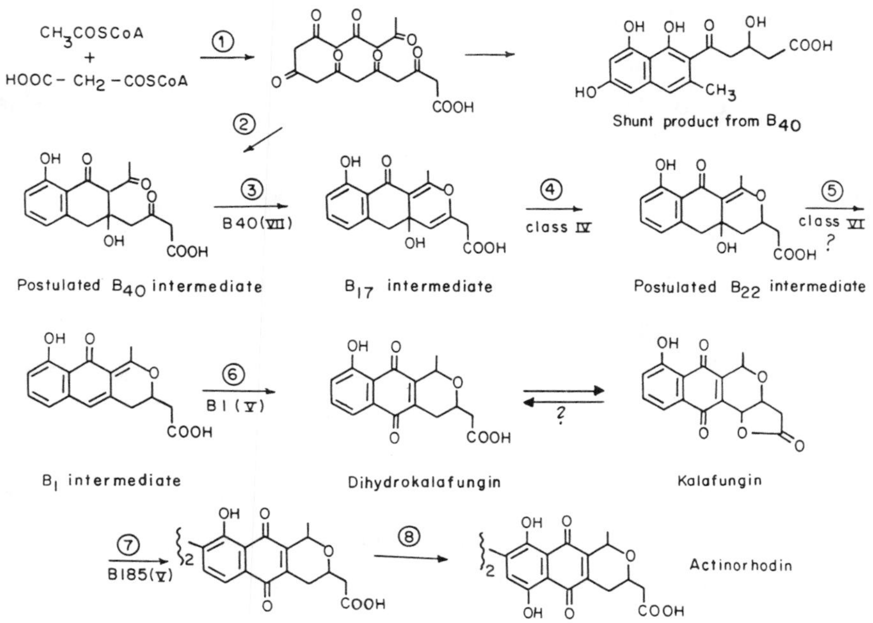

Fig. 17   Hypothetical pathway of actinorhodin biosynthesis

suggested for the B40 intermediate. Enolization of the 3-keto group, either to
the 2,3- or the 3,4-enol, addition of the 3-OH to the 15-keto group and loss of
water gives rise to the B17 intermediate. The $\Delta 3,4$ structure, as written, better
accommodates the spectroscopic data, whereas the alternative $\Delta 2,3$ structure would
account for the observed loss of one deuterium from C-2. Either way the pyran
ring oxygen would originate from C-3, as was demonstrated to be the case. Reduction of the $\Delta 3,4$ (or $\Delta 2,3$) double bond is proposed to precede dehydration to the
conjugated system because the B22 intermediate is colorless. Its predicted
allylic alcohol structure should undergo facile dehydration to the B1 intermediate,
which is then converted to dihydrokalafungin and/or kalafungin. Since there is
some evidence (55) that the remaining steps are insensitive to the stereochemistry
of the molecule, it is proposed that the dimerization occurs at the stage of
dihydrokalafungin or kalafungin, with control of the regiochemistry by the single
hydroxy group in the benzene ring, and that the remaining hydroxy group in each
half of the molecule is introduced last.

GENETICALLY ENGINEERED "HYBRID" STRUCTURES

Following the production and characterization of act mutants, Malpartida and Hopwood (59) constructed plasmids, derived from the S. coelicolor sex factor SPC2, carrying a thiostrepton selection marker and inserts of S. coelicolor DNA representing all or some of the genes coding for actinorhodin biosynthesis. Plasmid PIJ2303 was shown to carry all the actinorhodin genes by complementation of all available classes of act mutants and by production of actinorhodin by several actinorhodin non-producing streptomycetes, e.g., S. parvulus upon transformation with PIJ2303 (59). Mutation of S. violaceoruber (60) produced several gra mutants, some of which showed cosynthesis with act mutants. When one of these, B1140, which had a block equivalent to that of class IV act mutants, was transformed with PIJ2308 carrying a transcription unit which complements class IV act mutants, pigment production was restored. The pigments formed were identified as dihydrogranaticin and granaticin, indicating that at least one of the enzymes of actinorhodin biosynthesis can function in the granaticin pathway even though the substrate has different stereochemistry. Transformation with plasmids carrying other genes of the actinorhodin pathway did not restore pigment formation. When B1140 was transformed with PIJ2303, the resulting culture produced both granaticin and dihydrogranaticin (early in the fermentation) and actinorhodin (late in the fermentation). However, a transformant of the wild-type S. violaceoruber Tü22 carrying PIJ2303 produced, in addition to actinorhodin, a new compound, dihydrogranatirhodin, to the almost complete exclusion of granaticin and dihydrogranaticin. Dihydrogranatirhodin has the same molecular formula and very similar spectral properties as dihydrogranaticin, but showed significant upfield shifts of the proton NMR signals for H-3 and H-15. This is characteristic of compounds with cis arrangement of these two hydrogens (34). Observation of a 5.5% NOE at H-3 upon irradiation of H-15 confirmed that dihydrogranatirhodin is either the C-3 or the C-15 epimer of dihydrogranaticin (Fig. 18) (61).

Fig. 18   Dihydrogranatirhodin

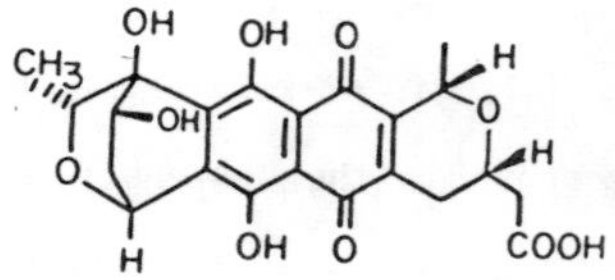

In a similar collaboration between the groups of Hopwood and Ōmura, transformation of <u>Streptomyces</u> sp. AM-7161, the producer of medermycin, with plasmids carrying DNA segments corresponding to the genes complementing class V <u>act</u> mutants led to the production of a new compound, mederrhodin A. This compound contains the entire medermycin structure plus an additional hydroxy group which is characteristic of actinorhodin (Fig. 19) (61). Mederrhodin and dihydrogranatirhodin are the

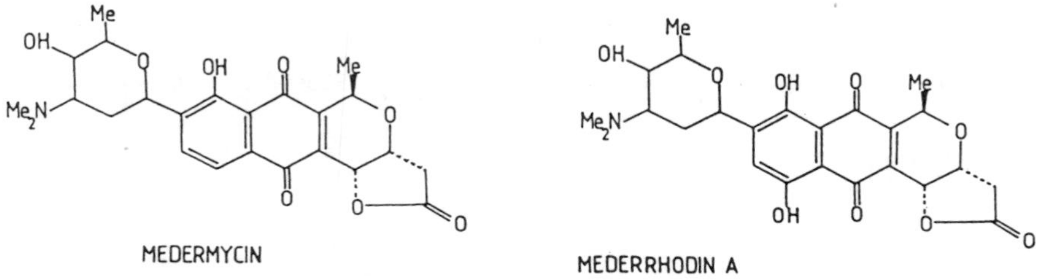

MEDERMYCIN   MEDERRHODIN A

Fig. 19

first and the second example of new hybrid structures produced by genetically engineered organisms containing and expressing genetic information from two different parents. The structural modifications achieved in these two examples are minor and probably of no practical importance. They demonstrate, however, an important principle. In the future, the classical approach of searching for new antibiotics by isolating metabolically unique new organisms from soil samples collected around the world will probably be complemented by a second approach in which genetically new organisms with unique new metabolic capabilities are created in the laboratory.

Acknowledgments The author is indebted to Professor David A. Hopwood, Norwich, and Professor Axel Zeeck, Göttingen, for productive collaborations, and to the National Institutes of Health (Grant AI 20264) and NATO for financial support.

REFERENCES AND NOTES

1. O.A. Mascaretti, C.-j. Chang, D. Hook, H. Otsuka, E.F. Kreutzer, H.G. Floss, Biochemistry 20 (1981) 919.

2. T.S.S. Chen, C.-j. Chang, H.G. Floss, J. Amer. Chem. Soc. 103 (1981) 4565.

3. T.S.S. Chen, C.-j. Chang, H.G. Floss, J. Org. Chem. 46 (1981) 2661.

4. S.W. Tsao, Ph.D. Thesis, Purdue University, 1983.

5. A. Nakagawa, T.-S. Wu, P.J. Keller, J.P. Lee, S. Ōmura, H.G. Floss, J.C.S. Chem. Comm. (1985) 519.

6. C.E. Snipes, C.-j. Chang, H.G. Floss, J. Amer. Chem. Soc. 101 (1979) 701.

7. C.P. Gorst-Allman, B.A.M. Rudd, C.-j. Chang, H.G. Floss, J. Org. Chem. 46 (1981) 455.

8. K. Schröder, H.G. Floss, J. Org. Chem. 43 (1978) 1438.

9. B. Krone, A. Zeeck, H.G. Floss, J. Org. Chem. 47 (1982) 472.

10. H. Hoeksema, W.C. Krueger, J. Antibiot. 29 (1976) 704; and references therein.

11. G.A. Ellestad, H.A. Whaley, E.L. Patterson, J. Amer. Chem. Soc. 88 (1966) 4109.

12. Y. Iwai, A. Kora, Y. Takahashi, T. Hayashi, J. Awaya, R. Masuma, R. Oiwa and S. Ōmura, J. Antibiot 31 (1978) 959.

13. H. Tanaka, Y. Koyama, T. Nagai, H. Marumo, S. Ōmura, J. Antibiot. 28 (1975) 868.

14. H. Tanaka, H. Marumo, T. Nagai, M. Okada, K. Taniguchi, S. Ōmura, J. Antibiot. 28 (1975) 925.

15. S. Ōmura, H. Tanaka, Y. Okada, H. Marumo, Chem. Comm. 1976, 320.

16. M. Sasai, K. Shirahata, S. Tshii, K. Mineura, H. Marumo, H. Tanaka and S. Ōmura, J. Antibiot. 32 (1979) 422.

17. Y. Iwai, K. Kimura, Y. Takahasi, K. Hinotozawa, H. Shimizu, H. Tanaka, S. Ōmura, J. Antibiot. 36 (1983) 1268.

18. N. Tsuji, M. Kobayashi, Y. Terui, K. Tori, Tetrahedron 32 (1976) 2207.

19. H. Brockmann and P. Christiansen, Chem. Ber. 103 (1970) 708.

20. H. Brockmann, H. Pini, Naturwissenschaften. 34 (1947) 190.

21. H. Brockmann, A. Zeeck, K. van der Merwe, W. Müller, Liebig's Ann. Chem. 698 (1966) 209.

22. B. Krone, A. Zeeck, Liebig's Ann. Chem. 1983 510.

23. P. Christiansen, Ph.D. dissertation, University of Göttingen, 1907.

24. L.F. Wright, D.A. Hopwood, J. Gen. Microbiol. 96 (1976) 289.

25. B.A.M. Rudd, D.A. Hopwood, J. Gen. Microbiol. 114 (1979) 35.

26. F. Malpartida, D.A. Hopwood, Nature 309 (1984) 462.

27. A. Zeeck, M. Mardin, Liebig's Ann. Chem. 1974 1063; A. Zeeck, H. Zähner, M. Mardin, Liebig's Ann. Chem. 1974 1100.

28. B. Krone, A. Zeeck, Liebig's Ann. Chem. 1983 471.

29. E. Egert, M. Noltmeyer, G.M. Sheldrick, W. Saenter, H. Brand, A. Zeeck, Liebig's Ann. Chem. 1983 503.

30. R. Carbaz, L. Ettlinger, E. Gäumann, J. Kalvoda, W. Keller-Schierlein, F. Kradolfor, B.K. Maunkian, L. Neipp, V. Prelog, P. Reusser, H. Zähner, Helv. Chim. Acta 40 (1957) 1262.

31. S. Barcza, M. Brufani, W. Keller-Schierlein, H. Zähner, Helv. Chim. Acta 49 (1966) 1736.

32. P. Soong, A.A. Au, Rep. Taiwan Sugar Expt. Station 29 (1962) 33; P. Soong, Y.Y. Jen, Y.S. Hsu, A.A. Au, ibid 34 (1964) 105.

33. C.-j. Chang, H.G. Floss, P. Soong, C.-t. Chang, J. Antibiot. 28 (1975) 156.

34. J. St. Pyrek, O. Achmatowicz and A. Zamojski, Tetrahedron 33 (1977) 673.

35. H. Maehr, H.V. Cuellar, J. Smallheer, T.H. Williams, G.J. Sasso, J. Berger, Mh. Chem. 110 (1979) 531.

36. W. Keller-Schierlein, M. Brufani, S. Barcza, Helv. Chim. Acta 51 (1968) 1257.

37. M. Brufani, M. Dobler, Helv. Chim. Acta 51 (1968) 1269.

38. A. Ogilvie, K. Wiebauer and W. Kersten, Biochem. J. 152 (1975) 511, 517.

39. P.F. Heinstein, J. Pharm. Sci. 71 (1982) 197; G.G. Clay, S.R. Bryn, P.F. Heinstein, J. Pharm. Sci. 71 (1979) 467.

40. A. Arnone, L. Camarda, R. Cardillo, G. Fronza, L. Merlini, R. Mondelli, G. Nasini, J. St. Pyrek, Helv. Chim. Acta 62 (1979) 30.

41. As a matter of convenience we use an arbitrary, biosynthetic numbering throughout this article, rather than the systematic IUPAC numbering.

42. O. Gabriel, "Carbohydrates in Solution", R. Gould, Ed., Adv. Chem. Ser. No. 117 (1973) 387.

43. C.E. Snipes, G.-U. Brillinger, L. Sellers, L. Mascaro, H.G. Floss, J. Biol. Chem. 252 (1977) 8113.

44. H.G. Floss, M.D. Tsai, Adv. Enzymol. 50 (1979) 243.

45. The added labeled glucose was diluted over 100-fold with unlabeled glucose in the medium, and a methyl group is only chiral if H, D and T are present in the same molecule.

46. C.C. Chang, C.-j. Chang, J.C. Vederas, H.G. Floss, unpublished work; cf ref. 47.

47. J.C. Vederas, Can. J. Chem. 60 (1982) 1637.

48. C.C. Chang, C.-j. Chang, G.A. McInnes, H.G. Floss, unpublished work.

49. S. Ōmura, Bacteriol. Rev. 40 (1976) 681.

50. C. Kitao, H. Tanaka, S. Minami, S. Ōmura, J. Antibiot. 33 (1980) 711.

51. S. Ōmura, S. Minami, H. Tanaka, J. Biochem. (Toyko) 90 (1981) 291.

52. S. Ōmura, H. Tanaka, S. Minami, I. Takahashi, J. Biochem. (Tokyo) 90 (1981) 355.

53. H. Tanaka, S. Minami-Kakinuma, S. Ōmura, J. Antibiot. 35 (1982) 1565.

54. X-G. He, H.G. Floss, unpublished work.

55. S.P. Cole, Ph.D. thesis, Purdue University, 1985.

56. S.P. Cole, B.A.M. Rudd, X.-G. He, H.G. Floss, unpublished work; see ref. 55.

57. A.D. Webb, T.M. Harris, Tet. Letters (1977) 1069.

58. T.M. Harris, C.M. Harris, Tetrahedron 33 (1977) 2159.

59. F. Malpartida, D.A. Hopwood, Nature 309 (1984) 462.

60. B.A.M. Rudd, H.G. Floss, unpublished work.

61. D.A. Hopwood, F. Malpartida, H.M. Kieser, H. Ikeda, J. Duncan, I. Fujii, B.A.M. Rudd, H.G. Floss, S. Ōmura, Nature, 314 (1985) 642.

Biosynthesis of Tylosin and its Regulation by Ammonium and Phosphate

Satoshi Ōmura and Yoshitake Tanaka

Kitasato University, The Kitasato Institute and School of Pharmaceutical Sciences,
5-9-1 Shirokane, Minato-Ku, Tokyo 108, Japan

SUMMARY

The biosynthesis of tylosin and its regulation in Streptomyces fradiae were studied using blocked mutants, by bioconversion, and by enzymatic reactions. Protylonolide, a precursor of the aglycone moiety, is constructed from acetate, propionate and n-butyrate. These building units were found to be supplied by the metabolism of valine, threonine and other amino acids, succinate, and higher fatty acids. The pathway after protylonolide was suggested by bioconversion studies using cerulenin as an aid. The result was confirmed at the enzyme level as follows: Protylonolide $\longrightarrow$ 5-$\underline{O}$-mycaminosylprotylonolide $\longrightarrow$ 20-hydroxy-5-$\underline{O}$-mycaminosylprotylonolide $\longrightarrow$ 20-oxo-5-$\underline{O}$-mycaminosyl-protylonolide $\longrightarrow$ 5-$\underline{O}$-mycaminosyltylonolide $\longrightarrow$ tylosin. Two α-keto-glutarate-dependent dioxygenases involved in the hydroxylations at C-20 and C-23 and a dehydrogenase with a broad substrate specificity responsible for the oxidation of C-20 hydroxyl to an oxo group were detected and characterized.

Tylosin production is inhibited by adding ammonium salts to fermentation media. It increases, however, with simultaneous reduction of ammonium levels in the media when ammonium-trapping agents such as natural zeolite were supplemented to the media. Studies with a co-synthetic pair of mutants, the secretor strain 261 and the convertor strain NP-10, showed that the effect of ammonium is directed toward steps prior to, but not beyond, protylonolide. Protylonolide production from valine or succinate by resting cells of strain 261 was much lower when the cells were previously grown under high-ammonium conditions than when grown under low-ammonium conditions. The inhibition of protylonolide production by ammonium was reversed by adding acetate + propionate + n-butyrate. These results point to amino acid and succinate metabolisms as possible targets of ammonium action. A cell-free study showed that valine dehydrogenase is one of such enzymes.

Phosphate inhibits both tylosin and protylonolide production. Unlike the case of the ammonium effect described above, phosphate interferes both protylonolide formation and its conversion to tylosin. The addition of phosphate-trapping agents such as Kanuma earth, an allophane-containing clay, increased production of both. Valine dehydrogenase was suggested to be one of the phosphate-sensitive enzymes.

It is concluded that high levels of ammonium and phosphate cause a limited supply of the building units acetate, propionate and n-butyrate to suppress protylonolide formation, leading consequently to a decrease of tylosin production.

1 INTRODUCTION

Tylosin, a 16-membered macrolide antibiotic produced by Streptomyces fradiae, is active against gram-positive and some gram-negative bacteria, anaerobic bacteria like Bacteroides, and Mycoplasma. The structure consists of a 16-membered lactone with an aldehyde group and three sugars attached to the lactone. The present authors have been interested in the biosynthesis, assembly of individual building units, and regulatory mechanisms involved in these processes. They provide a good model of formation of secondary metabolites, particularly the polyketide antibiotics.

Several review articles have appeared on the biosynthesis (1,2), genetic regulation (3), and chemical modification (4) of macrolide antibiotics. This paper presents recent progresses in tylosin biosynthesis and its regualtion. Simple fermentation techniques for release of regulations resulting in a marked increase of tylosin production are also described.

2 BIOSYNTHETIC PATHWAY TO TYLOSIN IN STREPTOMYCES FRADIAE

The biosynthetic pathway to tylosin can be divided into two parts: one is to afford protylonolide, an earliest lactonic precursor of the aglycone moiety, and the other is for the conversion of

protylonolide to tylosin. In the latter part the oxidation and
reduction occur on protylonolide moiety in association with the
attachment of three sugars to the lactone.

A pair of co-synthetic mutants of S. fradiae, strains 261 and
NP-10, were obtained (Fig. 1) (5). When grown individually, these
mutants do not produce tylosin, but can do so on mixed culture.
Strain 261, blocked in mycaminose biosynthesis, accumulates
protylonolide. This lactone is converted to tylosin by another mutant
NP-10, which is defective of protylonolide formation. Thus, the
pathways functioning in the two mutants correspond to the two parts of
tylosin biosynthesis described above. In the studies presented below,
these two mutants were successfully used.

2.1 Biosynthesis of Protylonolide

Early studies with ^{13}C-labeled precursors together with ^{13}C-NMR
spectroscopic analyses of resulting labeled tylosin showed that the
carbons of the aglycone moiety originate from acetate, propionate and
n-butyrate (6,7). It has been assumed that these lower fatty acids
are supplied by diversion from anabolic primary metabolism. Acetate
can arise from pyruvate, propionate or its biosynthetically equivalent
counterpart methylmalonate from succinate, and n-butyrate from two
acetates. In fact, the supplement of [1-^{13}C]acetate enriched C-5 and
19 with ^{13}C, the carbons also enriched by ^{13}C-labeled n-butyrate.
However, such observations do not rule out necessarily the possible
contribution of other routes in supplying the lower fatty acids.
Several observations were noted which can be regarded as evidence
suggesting the latter possibility.

Protylonolide production by S. fradiae strain 261 begins
with cessation of cell growth in both complex and chemically defined
media. It continues for a long duration, e.g. several days, in spite
that the activities of glycolysis and the tricarboxylic acid (TCA)
cycle decrease under such conditions. Animal and plant oils have a
promoting effect on production of protylonolide and tylosin. In
addition, protylonolide production was enhanced by the addition of
certain amino acids. The fermentation is often associated with a
pH-rise due to the generation of ammonia into media. These observations suggest that catabolic processes have a role in tylosin
biosynthesis, and that amino acids, as well as succinate and higher
fatty acids, are utilized for protylonolide biosynthesis.

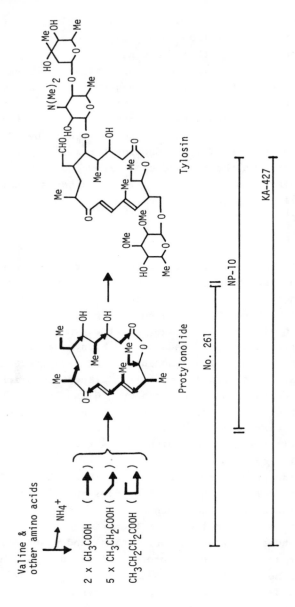

Fig. 1. Biosynthesis of tylosin in *Streptomyces fradiae* KA-427, and co-synthesis of tylosin by the mutant strains 261 and NP-10.

2.2 Sources of Lower Fatty Acids

To examine this possibility, a resting cell system was developed, in which short-term production of protylonolide was carried out with labeled compounds added as the substrates. After incubation, the supernatant solution of the reaction mixture was extracted with benzene, and the benzene layer, after being washed, was assayed for radioactivity. Protylonolide and 5-O-mycarosylprotylonolide were the only labeled products detected by autoradiography in the benzene extracts. The latter mycarosyl derivative is a shunt metabolite possibly formed from protylonolide. The production of protylonolide proceeds linearly for 6 hours under the conditions employed.

^{14}C-labeled valine, threonine, and succinate labeled pro-tylonolide most efficiently, followed by leucine and isoleucine, but lysine did not do so substantially (8). Because protylonolide is constructed only with acetate, propionate and n-butyrate, the formation of labeled protylonolide from labeled amino acids and succinate is a strong indication that the three lower fatty acids are supplied by the metabolism of valine and other amino acids, probably except for lysine, and of succinate.

The incorporation of valine carbons into protylonolide was confirmed by ^{13}C-NMR spectroscopy. Valine is metabolized to isobutyrate, which is oxidized further to methylmalonate in many microorganisms. [3,3'-^{13}C$_2$]Isobutyrate, synthesized chemically, was incubated with protylonolide producer, strain 261, and the resulting [^{13}C]protylonolide was subjected to ^{13}C-NMR spectrometry. As anticipated, propionate-derived methyl carbons (C-17, 18, 21, 22, and 23) were intensely enriched (Fig. 2) (9). In addition, carbons at 6- and 20-positions were also efficiently enriched by ^{13}C, which had been known to arise from n-butyrate. We suggest that the valine metabolism involves an interconversion of isobutyrate and n-butyrate, a reaction which have not been reported before. In an early paper, Ōmura et al. (6) showed that a small fraction of [^{13}C]n-butyrate was converted to [^{13}C]propionate in tylosin biosynthesis by S. fradiae, resulting in weak enrichment of normally propionate-originated carbons. They then explained this by a pathway of n-butyrate to succinate. Now we suggest another possible route: n-butyrate $\longrightarrow$ isobutyrate $\longrightarrow$ methylmalonate (Fig. 2). Recently, Vanek described a similar inter-conversion in monensin biosynthesis by S. cinnamonensis (10). The incorporation of amino acid carbons into protylonolide molecule is

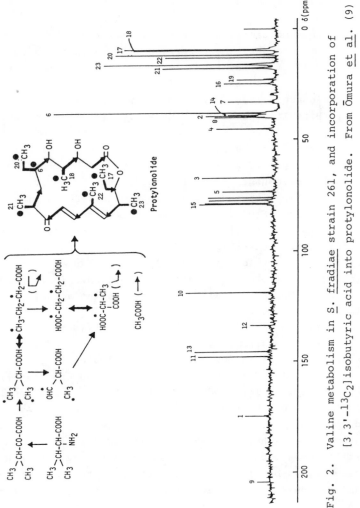

Fig. 2. Valine metabolism in S. fradiae strain 261, and incorporation of [3,3'-$^{13}C_2$]isobutyric acid into protylonolide. From Ōmura et al. (9)

supported by a recent paper of Dotzlaf et al. (11)

The incorporation of amino acid carbons into aglycones is not restricted to tylosin biosynthesis. The biosynthesis of the leucomycin aglycone by Streptoverticillium kitasatoensis was demonstrated to involve a similar metabolism of valine (9).

2.3 Biosynthesis after Protylonolide Formation

2.3.1 Cerulenin, a useful tool for biosynthetic studies

The conversion of protylonolide to tylosin requires oxidations of C-20 methyl to an aldehyde and C-23 methyl to a hydroxylmethyl giving rise to the tylosin aglycone, and glycosidation of the aglycone by the three sugars mycaminose, mycinose and mycarose. These sugars are synthesized in separate routes to be attached to the aglycone moiety. Methylations are also involved in the biosyntheses of the three sugars. The order of assembly of these building blocks in tylosin biosynthesis was studied by Ōmura et al. (12). They analyzed the bioconversion of possible intermediates into tylosin in the presence of cerulenin.

Cerulenin, an antifungal and antibacterial antibiotic produced by Cephalosporium caerulens, is a specific inhibitor of higher fatty acid biosynthesis. It inhibits β-ketoacyl acyl carrier protein synthetase (condensing enzyme) from Escherichia coli and other microbial and animal systems (13,14). The antibiotic inhibits also polyketide condensing enzyme probably by a mechanism analogous to the action on fatty acid biosynthesis. The cerulenin level required to inhibit polyketide formation is lower than that for interfering with growth of the polyketide-producing organisms. Therefore, when tylosin-producing S. fradiae KA-427 is grown in the presence of a low level (20-40 µg/ml) of cerulenin, it becomes unable to produce tylosin-related compounds due to the lack of protylonolide formation, but remains fully functional in the other parts of tylosin biosynthesis, which include methyl oxidation, sugar synthesis, its attachment, and methylation. In fact, the addition of protylonolide to a cerulenin-supplemented culture of S. fradiae results in tylosin production. Thus, cerulenin-supplemented cells provides a simple and convenient tool to examine whether or not a given lactone compound is an intermediate of tylosin biosynthesis.

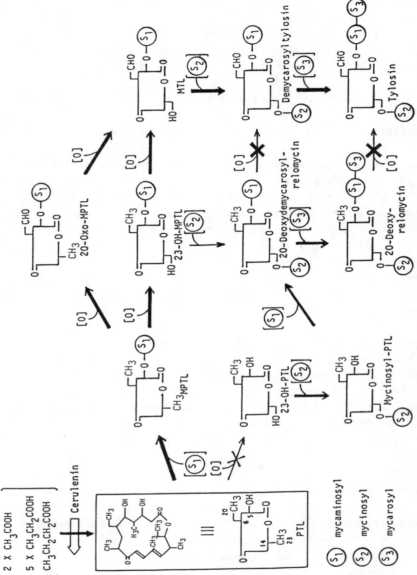

Fig. 3. Bioconversion of tylosin-related compounds and proposed pathway of tylosin biosynthesis in S. fradiae KA-427. From Ōmura et al. (12). PTL, protylonolide; MPTL, 5-O-mycaminosyl-PTL; MTL, 5-O-mycaminosyltylonolide.

2.3.2 Bioconversion studies using cerulenin

Glycosylated derivatives of protylonolide with its methyls being
oxidized at different levels were obtained chemically from protylonolide and from tylosin. They were subjected to bioconversion
studies with S. fradiae cells grown in the presence of cerulenin.
Products were separated by silica gel thin-layer chromatography,
followed by scanning at 283 nm. The results show the major pathway to
tylosin illustrated in Fig. 3 (12).

Protylonolide is first glycosylated to mycaminosyl-protylonolide
(MPTL), and is then oxidized at C-20 or at C-23. The C-20-hydroxyl
intermediate is further oxidized to a 20-oxo derivative, which is
hydroxylated at C-23 to mycaminosyltylonolide (MTL). MTL is thereafter glycosylated successively by mycinose, and finally by mycarose,
to afford tylosin. With protylonolide as the starting material, no
trace amount of 23-OH-PTL was detected. However, the use of the
latter compound as the substrate resulted in the production of a
triglycosylated compound 20-deoxyrelomycin, a tylosin analog with a
C-20 methyl instead of an aldehyde.

2.4 Enzymes Involved in Mycaminosyltylonolide (MTL) Formation from
    Mycaminosylprotylonolide (MPTL)

Details of the pathway from MPTL to MTL were studied using
cell-free extracts from S. fradiae KA-427 (15,16). The purpose of
this study was to clarify 1) which one of C-20 and C-23 methyls of
MPTL is oxidized earlier, and 2) properties of enzymes involved in the
oxidations of the two methyls. The cells of S. fradiae KA-427 were
disrupted by sonication, and centrifuged at 12,000 x g for 10 min.
The supernatant solution was used as the enzyme source with or without
dialysis for 2-3 hours. Overnight dialysis caused an entire loss of
enzyme activities. Restoration of the activities was unsatisfactory.
The incubation was carried out with shaking. HPLC allowed to identify
and quantify reaction products (Fig. 4).

2.4.1 20- and 23-Hydroxylases

Table 1 shows requirements for enzyme activities to oxidize C-20
and C-23 methyls. Both 20-hydroxylase and 23-hydroxylase absolutely
require α-ketoglutarate for activity (15). Additional supplements of
ascorbate and ferrous ions have a stimulating effect, although they
are not essential, as they are for other known dioxygenases. The two
hydroxylation reactions proceed only under aerobic conditions:

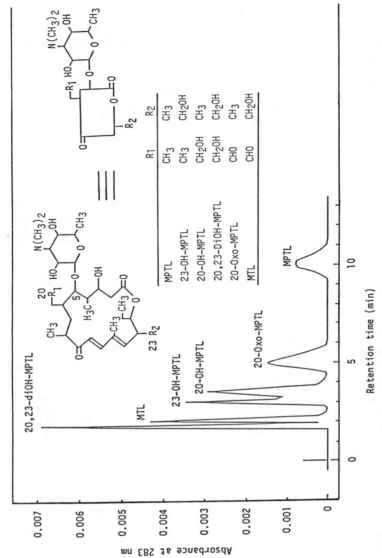

Fig. 4.   Separation of tylosin-related compounds by HPLC. The column material was Lichrosorb RP-18 (10 μm). The solvent was a mixture of acetonitrile:buffer (10 mM KH$_2$PO$_4$ plus 25 mM Na$_2$SO$_4$, pH 2.5 adjusted with H$_3$PO$_4$)=6:4.   20,23-DiOH-MPTL implys 20,23-dihydroxyl-5-$\underline{O}$-mycaminosylprotylonolide.   For other abbreviations, see Fig. 3.

Table 1. Requirements for MPTL 20- and 23-hydroxylases[a)] (15).

Addition (mM)				Relative activity (%)	
α-Keto-glutarate (1.0)	NADH (1.0)	Fe^{2+} (0.1)	Ascorbate (1.0)	20-Hydroxylase	23-Hydroxylase
−	−	−	−	10	0
+	−	−	−	100[b)]	100[c)]
−	+	−	−	18	6
−	−	+	−	16	2
−	−	−	+	15	0
+	+	−	−	—	100
+	−	+	−	98	122
+	−	−	+	107	104
+	+	−	−	41	57
−	−	+	+	11	0
−	+	+	+	—	0
+	−	+	+	81	118
+	+	−	+	—	100
+	+	+	−	—	105

a) The reaction mixture contained in a total volume of 0.1 ml: 10 mM phosphate buffer (pH 6.5), additions as indicated, enzyme protein 0.5-0.7 mg. The incubation was done at 27°C for 20 min. Reaction products were determined by HPLC as described in Fig. 4.
b) 20-OH-MPTL 56 μM was taken as 100%.
c) 23-OH-MPTL 69.7 μM was taken as 100%.

no product was formed under an atomosphere of nitrogen gas, suggesting the involvement of molecular oxygen in the reactions. The same was true for the oxidation of C-23. It is suggested that 20-oxo-MPTL receives one oxygen atom from molecular oxygen by the catalysis of 23-hydroxylase in the presence of α-ketoglutarate. Concomitantly, α-ketoglutarate is decarboxylated to succinate which bears another atom of molecular oxygen at one of two terminal carboxyl hydroxyls (Fig. 5). This hypothesis is supported, because the amount of labled

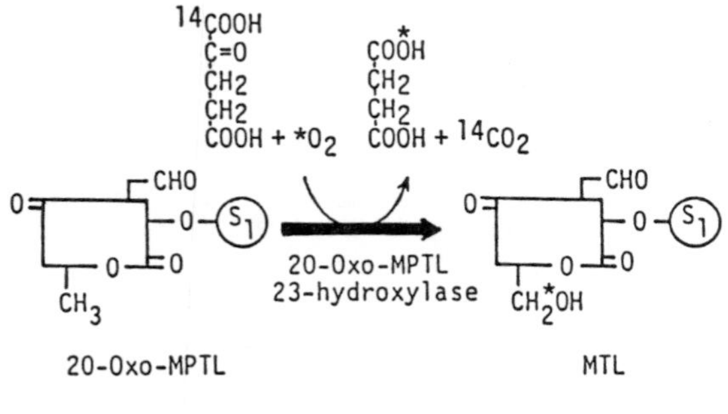

Fig. 5 Reaction mechanism of 20-oxo-MPTL 23-hydroxylase.

carbon dioxide generated from $1-[^{14}C]-\alpha$-ketoglutarate was proportional
to the amount of MTL formed enzymatically. Thus, 20- and 23-hydrox-
ylating enzymes are dioxygenases with different properties.

In cephalosporin biosynthesis by C. acremonium, ring expandase
(17), an enzyme responsible for the conversion of the 5-membered
penicillin N to the 6-membered deacetoxycephalosporin C, and
deacetoxycephalosporin C 3-methyl-oxidizing enzyme (18) were reported
to be α-ketoglutrate- and molecular oxygen-requiring dioxygenases. In
a plant system, flavanone 3-hydroxylase is such a dioxygenase.

Table 2 shows the substrate specificities of 20- and 23-hydroxyl-
ases. MPTL is the best substrate for 20-hydroxylation (15). 23-OH-
MPTL follows it, suggesting that 20,23-diOH-MPTL is formed if 23-OH-
MPTL is available intracellularly. Actually, however, this may not be
the case. 23-OH-MPTL is not synthesized enzymatically from MPTL, as
will be described later. In addition, a separate experiment with MPTL
as the substrate demonstrated that the ratio of 20-OH-MPTL over total
reaction products was higher (>70%) when the reaction period was
shorter. This indicates strongly that 20-OH-MPTL is the major product
formed from MPTL. An aminosugar attached at C-5 is necessary for
20-hydroxylation. Although not shown here, 5-O-mycaminosyl and
desosaminyl derivatives served as equally good substrates, but neutral
sugar-bearing 5-O-mycarosylprotylonolide was not oxidized at all.

Table 2. Substrate specificities of enzymes involved in the formation
of MTL from MPTL[a] (15).

MTPL 20-hydroxylase		20-OH-MPTL dehydrogenase		20-Oxo-MPTL 23-hydroxylase	
Substrate	Relative activity (%)	Substrate	Relative activity (%)	Substrate	Relative activity (%)
PTL	0	20-OH-MPTL	100[c]	20-Oxo-MPTL	100[d]
23-OH-PTL	0	20,23-diOH-MPTL	87	20-OH-MPTL	66
MPTL	100[b]	Demycarosyl-relomycin	36	MPTL	0
23-OH-MPTL	62	Relomycin	62	PTL	0
5-O-Mycarosyl-PTL	0				
23-O-Mycinosyl-PTL	0				
20-Deoxy-demycarosyl-relomycin	0				
20-Deoxy-relomycin	0				

a) For abbreviations, see Figs. 3 and 4.
b) 20-OH-MPTL at 25.4 μM was taken as 100%.
c) wo-Oxo-MPTL at 3.9 μM was taken as 100%.
d) MTL at 80.7 μM was taken as 100%.

Protylonolide moiety is preferred to platenolide moiety.   The optimal
pH was 6.5.

As to 23-hydroxylatin, 20-oxo-MPTL is the best substrate.
20-OH-MPTL served as a less good substrate, but MPTL was not oxidized.
This indicates again that MPTL is oxidized preferentially at C-20
rather than at C-23.   It appears that previous oxidation at C-20 is
necessary for 23-hydroxylation.   The optimal pH was 6.5.

2.4.2 20-Hydroxy-5-<u>O</u>-mycaminosylprotylonolide (20-OH-MPTL)
      20-dehydrogenase

20-OH-MPTL is dehydrogenated by a cell-free extract from <u>S</u>.
<u>fradiae</u> at the expense of NAD and, although at a slower rate, of NADP.
This enzyme is of broad substrate specificity (Table 2) (15).   20,23-
diOH-MPTL was oxidized to MTL almost at the same rate, thereby forming
a metabolic grid.

2.5 Summary of Biosynthetic Studies

The above results are in good accordance with the results obtained by bioconversion experiments described earlier (Fig. 3).   Where no
bioconversion was observed (with a mark X in Fig. 3), cell-free oxidation was not detected, either.   For example, protylonolide was not
oxidized either at C-20 or C-23.   The possibility of the first oxidation of protylonolide at C-20 followed by mycaminosylation at C-5 can
be ruled out.   Oxidations at C-20 of 20-deoxydemycarosylrelomycin and
of 20-deoxyrelomycin was not suggested by bioconversion studies (Fig.
3), and by cell-free studies (Table 2).   The only discrepancy is on
the route from MPTL to 23-OH-MPTL, which was indicated by bioconversion studies, but was not shown to occur by cell-free studies (Table
2).   The reason for this is not known.

All the results of cell-free studies described above together
with those of bioconversion studies suggest the pathway to tylosin, as
shown in Fig. 6.

Recently, genetic studies on tylosin biosynthesis led Baltz <u>et</u>
<u>al</u>. (19,20) to propose a preferred pathway to tylosin in <u>S</u>. <u>fradiae</u>.
The proposed pathway is essentially identical with that obtained by
our experiments, but the steps of methylation occurring on the
mycinose moiety were clarified.   According to these authors, the
second sugar attached to MTL is not mycinose itself, but its demethyl
derivative deoxyallose.   To the diglycosylated intermediate is tied
the third sugar mycarose forming demethylmacrocin, which is methylated
successively on the hydroxyls at C-2 and C-3 of the deoxyallose moiety

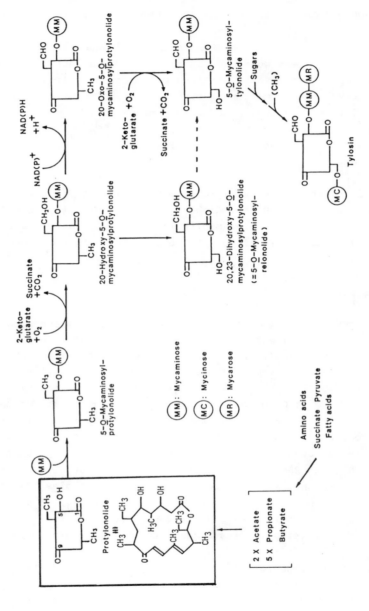

Fig. 6. Proposed biosynthetic pathway to tylosin in S. fradiae KA-427, and enzymes involved in it. From Ōmura et al. (15,16)

to complete tylosin biosynthesis.   The biosynthesis of the mycarose
moiety, bearing a methionine-derived methyl at C-3, appears to be
completed before its attachment to mycaminose (21).

3 NITROGEN CATABOLITE REGULATION OF TYLOSIN BIOSYNTHESIS

Tylosin biosynthesis by S. fradiae is regulated by several
mechanisms which are also involved in the biosynthesis of other
secondary metabolites.   These include induction, carbon and nitrogen
catabolite regulation, phosphate regulation, and feedback inhibition.
Resistance of the producing organism to the action of its own
antibiotic is an important prerequisite. In some cases, mechanisms of
regulation are suggested at the enzyme level.   Of these regulatory
mechanisms, nitrogen catabolite regulation was least understood before
we began to study it.

Table 3 lists antibiotics whose synthesis is controlled by
nitrogenous compounds. It is noted that this type of regulation is
not limited either to the biosynthesis of nitrogen-containing
antibiotics or to nitrogen-involving biosynthetic reactions such as
transamination.

The occurrence of nitrogen catabolite regulation of tylosin
biosynthesis was observed in the course of study on macrolide
fermentation with the use of ammonium-trapping agents.

Table 3. Nitrogen catabolite regulation in antibiotic biosynthesis

Antibiotic	Producing organism	Target of action	Reference
Cephamycin	Streptomyces clavuligerus	Cyclase & ring expanding enzyme	(22)
Cephalosporin	Cephalosporium acremonium	Ring expanding enzyme & cyclase	(23)
Tylosin	S. fradiae	Valine dehydrogenase	(24)
Leucomycin	Streptoverticillium kitasatoensis	Valine dehydrogenase	
Patulin	Penicillium urticae	m-Hydroxybenzyl alcohol dehydrogenase	(25)

3.1 Effect of Ammonium-Trapping Agents on Antibiotic Production and the Relevance to Nitrogen Catabolite Regulation

In an early paper, we reported a stimulatory effect of magnesium
phosphate on leucomycin production by Stv. kitasatoensis (26,27).   The

Table 4. Enhancement of antibiotic production by ammonium ion-trapping agents.

Organism	Antibiotic	NH$_4^+$-Trapping agent	Amount added (%)	Maximum antibiotic titers (µg/ml) No addition	Maximum antibiotic titers (µg/ml) Addition	References
Streptoverticillium kitasatoensis	Leucomycin	Magnesium phosphate (MgP)	1.0	700	3800	(26-28)
Streptomyces ambofaciens	Spiramycin	Sodium phosphotungstate	0.5	150	450	(28)
S. fradiae	Tylosin	Natural zeolite (ZL)	1.0	59	149	(29)
Cephalosporium acremonium	Cephamycin	MgP	1.0	400	1600	(23)
Streptomyces sp.	Dihydrostreptomycin	MgP	1.0	55	145	
Streptomyces sp.	Chloramphenicol	MgP	1.0	7	32	
S. aureofaciens	Tetracycline	MgP	1.0	28	45	
S. rosa subsp. notoensis	Nanaomycin	NH$_4^+$-satd. ZL	0.2	85	750	(31)
C. caerulens	Cerulenin	ZL	1.0	40	280	(30)

enhancement of antibiotic yield was associated with a marked reduction of ammonium in the supplemented media. The mechanism was assumed as follows. Magnesium phosphate captures ammonium and reduces the concentration in the medium down to a threshold level. This causes a release of the leucomycin-producing machinery from inhibition by ammonium, leading to promotion of antibiotic production.

Magnesium phosphate and other ammonium-trapping agents enhanced production of other macrolides such as spiramycin (28) and tylosin (28,29) (Table 4). Aminoglycosides, β-lactams (23), and cerulenin (30) are also among such antibiotics. Two- to ten-fold increases in titers were brought about, although the extent of enhancement depended on trapping agents, producing organisms, and media employed. Not every antibiotic production examined was increased by only one of the trapping agents used. Magnesium phosphate was effective in one case, but natural zeolite was desirable in the other.

Not every antibiotic production which was enhanced by an ammonium-trapping agent had not been reported to be sensitive to the ions, but many cases were demonstrated later to be so. These include leucomycin production by Stv. kitasatoensis promoted by magnesium phosphate (27), spiramycin production by S. ambofaciens increased by sodium phosphotungstate, and cerulenin productin by C. caerulens enhanced by natural zeolite (30). Exceptional is nanaomycin production, which is apparently stimulated by a small amount of ammonium (31). Thus, the use of ammonium-trapping agents is not only a convenient method to improve significantly macrolide and other antibiotic yields, but its results, that is, an enhancement of antibiotic production, can be regarded as an evidence suggesting that nitrogen catabolite regulation is an underlying factor that affects production of the antibiotics.

Tylosin production by S. fradiae was not promoted by magnesium phosphate possibly due to phosphate inhibition. However, it increased four-fold when ammonium magnesium phosphate, a water-insoluble material, was used as sole nitrogen source in place of soluble ammonium salts (28). In addition, the supplement of a mordenite-containing natural zeolite, which is known as an ammonium-trapping agent, resulted in a three-fold increase of the tylosin titer with simultaneous reduction of ammonium levels in the supplemented media (29). Such increases indicates the operation of nitrogen catabolite regulation of tylosin biosynthesis in S. fradiae. The mechanism was studied below.

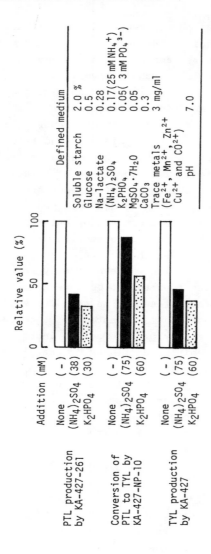

Fig. 7.   Effects of $(NH_4)_2SO_4$ and K_2PHO_4 on tylosin (TYL) and protylonolide (PTL) production, and on conversion of PTL to TYL by *S. fradiae* KA-427 and its mutants in a defined medium.

Possible blocked steps in the two mutants are shown in Fig. 1. The two mutants and the parent strain KA-427 were grown in the defined medium given, to which $(NH_4)_2SO_4$ and K_2HPO_4 were supplemented as indicated. Relative amounts of products are shown. From Ōmura et al. (32).

3.2 Sites of Ammonium Action

Two blocked mutants of S. fradiae, strains 261 and NP-10, and the parent strain KA-427 were used to study the site of action of ammonium. As described earlier, these two mutants function in an earlier and a later part of tylosin biosynthetic pathway. Therefore, whether ammonium affects the earlier or later part of the pathway can be indicated by responses of the mutants to the ions. A chemically defined medium was developed in which the parent strain KA-427 produces tylosin, whereas strain 261 accumulates protylonolide, and strain NP-10 converts added protylonolide to tylosin.

Figure 7 shows that the addition of ammonium sulfate to the defined medium decreases tylosin production by KA-427. This decrease was found to be due to suppression of protylonolide formation, as can be seen from the inhibitory effect of ammonium on protylonolide production by strain 261, while only a weak effect on the conversion of protylonolide to tylosin by strain NP-10 (32).

Protylonolide biosynthesis starts with metabolism of amino acids, succinate, or of higher fatty acids to supply lower fatty acids (see Section 3). We focused our attention on the amino acid metabolism as a possible site of ammonium action. The rationale is as follows. According to Magasanik (33), the degradation of glutamine, asparagine, proline and histidine is controlled by extracellular ammonium levels in enteric bacteria. The enzyme protein of glutamine synthetase plays a central role in this control mechanism. Such a mechanism has been demonstrated to occur also in thienamycin-producing S. cattleya (34). The present authors showed the involvement of ammonium and glutamine synthetase as effectors regulating glycine decarboxylase synthesis in Nocardia butanica (35).

Short-term production of protylonolide by resting cells of strain 261 was monitored by radioisotope and HPLC analyses. Strain 261 was grown under high- and low-ammonium conditions. Figure 8 shows that the incorporation of carbons from labeled valine and threonine into protylonolide decreased considerably when strain 261 was previously grown in 75 mM ammonium, as compared to the cells previously grown in 25 mM ammonium (8). Unexpectedly, a similar decrease was observed when labeled succinate was used as the substrate. HPLC analysis, determining the amount of protylonolide produced instead of the radio-activity, gave similar results.

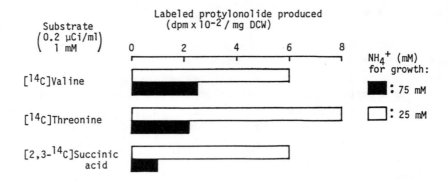

Fig. 8 Labeled protylonolide production by resting cells of S. fradiae
        strain 261 previously grown under two NH₄⁺ conditions.

Cells of two-day cultures were incubated with the indicated
substrates at 27 °C for 5 hours in 0.1 M MOPS (pH 7.8). Radioactivity
of protylonolide formed is shown.

The pathway to protylonolide was divided tentatively into two
parts: one was the metabolism of sources of lower fatty acids
supplying acetate, propionate and n-butyrate, and the other one was
for their condensation and post-condensation processes to afford
protylonolide. To examine which one of the two is the site of
ammonium action, the reversal effect of lower fatty acids on
inhibition by ammonium was studied. Figure 9 indicates that under
conditions in which ammonium sulfate inhibits protylonolide formation
by about 50% or more, the addition of the three acids acetate,
propionate and n-butyrate reversed ammonium inhibition almost
completely (8). It is worthy to note that isobutyrate and/or
α-keto-isovalerate, which are to be derived from valine metabolism,
had a similar reversing effect. These observations suggest that the
action of ammonium is directed at least toward steps between valine
and isobutyrate, and between threonine and propionate, but is not so
toward steps after formation of the building units for protylonolide
biosynthesis, involving the condensation reaction.

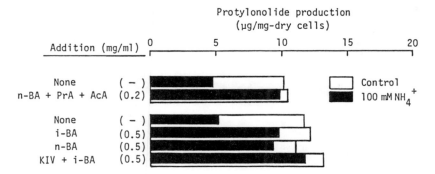

Fig. 9 Inhibitory effect of ammonium on protylonolide production by S. fradiae strain 261, and its reversal by valine-derived lower fatty acids.

Strain 261 was grown in a defined medium (see Fig. 7) supplemented with one or both of 100 mM ammonium and the indicated fatty acids. From Ōmura et al. (8)

3.3 Valine Dehydrogenase as One of the Targets of Nitrogen Catabolite Regulation

Valine dehydrogenase, an enzyme catalysing a deaminating reaction converting valine to α-keto-isovalerate, was singled out to examine if it is one of the targets of ammonium action. Protylonolide producing mutant, strain 261, was grown in defined media containing ammonium ranging from 25 to 100 mM. Cell-free extracts were prepared from these cells. The protylonolide titers decreased as the increase of ammonium levels. Valine dehydrogenase activity in the cell extracts decreased in parallel to the decline of protylonolide titers (24). A similar result was obtained when cell-free extracts prepared from the tylosin producer KA-427 previously grown with or without ammonium supplements were used (Table 5). Alanine dehydroganase activity did not correlate with the tylosin titers, suggesting that the variations in valine dehydrogenase is not a general response to ammonium, but is surely relevant to tylosin biosynthesis.

Although not shown here, threonine deaminase activity varied just as valine dehydrogenase did in cell-free extracts, but glutamine synthetase activity did not correlate with tylosin production. It appears that the fine mechanism involved in the regulation of tylosin biosynthesis by ammonium is different from those of the general amino acid metabolism in enteric bacteria.

Table 5. Effects of various compounds on the production of tylosin,
          valine dehydrogenase (VDH) and alanine dehydrogenase (ADH).

Effector	Amount added (mM)	pH	Specific TYL production (µg/mg-dry cells)	VDH (U/mg-P)	ADH (U/mg-P)
None	–	7.2	8.5	11.7	15.3
Glucose	55	6.2	8.4	12.9	26.4
$(NH_4)_2SO_4$	75	6.2	5.6	0	42.5
K_2HPO_4[a]	62	5.6	1.3	2.1	11.1

a) K_2HPO_4; KH_2PO_4 (0.3%) + K_2HPO_4 (0.7%)
   Added at the 2nd day: 4-day culture in defined medium

4 PHOSPHATE REGULATION OF TYLOSIN BIOSYNTHESIS

4.1 Phosphate Regulation of Antibiotic Production, and Effect of Phosphate-Trapping Agents

Inorganic phosphate is one of the important regulatory effectors
in microbial secondary metabolite formation. Enzymatic mechanisms of
phosphate regulation were suggested in cephalosporin (36), streptomycin (37), candicidin (41), and tetracycline (42) biosyntheses (Table
6). It is expected that such regulation is released by reducing
phosphate levels in media, resulting in an increase of antibiotic
production. By analogy with the ammonium-trapping agents described
earlier, phosphate depression may be accomplished by adding phosphate-
trapping agents. We found that Kanuma earth is effective as one of
such agents. Kanuma earth is a clay found around volcanic mountains
like Kanuma district, Tochigi, Japan. It contains the mineral
allophane, an amorphous hydrogel composed of silica gel and alumina
gel, and possesses a potent phosphate-trapping capacity. The
mechanism of the phosphate-trapping reaction is not known. Table 7
summarizes enhanching effects of Kanuma earth on production of various
antibiotics. Tylosin production was increased two-fold (Fig. 10),
and nanaomycin production five-fold. These increases are assumed to
be a consequence of release from phosphate regulation when the
regulation is already known, or an indication of its occurrence if it
has not been suggested.

Table 6. Phosphate regulation in antibiotic biosynthesis.

Antibiotic	Producing organism	Target of action	Reference
Cephalosporin	Cephalosporium acremonium	Ring expanding enzyme	(36)
Streptomycin	Streptomyces griseus	SM-P phosphatase	(37)
Neomycin	S. fradiae	NM-P phosphatase	(38)
Tylosin	S. fradiae	TDP-Glucose 4,6-dehydratase	(39)
		TDP-Mycarose-forming enzyme	(39)
		Macrocin O-methyltransferase	(39)
		Valine dehydrogenase	
		Methylmalonyl-CoA carboxytransferase	(40)
		Propionyl-CoA carboxylase	(40)
Candicidin	S. griseus	p-Aminobenzoate synthetase	(42)
Tetracycline	S. aureofaciens	Anhydrotetracycline oxygenase	(43)

Table 7. Enhancement of antibiotic production by Kanuma earth, a phosphate-trapping agent.

Organism	Antibiotic	Antibiotic titers(µg/ml)	
		Not added	Kanuma earth added (0.5%)
Streptomyces fradiae	Tylosin	70	130
S. fradiae	Protylonolide	56	122
S. erythraeus	Erythromycin	29[a]	46[a]
S. rosa subsp. notoensis	Nanaomycin	110	560
S. orientalis	Vancomycin	14.5[b]	18.3[b]
Pseudonocardia azurea	Azureomycin	trace	15.0[b]
Micromonospora echinospora subsp. echinospora	Gentamicin	3	18

a) Titers at day 4. At day 5, ca. 100 µg/ml was reached in both conditions.
b) Diameter (mm) of inhibition zone.

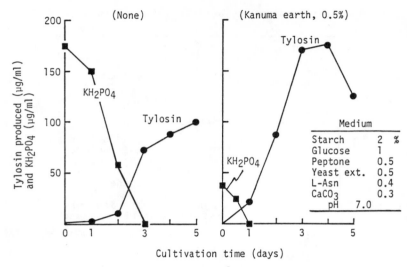

Fig. 10 Effect of Kanuma earth, a PO_4^{3-}-trapping aget, on tylosin
production by S. fradiae KA-427 and PO_4^{3-} concentration in the
medium.

4.2 Mechanism of Phosphate Regulation of Tylosin Biosynthesis in S. fradiae

Pape (39), and Vu-Trong (40) studied phosphate regulation of
tylosin biosynthesis at the enzyme level (Table 6). Our findings
shown in Fig. 7 are in support of their results, indicating that
phosphate inhibits tylosin biosynthesis by affecting both protylonolide formation and its conversion to tylosin. Table 5 shows
that valine dehydrogenase activity decreases in dependence on the
amount of added phosphate, while alanine dehydrogenase activity does
not do so. It is suggested that, in addition to the already reported
sites, valine dehydrogenase is another target of phosphate action in
tylosin biosynthesis.

5 SUMMARY OF STUDIES ON REGULATION

The results of our studies presented above are summarized in Fig.
11. It is concluded that ammonium and phosphate cause a limited
supply of building units to suppress protylonolide construction,
leading subsequently to a reduction of tylosin biosynthesis. It is

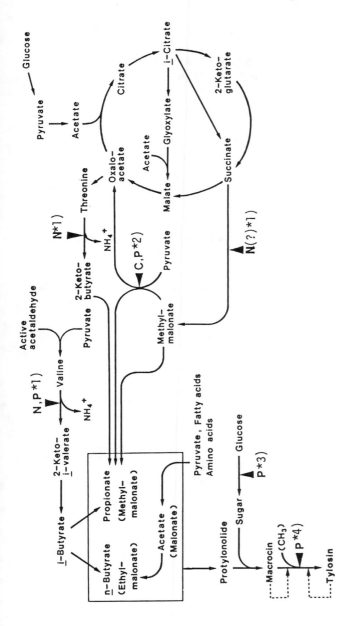

Fig. 11. Proposed sites (▼) of carbon (C), nitrogen (N) and phosphate (P) regulation and feedback inhibition (-----) in the pathway to tylosin in S. fradiae. *1), Present study; *2), Vu-Trong et al. (41); *3), Madry and Pape (30); *4), Seno and Baltz (20).

emphasized that amino acid metabolism is important both in supplying lower fatty acids and as the targets of ammonium and phosphate regulation. This mechanism appears to be of general significance in the biosynthesis of other types of polyketide antibiotics, and suggests that mutations for potentiating both the synthesis and degradation of relevant amino acids are beneficial for improving production of the antibiotic.

Carbon and nitrogen catabolites, and phosphate affect tylosin production at multiple steps. Release from the regulation by mutation may require multi-step trials, but that by trapping agents is accomplished by a single addition of them. This explains why a marked increase in antibiotic titers is brought about by the latter technique. This method is applicable to the improvement of antibiotic fermentation, and to the search for new antibiotics. The usefulness has been proved. Details will be described elsewhere.

It is unlikely that ammonium and phosphate interact directly with resonsible genes to control their expression. Intracellular chemical messengers have to be postulated, but the nature of such messengers and fine regulatory mechanims at the molecular level await further investigations. Stringent responses in tylosin biosynthesis is also a subject of future studies.

6 REFERENCES

(1)   S. Ōmura, Y. Tanaka, in Macrolide Antibiotics. Chemistry, Biology and Practice (S. Ōmura, ed.), Academic Press, Orlando 1984, pp. 199–229.

(2)   S. Ōmura, A. Nakagawa, in Antibiotics, Vol. 4 (J. W. Corcoran, ed.), Academic Press, New York 1981, pp. 175–192.

(3)   S. Ōmura, Y. Tanaka, in Biochemistry and Genetic Regulation of Commercially Important Antibiotics (L. C. Vining, ed.), Addison-Wesley, Massachusetts 1983, pp. 179–206.

(4)   H. Sakakibara, S. Ōmura in (1), pp. 85–125.

(5)   S. Ōmura, C. Kitao, H. Matsubara, Chem. Pharm. Bull., 29 (1980) 1963–1965.

(6)   S. Ōmura, H. Takeshima, A. Nakagawa, N. Kanemoto, G. Lukacs, Bioorg. Chem. 5 (1976) 451–454.

(7)   S. Ōmura, A. Nakagawa, A. Neszmelyi, S. D. Gero, A.-M. Sepulchre, F. Piriou, G. Lukacs, J. Am. Chem. Soc. 97 (1975) 4001–4009.

(8)   S. Ōmura, A. Taki, K. Matsuda, Y. Tanaka, J. Antibiot. 37 (1984) 1362–1369.

(9)   S. Ōmura, K. Tsuzuki, Y. Tanaka, H. Sakakibara, M. Aizawa, G. Lukacs, J. Antibiot. 36 (1983) 614–619.

(10) S. Pospíšil, P. Sedmera, M. Havránek, V. Krumphanzl, Z.
     Vanek, J. Antibiot. 36 (1983) 617-619.

(11) J. E. Dotzlaf, L. S. Metzger, M. A. Foglesong, Antimicrob. Agents
     Chemother. 25 (1984) 216-220.

(12) S. Ōmura, N. Sadakane, H. Matsubara, Chem. Pharm. Bull. 30 (1982)
     223-229.

(13) S. Ōmura, Bacteriol. Rev. 40 (1976) 681-697.

(14) S. Ōmura, in Methods in Enzymology. Vol. 72 (J. M. Lowenstein,
     ed.), Academic Press, New York 1981, pp. 520-532.

(15) S. Ōmura, H. Tomoda, S. Yamamoto, M. Tsukui, H. Tanaka, Biochim.
     Biophys. Acta 802 (1984) 141-147.

(16) S. Ōmura, H. Tanaka, M. Tsukui, Biochem. Biophys. Res. Commun.
     107 (1982) 554-560.

(17) J. Kupka, Y.-Q. Shen, S. Wolfe, A. L. Demain, Can. J. Microbiol.
     29 (1983) 488-496.

(18) M. K. Turner, J. E. Farthing, S. J. Brewer, Biochem. J. 173
     (1978) 839-850.

(19) R. H. Baltz, E. T. Seno, J. Stonesifer, G. M. Wild, J. Anti-
     biot. 36 (1983) 131-141.

(20) E. T. Seno, R. H. Baltz, Antimicrob. Agents Chemother. 21 (1982)
     758-763.

(21) H. Pape, G. U. Brillinger, Arch. Microbiol. 88 (1973) 25-35.

(22) A. L. Demain, this volume.

(23) Y.-Q. Shen, J. Heim, N. A. Solomon, A. L. Demain, J. Antibiot. 37
     (1984) 503-511.

(24) S. Ōmura, Y. Tanaka, H. Mamada, R. Masuma, J. Antibiot. 36 (1983)
     1972-1974.

(25) J. W. D. Grootwassink, G. M. Gaucher, J. Bacteriol. 141 (1980)
     443-455.

(26) S. Ōmura, Y. Tanaka, C. Kitao, H. Tanaka, Y. Iwai, Antimicrob.
     Agents Chemother. 18 (1980) 691-695.

(27) Y. Tanaka, Y. Takahashi, R. Masuma, Y. Iwai, H. Tanaka, S. Ōmura,
     Agric. Biol. Chem. 45 (1981) 2475-2481.

(28) S. Ōmura, Y. Tanaka, H. Tanaka, Y. Takahashi, Y. Iwai, J.
     Antibiot. 33 (1980) 1568-1569.

(29) R. Masuma, Y. Tanaka, S. Ōmura, J. Ferment. Technol. 61 (1983)
     607-614.

(30) R. Masuma, Y. Tanaka, S. Ōmura, J. Antibiot. 35 (1982) 1184-
     1193.

(31) Y. Tanaka, R. Masuma, S. Ōmura, J. Antibiot. 37 (1984) 1370-1375.

(32) S. Ōmura, Y. Tanaka, H. Mamada, R. Masuma, J. Antibiot. 37 (1984)
     494-502.

(33) B. Magasanik, Annu. Rev. Genet. 16 (1982) 135-168.

(34) S. L. Streicher, B. Tyler, Pro. Natl. Acad. Sci. USA 78 (1981) 229-233.

(35) Y. Tanaka, S. Ōmura, K. Araki, K. Nakayama, Agric. Biol. Chem. 45 (1981) 2661-2664.

(36) J. F. Martín, G. Revilla, D. M. Zanca, M. J. Lopez-Nieto, in Trends in Antibiotic Research (H. Umezawa et al. eds.), Japan Antibiot. Res. Assoc., Tokyo 1982, pp. 258-268.

(37) M. S. Walker, J. B. Walker, J. Biol. Chem. 246 (1971) 7034-7040.

(38) M. K. Majumdar, S. K. Majumdar, Folia Mirobiol. 16 (1971) 285-292.

(39) N. Madry, H. Pape, Arch. Microbiol. 131 (1982) 170-173.

(40) K. Vu-Trong, S. Bhuwapathanapun, P. P. Gray, Antimicrob. Agents Chemother. 19 (1981) 209-212.

(41) ibid. 17 (1980) 519-525.

(42) J. F. Martín, G. Naharro, P. Liras, J. R. Villanueva, J. Antibiot. 32 (1979) 600-606.

(43) V. Běhal, J. Grégrová-Prušáková, Z. Hošťálek, Folia Microbiol. 27 (1982) 102-106.

Productivity of Aminoglycoside Antibiotics With Reference to Antibiotic Resistance of the Producer

Yoshiro Okami

Microbial Chemistry Research Foundation, Institute of Microbial Chemistry, 3-14-23, Kamiosaki 3-chome, Shinagawa-ku, Tokyo, Japan

SUMMARY

   Aminoglycoside antibiotic producers were found to be resistant to multiple aminoglycoside antibiotics, including the antibiotics produced. The inactivation by enzymes, ribosomal resistance and the permeability of the cell surface barrier are major mechanisms for the resistance of target clinical bacteria for antibiotics, but the resistance of amino-glycoside antibiotic producers to aminoglycoside antibiotics is sometimes complex with a combination of the above major mechanisms. However, antibiotic resistance as a phenotype is very useful for the selection of desired clones after genetic manipulations. Fusion treatment and protoplast regeneration of aminoglycoside antibiotic producers offered possibility for generation of new antibiotic productions after selection of clones by the resistance to aminoglycoside antibiotics as the selective markers. The streptomycin (SM) resistance gene was cloned and mapped by restriction enzymes, and was found to encode in cluster with the SM synthesis gene within a short DNA fragment. The producer of an aminoglycoside antibiotic, istamycin (IM), produced several related metabolites simultaneously in the fermented broth. The regula-tion for the production of IM was studied both by experiments of environmental manipulations of the producer and by conversion experiments of their products as the substrates for the growing cell of the producer. Based on the results of conversion experiments, a biosynthetic pathway is presumed, even without employing blocked mutants and radioisotopic tracers. The regulatory manipulation for the yield of each product in the fermentation broth is discussed.

1 ANTIBIOTIC RESISTANCE OF ANTIBIOTIC PRODUCER

Resistance of clinical isolates to aminoglycoside antibiotics has been studied intensively and the plasmid-determined inactivating enzymes were found to play a major role in the resistance. On the other hand, the antibiotic resistance of the producers seems not to be analogous to the above, though studies have not been deep, in comparison with those performed on clinical pathogens. There is an idea that the resistance determinant in clinical pathogen may have originated from antibiotic-producing organisms (1). In this regard, it was reported that the inactivating enzymes of aminoglycoside antibiotics in clinical pathogens had considerable homologies with those of aminoglycoside-producing organisms. However, immunological cross-reactions were not found between the inactivating enzymes of pathogenic bacteria and those of aminoglycoside antibiotic-producing organisms. In spite of accumulated evidences that the lack of inactivating enzymes in some producers corresponded to the reduction of the antibiotic productivity (2,3) and that increased antibiotic production often corresponded with increases of the inactivating enzymes in the producers (4), the precise role of those inactivating enzymes in the antibiotic producers has not been yet made clear.

To yield sufficient amount of antibiotic in the fermented broth, an antibiotic producer must be protected from the inhibitory action of its own antibiotic produced (self-resistance) to avoid suicide (5). For this protection mechanism, the inactivating enzymes may have a possible role in the resistance, since inactivated products of the antibiotics by acetylation or phosphorylation have been found in the course of fermentation. Even so, the inactivation by enzymes may not be the sole mechanism for the protection from suicide. Decrease of inward permeability of antibiotic (6), adsorption of the antibiotic on the cell wall which protects the inward penetration of the excreted inhibitory products (6) or resistance of target ribosomes to antibiotics (7,8) are the other possible mechanisms for resistance of the producer to aminoglycoside antibiotics.

As observed in the biosynthesis of streptomycin (SM), SM is phosphorylated and inactivated by SM-phosphorylase before the excretion from the producer cells (9). Accordingly, it was suggested that such inactivation by enzymes may be involved in the biosynthesis of amino-glycoside antibiotics. As it is, when the DNA of neomycin (NM)-producing S. fradiae was ligated with plasmid and introduced into S. lividans, the recipient became resistant to NM, but the production of NM was not expressed (10). Thus, the relationship between the inacti-vating-enzyme, the resistance and the production of NM failed to be revealed.   Up to now, the direct relationship between the self-resistance and the antibiotic production is revealed merely in methylenomycin, which is not aminoglycoside antibiotic, and the gene of which is encoded in plasmid SCP_1 (11).

Table 1. Antibiotic resistance of antibiotic producing actinomycetes.

Organisms	Antibiotics produced	Resistance* to 50 µg/ml of														
		Aminoglycosides											Others**			
		SM	KM	DK	GM	RM	BT	NM	PR	LV	NE	IS	TC	CP	EM	AC
Streptomyces tenebrarius ISP5477	Nebramycins	●	●	●	●	●	●	●	●	●	●	●		●	●	●
S. spectabilis ISP5512	Spectinomycin	●	○	●	◐	●	●	●	●	●	●	●		●	●	●
S. kasugaensis MB273	Kasugamycin	●	●	◐	◐	●	◐	●	●	●	●	●	NT***	NT	NT	NT
S. tenjimariensis SS-939	Istamycins	●	●	●	●	●	●	●	●	●	●	●		●		
S. kanamyceticus ISP5500	Kanamycins	●	●	●	●	●	●	●	●	●	●		◐			
S. fradiae ISP5063	Neomycins	○	○	●	●	●	○	●	●	●						
Micromonospora sp. SS-1853	Gentamicins	●	●	●		●						●				
S. catenulae ISP5258	Paromomycin					●			●				○	●		●
S. griseus ISP5236	Streptomycins	●													◐	◐
S. aureofaciens ISP5127	Chlortetracycline												●	●		
S. venezuelae ISP5230	Chloramphenicol												●	●		
S. omiyaensis ISP5552	Chloramphenicol															●
S. antibioticus ISP5234	Actinomycins														●	
S. erythreus ISP5517	Erythromycin									●				●	●	●
S. griseinus ISP5047	Grisein	●			●					●	●					●
S. griseochromogenes ISP5499	Blasticidins	●			●	●				●	●		●	●	●	●

* Solid circle, half solid circle, open circle and no indication refer to good growth, retarded growth, variable growth, and no growth, respectively.

** TC: tetracycline,   CP: chloramphenicol,   EM: erythromycin,   AC: actinomycin D.

*** NT: Not tested.   Abbreviation of aminoglycosides refer in the text.

In spite of the lack of direct verification for the relationship between antibiotic resistance and antibiotic productivity of the aminoglycoside antibiotic-producing organisms, the relation of antibiotic resistance to the productivity of aminoglycoside antibiotics offered interesting subjects to be studied, as follows. When actinomycetes capable of producing various antibiotics were tested for their resistance to 11 kinds of aminoglycoside antibiotics together with 4 other antibiotics which are not aminoglycoside antibiotics, the aminoglycoside antibiotic-producing actinomycetes showed a wide range in spectrum of resistance to the various antibiotics, except for SM-producing S. griseus. Actinomycetes producing other antibiotics than aminoglycoside antibiotics showed no or few resistances to aminoglycoside antibiotics, as shown in Table 1 (12,13). In addition, the results demonstrated that each antibiotic-producing actinomycete has an individual profile, different in antibiotic resistance spectrum depending on the type of antibiotic produced. Therefore, it is expected that the selection of new actinomycetes with new patterns of resistance spectrum may result in the discovery of new antibiotic productivity.

The above expectation led us to screen about 100 strains of actinomycetes newly isolated from coastal sea muds with reference to unique profile of antibiotic resistance spectrum. A strain designated as SS-939 which showed an unique profile of the resistance spectrum was found to produce a new aminoglycoside antibiotic named istamycin (IM). The producer was identified to be a new species, Streptomyces tenjimariensis (14).

S. tenjimariensis SS-939 was highly resistant not only to its own antibiotic, IM, but also to neamine (NE), ribostamycin (RM), kanamycin (KM), and butirosin (BT). Protein synthesis in this strain was not inhibited by its own antibiotic and no inactivating enzyme was found. In order to know the mechanism of antibiotic resistance of this strain, in vitro phenylalanine synthesizing system was successfully prepared by cell-free extract of the strain and the inhibition caused by antibiotics was examined by a reciprocal reconstitution between S150 and ribosomal fractions of this strain, as well as with a strain of S. griseus which was sensitive to IM. Polyphenylalanine synthesis in the systems containing ribosome of S. tenjimariensis was found to be resistant to IM regardless of the origin of S150 fractions, while the synthesis in the systems containing ribosome of S. griseus was sensitive to IM regardless of S150 fraction origin, and the synthesis was resistant to SM only in the presence of the S150 fraction of S. griseus, in which SM-inactivating enzyme was found. To exclude the possibility that the S150 fraction of S. tenjimariensis might possess ATPase or other factors interfering with inactivating enzymes, the S150 fraction was further fractionated by gel filtration on Sephadex G-200 superfine and the eluate was tested for inactivating activity. No enzymic inactivation was confirmed. Thus, ribosomal resistance to the anti- biotics of S. tenjimariensis was confirmed as the first case among aminoglycoside antibiotic-producing streptomycetes (7).

2 ANTIBIOTIC PRODUCTION AND RESISTANCE IN RELATION TO PLASMIDS

Several strains which were identical with S. tenjimariensis in taxonomic features and in IM production were isolated during 3 years at the same place in a coastal sea area. They were found to harbor multiple plasmids in each strain, and the profile of the plasmids on gel-electrophoresis was different among the 3 isolates which were obtained in 3 different years (15). Some of the plasmids were eliminated by plasmid-curring agents, such as acriflavin, but all were never curred. The elimination treatment responded the decrease of antibiotic productivity, suggesting the involvement of plasmids in the productivity. However, which plasmids are involved directly in the antibiotic produc- tivity is not certain. In addition, the elimination of plasmids was not responded to the antibiotic resistance, since the resistance was unchanged by the elimination treatment.

Each of the plasmids was isolated and fragmented by various rest- riction enzymes. The maps of each plasmid based on the restriction sites showed that some plasmids were related in part but others were not entirely related, suggesting they are almost independent from each other. In addition, it was found that the plasmids are compatible with each other within a strain when the strains having different plasmids were protoplasted and treated with fusion treatment in the presence of polyethyleneglycol. It seemed possible that the difference in plasmids between the strains may have occurred during subculture of the strains after their isolation from soil. However, such plasmid changes may not be probable, because no change of plasmids was observed during several subcultures of the strains. Therefore, it is likely that such plasmid changes occurred in the natural environment, where they survived. Furthermore, the strains having different plasmids exhibited the same productivity of IM and also the same antibiotic resistance spectrum, suggesting the relationship between plasmid existence, antibiotic productivity and antibiotic resistance is not a direct one. Accordingly, plasmids in this antibiotic producer may not directly govern the antibiotic productivity of IM nor the ribosomal resistance to antibiotics.

3 GENERATION OF A NEW ANTIBIOTIC PRODUCTIVITY BY FUSION TREATMENT WITH USE OF ANTIBIOTIC RESISTANCE AS A SELECTIVE MARKER

Natural resistance of S. tenjimariensis SS-939 is reciprocal with that of S. griseus SS-1198 in terms of KM and SM (the former is resistant to KM and sensitive to SM), as shown in Table 2. With reference

Table 2. Resistance of S. tenjimariensis SS-939 and S. griseus ISP5236 to aminoglycoside antibiotics.

Antibiotic	Resistance* (μg/ml)	
	S. tenjimariensis SS-939	S. griseus ISP5236
Istamycin A	3,000	< 2
Istamycin B	3,000	< 2
Kanamycin A	3,000	< 2
Neamine	1,200	10
Ribostamycin	500	2
Butirosin A	500	< 2
Neomycin B	20	< 2
Lividomycin A	10	< 2
Streptomycin	1	400

Both strains were incubated at 27°C for 3 days in TSB medium.
*Maximal concentrations permitting growth.

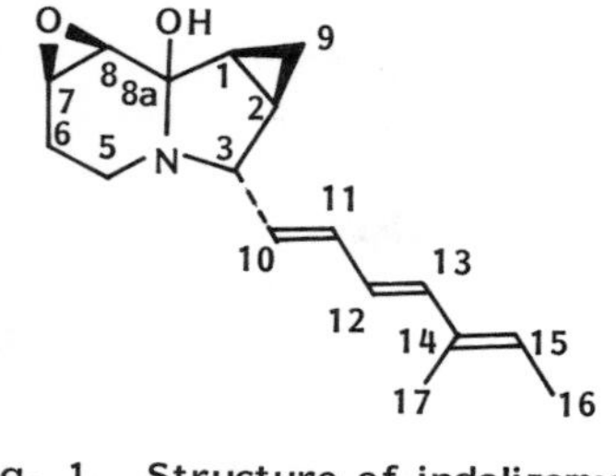

Fig. 1. Structure of indolizomycin.

to this reciprocal resistance as a selective marker, the above two strains belonging to different species were subjected to an interspecies fusion treatment (16,17). Antibiotic non-producing mutants (NP1-1 of S. tenjimariensis and NM16 of S. griseus) were obtained by UV irradiation and fusion treatment with these two mutants resulted in obtaining the clones resistant to both antibiotics (KM^r and SM^r) (18). Certain of these clones generated a new antibiotic productivity and one of the active principles in the fermented broth of SK2-52 clone was extracted, yielding a purified substance indolizomycin, of which structure was

entirely different from the parental antibiotics, as shown in Fig. 1.
It is of great interest that the generation of antibiotic productivity
was exhibited only by clones resistant to 400 µg SM and 20-50 µg KM
(but not by those to 400 µg SM and 10 µg or 40 µg KM), as shown in
Table 3. SM^{r}KM^r clones obtained by self-fusion of each strain did not
give antibiotic production and also prototrophic clones obtained after

Table 3. Antibiotic productivity of SM^{r}KM^r clones.

Strains* used for fusion treatment	Resistance**		Resistant		Antibiotic producer***	
	SM	KM	No./Total	%	No./Total	%
NP1-1 + NM16	400	10	176/1,045	16.8	0/176	0
	400	20-50	831/1,045	79.6	604/831	72.7
	400	400	38/1,045	3.6	0/ 38	0
NP1-1	400	10	259/ 736	35.2	0/259	0
	400	20-50	440/ 736	59.8	0/440	0
	400	400	37/ 736	5.0	0/ 37	0

* NP1-1: S. griseus NP1-1; NM16: S. tenjimariensis NM16
** Upper limit of resistance to streptomycin and kanamycin A (µg/ml).
*** SM^{r}KM^r strains which showed 10.0 mm or larger inhibition zone against
B. subtilis PCI219 by agar cylinder method.

the interspecies fusion treatment between auxotrophic mutants of the
two strains did not generate antibiotic productivity. Therefore, it
can be concluded that the selection of clones by natural resistance
after the interspecies fusion treatment was the successful aspect in
obtaining a novel antibiotic-producing clones. The new antibiotic
producers thus obtained showed a yellow-colored growth appearance
which is identical with S. griseus, but they showed an unique resistance
pattern to multiple aminoglycoside antibiotics which was different
from the profile of the parental S. griseus and also from any profiles
of naturally occuring streptomycetes. In fact, the new indolizomycin-
producing clone was found to be sensitive to IM to which S. tenjimariensis
SS-939 was resistant, and resistant to multiple aminoglycoside antibiotics in addition to SM, to which S. griseus SS-1198 was resistant,
as shown in Table 4. This multiple resistance [KM, dibekacin (DK),
RM, paromomycin (PR), lividomycin (LV) and NE] of SK2-52 were due to
acetylating enzymes, as shown in Table 5. Although there is a report
by Weisblum et al. (19) that resistance to certain antibiotics of
certain streptomycetes and the enhanced antibiotic yield were induced
by direct contact of the organisms with the antibiotics, the present
experiment insured that the organisms had no chance for contact with

Table 4. Resistance of parents and SK2-52 to various aminoglycoside antibiotics.

Organisms	Concentration (μg/ml)	Resistance* to										
		SM	KM	DK	GM	RM	BT	NM	PR	LV	IM	NE
<u>S</u>. <u>griseus</u>												
SS-1198	50	++										
NP1-1	50	++										
<u>S</u>. <u>tenjimariensis</u>												
SS-939	50		++	++		++	++				++	++
NM16	50		++	++		++	++				++	++
SK2-52	50	++	++	++	±	++	+		+	+		++

* SM: streptomycin, KM: kanamycin A, DK: dibekacin, GM: gentamicin C complex, RM: ribostamycin, BT: butirosin A, NM: neomycin B, PR: paromomycin, LV: lividomycin A, IS: istamycin B, NE: neamine. Concentrations as free base.
++: good growth, +: retarded growth, ±: very weak growth, no indication: no growth

Table 5. Acetylation of various aminoglycoside antibiotics by cell free extract.

Antibiotics	SK2-52	
	Resistance*	dpm
Streptomycin	R	0
Kanamycin	R	5,757
Dibekacin	R	4,754
Gentamicin C	S	885
Ribostamycin	R	3,813
Butirosin A	WR	859
Neomycin B	S	866
Paromomycin	R	3,808
Lividomycin A	R	2,549
Neamine	R	2,759
Istamycin B	S	217

Incorporation of [^{14}C]acetyl CoA (dpm) into an antibiotic (100 μg/ml) was measured after reaction mixtures were incubated at 37°C for 60 minutes. Blank values were subtracted.

* Resistance <u>in vivo</u> to 50 μg/ml of antibiotics.

R: resistant, WR: weakly resistant, S: susceptible.

the antibiotics to induce antibiotic productivity and resistance, except with SM, KM and IM, during the experimental procedures. In relation to the protoplast regeneration procedure, it is worthy to note a report by Sugiyama et al. (20) that when S. griseus which was sensitive to SM due to the lack of SM-kinase was treated with protoplast regeneration process, resistance to SM was generated due to the generation of a phosphorylating enzyme. However, $SM^r KM^r$ clones which were obtained by self-fusion treatment between S. griseus NP1-1 and S. tenjimariensis NM16, after the protoplast regeneration process and the selection by both SM and KM, had shown the same growth appearance and antibiotic resistance as those of the ancestor strains (21).

Summarizing the above, it seems likely that the multiple aminoglycoside antibiotic resistance of the new antibiotic producer, SK2-52 clone, was originated partly from a parental strain of S. griseus and partly from another parental strain of S. tenjimariensis, and also had added resistances generated by acetylating enzymes of LV and PR, which were not significant in both the parental strains.

The multiple aminoglycoside antibiotic resistance of SK2-52 clone was stable, while the new antibiotic productivity of the clone was unstable and the productivity was easily reduced with the increased segregation of large colony-forming clones by subcultures, without change of growth appearance of S. griseus. This fact implies that the generation of the new antibiotic productivity was not caused by a genetic change in the generation of antibiotic resistance. Consequently, it seems likely that the interspecies fusion treatment between S. griseus and S. tenjimariensis in this experiment caused specific genetic changes in the former to induce expression of gene(s) for a new antibiotic productivity and independently resistance to certain antibiotics which were criptic in the parental strains.

4 CLUSTER OF GENES RELATING TO ANTIBIOTIC SYNTHESIS AND RESISTANCE

As above, antibiotic resistance is a useful marker for the selection of clones in genetic experiments with antibiotic producing organisms. The cloning of antibiotic resistance genes in antibiotic-producing organisms is important for genetic technology of antibiotic production. If the gene is suitably cloned by encoding it in a reasonably short fragment of DNA and ligated with a certain suitable vector DNA, the vector connected with such antibiotic marker would be extremely useful in genetic studies. Since compatible plasmids of S. tenjimariensis were successfully isolated and mapped by restriction enzymes, a plasmid with reasonably small size (5.8 Md) is expected to be a useful vector

DNA, if the plasmid is connected with a DNA fragment having certain antibiotic resistance marker. The resistance genes of NM, viomycin, methylenomycins, thiostrepton (TP), erythromycin, RM, KM, novobiocin, destomycin and racemomycin have been already cloned, but the SM resistance gene has not been cloned yet. Since S. tenjimariensis as the host is sensitive to SM, a SM resistance determinant which encodes SM-phosphotransferase was cloned from a SM-producing S. griseus to facilitate the development of host-vector system with SM resistance as a selective marker. At first, S. griseus ISP 5236 was employed as the donor of SM resistance gene, and S. lividans as the recipient, and its suitable vectors such as pIJ 702 were kindly supplied by Dr. C. Thompson. Growth conditions and preparation of chromosomal and plasmid DNA were those described by Chater et al. (22). Total DNA of S. griseus was digested with each of Sph I, Sst I and Bgl II for the ligation into the corresponding site within the tyrosinase gene of pIJ 702 (23). Vector and donor DNA were mixed and digested with restriction enzymes then ligated with T4 DNA ligase. Preparation of protoplast and transformation of S. lividans were as described by Chater et al. (22). After plating for 16 hours, R2YE plates were overlaid with R2YE containing thiostrepton (TP). Clones resistant to TP were replicated to ISP No. 4 plates containing 0.1% yeast extract and 20 or 50 µg/ml SM. Preparation of cell-free extract and inactivation of SM were as described by Nimi et al. (24) with the following modification; SM resistance clones were grown in YEME (22) medium containing 5 µg/ml SM. Ten grams of the mycelium was washed and suspended in 40 ml reaction buffer (125 mM Tris-malate and 12.5 mM $MgSO_4$, pH 7.0). The mycelium was disrupted with an ultrasonic oscillator in an ice bath. After centrifugation at 16,000 rpm for 10 minutes, 600 mg ATP, 200 mg SM sulfate and 1 ml toluene were added to the supernatant. Reactions were carried out at 37°C for 16 hours.

SM resistance clones only appeared in transformants of S. lividans with recombinant plasmids inserted with Bgl II fragments of the total DNA of S. griseus. Such clones failed to appear in transformations

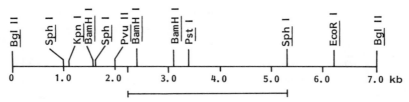

Fig. 2.   Restriction map of SM resistance fragment.

with Sph I and Sst I fragments. Accordingly, Bgl II fragments of S. griseus and pIJ 702 linearized with Bgl II were ligated and gave the recombinant plasmid, pST 141, after transformation into S. lividans. Recombinant plasmid pST 141 was digested with restiction endonucleases and analyzed by agarose gel electrophoresis. It was found that a 7.0 Kb Bgl II fragment of S. griseus encoded the SM resistance determinant. A restriction map of the fragment is shown in Fig. 2.

The recombinant plasmid pST 141 was able to re-transform S. lividans 1326 protoplasts to TP and SM resistance, and the resistance to TP and SM was cured simultaneously when transformants were incubated without selection at 37°C.

The resistance level of the transformants is shown in Table 6 as

Table 6. MIC of streptomycin (μg/ml) on S. lividans transformant and S. griseus.

Strain	Plasmid	MIC* (μg/ml)
S. lividans 1326	None	3
3131	pIJ 702	12
4-1	pST 141	200
S. griseus ISP 5236	None	100

* Agar dilution method.

minimum inhibitory concentration (MIC) to SM. S. lividans 4-1 harboring pST 141 and S. griseus ISP 5236 (donor strain) were resistant to SM, while S. lividans 1326 (recipient strain) and 3131 harboring pIJ 702 were sensitive. The susceptibility to SM in SM resistant clones of S. lividans was increased 10 fold or more over that of SM sensitive hosts.

Inactivated SM was isolated from a cell-free reaction mixture, purified by column chromatography on CM-Sephadex C-25 and LH-20, then subjected to ^{13}C NMR and SI-MS analysis. It gave positive color reaction with the ammonium molybdate-perchloric acid reagent. SI-MS, m/z 662 (M+1)$^{+}$, showed the presence of phosphorus in this molecule. From ^{13}C NMR spectrum the signal of 6-C (25) was shifted to lower field by 3.6 ppm and split by coupling with the phosphorus group. Therefore, it was identified as SM 6-O-phosphate (26).

It was presumed that Bgl II fragments encoding SM resistance of S. griseus are too long to be stable in the host when inserted into pIJ 702. Similarly, the SM resistance transformants harboring pST 141

(12.5 Kb) frequently lost their plasmids. Therefore, subcloning of
the Bgl II fragment containing the SM O-phosphotransferase gene will
be necessary to stabilize recombinant plasmid in the host. The Bgl II
fragment has three Sph I sites but since no resistance transformant
appeared when Sph I fragments from S. griseus were cloned, this suggests
that at least one of these sites may be within the resistance gene
(27). This Bgl II fragment (7.0 Kb) is almost identical with the Bgl
II fragment (7.4 Kb) which was cloned to encode SM synthesis of strep-
tidine formation (guanidine-streptamine) and streptidine-streptose
formation by Imanaka et al. of Osaka University (personal communication).
If the above is supposed, the SM resistance gene and the SM synthesis
gene are clustered within the above fragment. As reported in other
antibiotics, the clarification of the regulatory mechanism of expression
for the resistance and the antibiotic synthesis is of great interest.

5 REGULATION OF BIOSYNTHESIS AND CONVERSION OF PSEUDODISACCHARIDE ANTIBIOTICS WITH REFERENCE TO ANTIBIOTIC RESISTANCE

Although it was not successful to obtain blocked mutants available
for studies on biosynthetic pathway of IM, various IMs were found and
isolated from the fermentation broths, as shown in Fig. 3, and the
study on the relationship between those IMs will be helpful to know
the biosynthetic pathway and the regulation of IMs, of which chemical
structures are shown in Fig. 4. Some of these IMs are too small in
amount of the production, but some are available for the substrates of
conversion experiments with growing cells of the IM producer. Since
the IM producer was sufficiently resistant to the following substances
as substrates for the growing cell, conversion experiments were carried
out. Those substrate substances were IM and its related substances ·
including IM-X_0 and -Y_0, IM-A_0 and -B_0, IM-A and -B (=glycyl-IM-A_0
and -B_0), formimidoyl (FID)-IM-A and -B (=FID-glycyl-IM-A_0 and -B_0),
fortimicin (FM)-A (=glycyl-FM-B) and FM-B.

100 ml of medium P-5 (consisting of corn meal 6.0%, wheat germ
2.0%, $CaCO_3$ 0.6% and $MgSO_4 \cdot 7H_2O$ 0.05%, pH 7.0) in 500 ml flask was
inoculated with the antibiotic non-producing mutant (No. U-41) and was
fermented by rotary shaking for 72 hours at 27°C. To this broth, 100
or 200 μg of each substrate per ml of the medium was added and fermented
further for 9-10 days. The final broth was adjusted to pH 2.0 with
HCl, filtered, then adjusted to pH 7.0 with NaOH. This filtrate was
subjected to IRC-50 resin (NH_4^+), eluted with 1N NH_4OH, concentrated
in vacuo and applied to TLC or HPLC for de-formimidoyl type of IMs.
In order to detect formimidoyl type of IMs, IRC 50 (Na^+) was employed

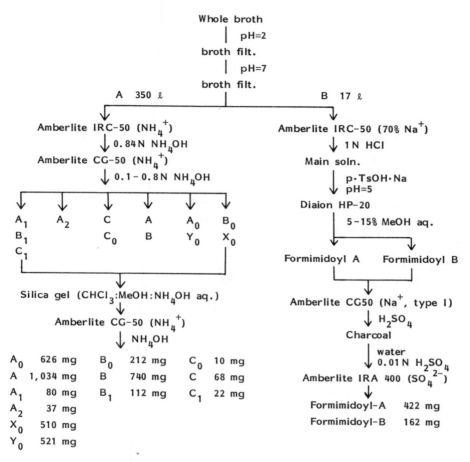

Fig. 3. Yield of istamycins in the broth (A=IM-A and so forth).

and eluted with 0.5N H_2SO_4, adjusted to pH 5.0 with NaOH and subjected
to HP_2C. TLC employed Kiesel gel $60F_{254}$ and the following solvents; A
$(CH_3Cl_3$:Methanol:NH_4OH=20:15:8), B $(CH_3Cl_3$:Methanol:28% NH_4OH=2:1:1)
and C $(CH_3Cl_3$:Methanol:Ethanol:28% NH_4OH=1:1:1:1). The products were
detected by ninhydrin reaction and bioautogram with B. subtilis PCI219.
HPLC of the eluate with H_2SO_4 employed YMC gel (Yamamura Chemical Co.)
for the column, aqueous solution (acetonitril 5.5%, acetic acid 0.1%,
1-pentasulfonic acid-Na 0.02 M and sodium sulfate 0.2 M) for the
solvent and UV adsorption at 344 nm by O-phthalaldehyde reaction in pH
10 boric buffer.

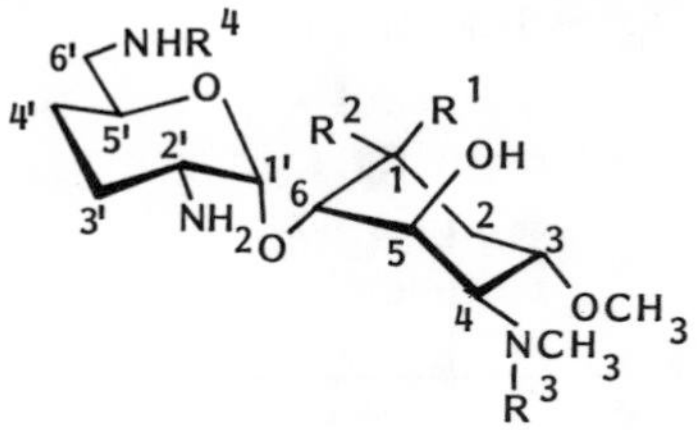

Istamycin (IM)	R^1	R^2	R^3	R^4	B. sub.%*
A_0	NH_2	H	H	CH_3	0.4
A	NH_2	H	$COCH_2NH_2$	CH_3	76
A_1	NH_2	H	$COCH_2NHCHO$	CH_3	3
A_2	NH_2	H	$COCH_2NHCONH_2$	CH_3	45
2"-N-Formimidoyl A	NH_2	H	$COCH_2NH-CH=NH$	CH_3	66
B_0	H	NH_2	H	CH_3	1
B	H	NH_2	$COCH_2NH_2$	CH_3	100
B_1	H	NH_2	$COCH_2NHCHO$	CH_3	9
2"-N-Formimidoyl B	H	NH_2	$COCH_2NH-CH=NH$	CH_3	73
C_0	NH_2	H	H	C_2H_5	0.3
C	NH_2	H	$COCH_2NH_2$	C_2H_5	68
C_1	NH_2	H	$COCH_2NHCHO$	C_2H_5	3
X_0	NH_2	H	H	H	
Y_0	NH_2	H	H	H	

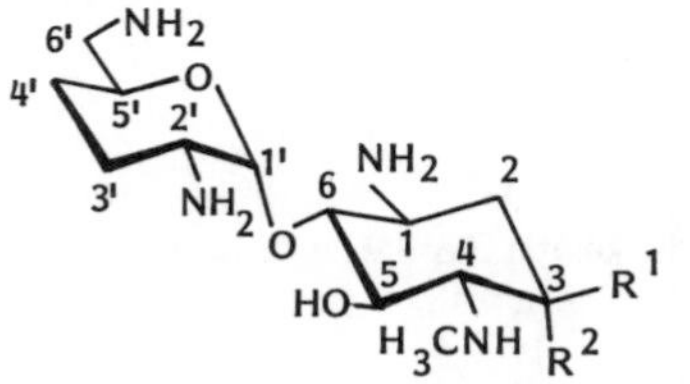

Istamycin (IM)	R^1	R^2	B. sub.%*
X_0	H	OCH_3	5
Y_0	OCH_3	H	0.3

* Inhibitory activity: IM-B as 100%.

Fig. 4.   Structure of istamycins.

Table 7. Conversion and products of istamycins.

Substrates	Products of IM							
	IM-X$_0$	IM-Y$_0$	IM-A$_0$	IM-B$_0$	FID-IM-A	FID-IM-B	IM-A	IM-B
IM-X$_0$		0	+	+	+	+	+	+
IM-Y$_0$	+		+	+	+	+	+	+
IM-A$_0$	0	0		+	+	+	+	+
IM-B$_0$	0	0	0		0	+	0	+
FID-IM-A (FID-gly-IM-A$_0$)	0	0	+	+		+	+	+
FID-IM-B (FID-gly-IM-B$_0$)	0	0	0	+	+		+	+
IM-A	0	0	0	0	0	0		0
IM-B	0	0	0	0	0	0	0	

IM: istamycin.

As shown in Table 7, IM-X$_0$ did not give IM-Y$_0$, while IM-Y$_0$ gave IM-X$_0$. IM-A$_0$ gave FID-IM-A and IM-A, while IM-B$_0$ did give FID-IM-B and IM-B. FID-IM-A gave IM-A$_0$, while FID-B did not, but gave IM-B$_0$, FID-IM-A, IM-A and IM-B. IM-A and IM-B did not give any products.

Capulating the above, the relation between the products is presumed to be as shown in Fig. 5. Since FID-glycine can be easily removed from FID-glycyl-IM-A$_0$ or -B$_0$ at alkaline pH of the broth, IM-A and -B are regarded as the products from FID-IM-A and -B by chemical reaction. As seen in Table 8, epimerization between A type (NH$_2$ is equatorial at 1 carbon of aminocyclitol moiety) and B type (NH$_2$ is axial) occurred

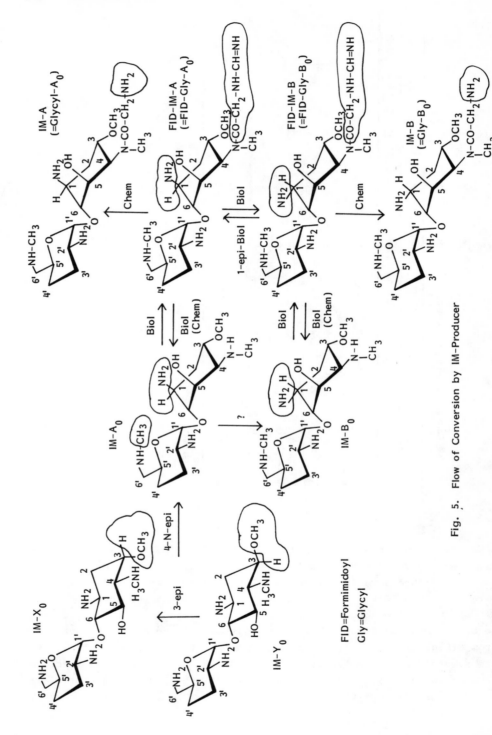

Fig. 5.   Flow of Conversion by IM-Producer

Table 8. Conversion by growing cell of S. tenjimariensis U-41.

Substrates	Conversion			
	Acet	Gly	FID	Epi
IM-A (=A_0-gly)	–		–	–
IM-B (=B_0-gly)	–		–	–
IM-A_0	–	+ (IM-A)	+ (FID-IM-A)	+ (FID-IM-B)
IM-B_0	–	+ (IM-B)	+ (FID-IM-B)	–
FID-IM-A (FID-gly-IM-A_0)	–			+ (FID-gly-IM-B_0) (IM-B_0)
FID-IM-B (FID-gly-IM-B_0)	–			+ (FID-gly-IM-A_0) (IM-A_0)
FM-A (Sugar-Fortamin-gly)	–		–	–
FM-B (Sugar-Fortamin)	–	+	+	+ (1-epi-FID-gly- FM-B) (1-epi-FM-B)
Neamine	+	–	–	–
KM-B	+	–	–	–

Acet: acetylation, Gly: glycylation, FID: formimidoylation,
KM-B: kanamycin B, Epi: epimerization, FM: fortimicin, IM: istamycin
+: present, –: absent

only when IM-A_0, IM-B_0, FID-IM-A and FID-IM-B were the substrates.
Accordingly, it is presumed that glycylation or formimidoylglycylation
was required before the epimerization. A similar situation was observed
in case of another pseudodisaccharide antibiotic, the fortimicins
(fortimicin A is called astromicin). Fortimicin (FM)-A which is
already glycylated form of FM-B was not epimerized 1-epi-FM-A, while
FM-B can be formimidoyl-glycylated to yield FID-gly-FM-B (FID-FM-
A=dactimicin) and epimerized to yield 1-epi-FID-glycyl-FM-B, of which
structures, naming and the flow of possible conversion are indicated
in Fig. 6.

When IM-A_0 was substrate, FID-IM-A and -B, IM-A and -B and IM-B_0
were the observed products, while when IM-B_0 was given as substrate,
only FID-IM-B and IM-B were observed as products. Similarly, when
FID-IM-A was substrate, IM-A_0 and -B_0, FID-IM-A and -B, IM-A and -B
were observed, while when FID-IM-B was substrate, IM-B_0, FID-IM-A, IM-

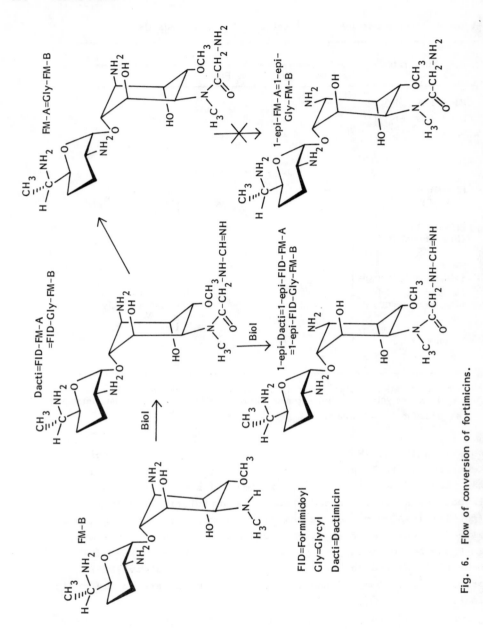

Fig. 6.   Flow of conversion of fortimicins.

A and -B were the products. This suggested that the flow of conversion
seemed to be easy from A type substances toward B type but not from B
type toward A type. Consequently, $IM-A_0$ gave $IM-B_0$, while $IM-B_0$ did
not give $IM-A_0$ and thus, the biosynthetic pathway of A type and B type

would not be a grid structure and B type would be positioned in down stream of the biosynthesis, as indicated in Fig. 5, if it is supposed that B type substances are lessly excreted from cell than A type. Before the flow of biosynthesis and its regulation are presumed, many problems remained for further studies. At least, experiments on permeability of substrates into growing cells, conversion experiments by cell-free extracts or radioisotopic trace of biosynthesis will be necessary. As reported by Itoh <u>et al</u>. (28,29), the FM (=astromicin)-producer afforded many blocked mutants by which the biosynthetic pathway was able to be confirmed. However, we were not successful in obtaining blocked mutants of the IM-producer, and thus the above biosynthetic pathway proposal could not be a conclusive one.

So far, supposed B type compounds are positioned in down stream of the biosynthetic pathway after the synthesis of A type compounds (as illustrated in Fig. 5), therefore, the regulation for selective production of A type compounds will be easier than that for the selective production of B type compounds. In fact, the production of A type compounds in the fermented broth of the IM-producer usually was much higher than that of B type compounds. On the other hand, the increased temperature (up to 32°C from 27°C) of the fermentation course resulted in higher yield of the B type compounds than of the A type, as shown in Fig. 7.

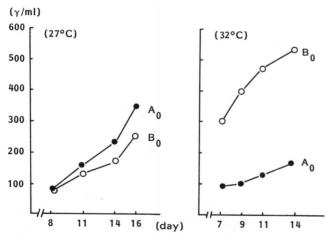

Fig. 7. Temperature effect to IM-production of A Type and
         B Type (as A_0 and B_0)

The regulatory mechanism for the production of IM is not known in detail, but the glucose effect was observed and the controls of nitrogen source in the medium had significant effect to the total production of IMs. The addition of Mg^{2+} or surfactants exhibited an increase of production in the broth, probably due to release of the antibiotics from the cell wall or surface, to which the antibiotics were adsorbed. These environmental manipulations gave some significant influences on the total production of the antibiotics, but they were not markedly influencial to the ratio between the yields of A type and B type IMs. In comparison with the influences of such environmental manipulations, mutations or single colony selections afforded clones with varied ratio of the yield between two types of IMs.

The author acknowledges the works in this article due greatly to the cooperations and contributions of K. Hotta, S. Kurasawa, F. Yamashita T. Shigyo, H. Tohyama, A. Takahashi, N. Saito, H. Yamamoto, S. Kondo, H. Naganawa, D. Ikeda, S. Gomi and M. Morioka of the author's laboratory.

6 REFERENCES

(1) R. Venviniste, J. E. Davis, Proc. Nat. Acad. Sci. U.S.A 70 (1973) 2276-2279.

(2) P. D. Shaw, J. Piwowarski, J. Antibiot. 30 (1979) 404-408.

(3) M. Yagisawa, T.-S. R. Huang, J. E. Davis, J. Antibiot. 29 (1978) 809-813.

(4) K. Komatsu, J. Leboul, S. Hartford, J. E. Davis, Microbiology-1981, Proceedings of Amer. Soc. Microbiol., Washington, D.C. (1981) p. 384-387.

(5) A. Demain, Ann. N. Y. Acad. Sci. 235 (1974) 601-602.

(6) K. Hotta, Y. Okami, J. Ferment. Technol. 54 (1976) 563-579; 572-578.

(7) H. Yamamoto, K. Hotta, Y. Okami, H. Umezawa, Biochim. Biophys. Res. Commun. 100 (1981) 1396-1401.

(8) H. Yamamoto, K. Hotta, Y. Okami, H. Umezawa, J. Antibiot. 35 (1982) 1020-1025.

(9) O. Nimi, G. Ito, S. Sueda, R. Nomi, Agric. Biol. Chem. <u>35</u> (1971)
     848-855.

(10) C. J. Thompson, J. M. Ward, D. A. Hopwood, Nature <u>286</u> (1980) 525.

(11) C. J. Thompson, R. H. Skinner, E. Candriffe, Eur. J. Bact. <u>151</u>
     (1982) 678.

(12) K. Hotta, A. Takahashi, N. Saito, Y. Okami, H. Umezawa, J. Antibiot.
     36 (1983) 1748-1754.

(13) K. Hotta, A. Takahashi, Y. Okami, H. Umezawa, J. Antibiot. <u>36</u>
     (1983) 1789-1791.

(14) Y. Okami, K. Hotta, M. Yoshida, D. Ikeda, S. Kondo, H. Umezawa,
     J. Antibiot. <u>32</u> (1979) 964-966.

(15) T. Shigyo, K. Hotta, Y. Okami, H. Umezawa, J. Antibiot. <u>37</u> (1984)
     635-640.

(16) F. Yamashita, K. Hotta, S. Kurasawa, Y. Okami, H. Umezawa, J.
     Antibiot. <u>38</u> (1985) 58-63.

(17) K. Hotta, F. Yamashita, Y. Okami, H. Umezawa, J. Antibiot. <u>38</u>
     (1985) 64-69.

(18) S. Gomi, D. Ikeda, H. Nakamura, H. Naganawa, F. Yamashita, K.
     Hotta, S. Kondo, Y. Okami, H. Umezawa, J. Antibiot. <u>37</u> (1984)
     1491-1494.

(19) B. Weisblum, Y. Fujisawa, S. Horinocuhi, Trends in Antibiotic
     Research, Japan Antibiotic Research Association, Tokyo 1982, p.
     73-78.

(20) M. Sugiyama, T. Katoh, H. Mochizuki, O. Nimi, R. Nomi, J. Ferment.
     Technol. <u>61</u> (1983) 347-351.

(21) F. Yamashita, K. Hotta, Y. Okami, H. Umezawa, J. Antibiot. <u>38</u>
     (1985) 126-127.

(22) K. F. Chater, D. A. Hopwood, T. Kiese, C. J. Thompson, Curr.
     Topics Microbiol. Immunol. <u>96</u> (1981) 59-65.

(23) E. Katz, C. J. Thompson, D. A. Hopwood, J. Gen. Microbiol. <u>129</u> (1983) 2703-2714.

(24) O. Nimi, G. Ito, S. Sueda, R. Nomi, Agric. Biol. Chem. <u>35</u> (1971) 848-855.

(25) M. H. G. Munro, R. M. Stroshane, K. L. Reihart, J. Antibiot. <u>35</u> (1982) 1331-1337.

(26) M. Sugiyama, H. Mochizuki, O. Nimi, R. Nomi, J. Antibiot. <u>34</u> (1981) 1183-1188.

(27) H. Tohyama, T. Shigyo, Y. Okami, J. Antibiot. <u>37</u> (1984) 1736-1737.

(28) S. Itoh, Y. Odakura, H. Kase, K. Takahashi, K. Iida, K. Shirahata, K. Nakayama, J. Antibiot. <u>37</u> (1984) 1664-1669.

(29) Y. Odakura, H. Kase, S. Itoh, S. Satoh, S. Takasawa, K. Takahashi, K. Shirahata, K. Nakayama, J. Antibiot. <u>37</u> (1984) 1670-1680.

Induction and Regulation of Phytoalexin Synthesis in Soybean

Hans Grisebach

Albert-Ludwigs-Universität, Institut für Biologie II/Biochemie der Pflanzen, Schänzlestr. 1, D-7800 Freiburg, FRG

Abstract

Upon infection of soybean seedlings with Phytophthora megasperma f.sp. glycinea (Pmg), pterocarpanoid phytoalexins (glyceollins) accumulate at the infection site. Induction of glyceollin accumulation in seedlings or in cultured soybean cells is also caused by treatment with a glucan elicitor of this fungus. Large increases and subsequent decreases of a number of enzymes involved in glyceollin biosynthesis occur after infection or elicitor treatment. Increases in enzyme activities are due to de novo synthesis and are reflected in increased activities and amounts of corresponding mRNAs. It can therefore be concluded that glyceollin accumulation is very probably controlled at the level of gene transcription. Effects of elicitor treatment of cell cultures on phosphatidylinositol turnover and phosphate distribution as well as the influence of Ca^{2+} ions on glyceollin accumulation and enzyme induction are described and the possible involvement in signal transduction is discussed.

1. Introduction

This chapter deals with the formation of antimicrobial substances in higher plants. Phytoalexins (alexin: Greek for a "warding-off compound") are defined as secondary metabolites with antimicrobial properties which are produced postinfectionally by the plant (1). Phytoalexins are not a uniform class of natural products, but include isoflavonoids, stilbenes, dihydrophenanthrenes, polyacetylenes, various terpenoids, and miscellaneous other compounds.

The role of phytoalexins in specific resistance of plants against potential pathogens has been studied in several systems (1). In this chapter I will describe studies on phytoalexin accumulation in soybean caused by infection with the Oomycete Phytophthora megasperma f.sp. glycinea. Studies in which induction of phytoalexin synthesis in soybean cell suspension cultures was effected by a glucan elicitor from this fungus will also be discussed. This work has been partly covered in reviews (2,3).

2. Soybean - Phytophthora megasperma f.sp. glycinea

Phytophthora root and stem rot caused by P. megasperma f.sp. glycinea (Pmg) is a very destructive disease in susceptible soybean cultivars. Pmg exists in different physiological races which are distinguishable only by their host-parasite interaction. For example, the soybean cultivar Harosoy 63 is resistant against race 1 of Pmg (incompatible interaction) but susceptible to race 3 (compatible interaction).

2.1 Accumulation of soybean phytoalexins

The structures of the major soybean phytoalexins (glyceollins) which accumulate at the infection site are shown in Fig. 1.

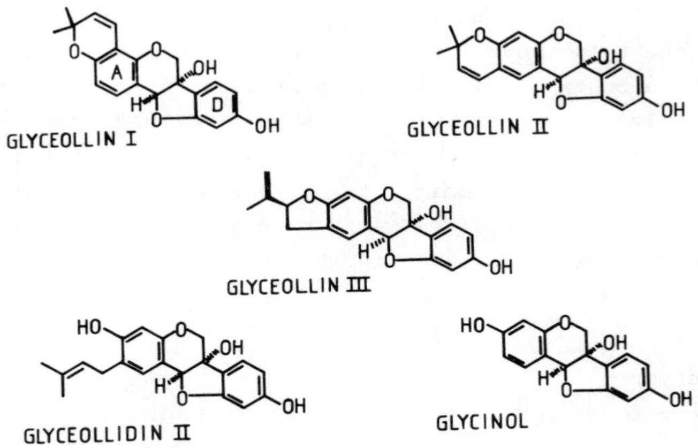

GLYCEOLLIN I   GLYCEOLLIN II

GLYCEOLLIN III

GLYCEOLLIDIN II   GLYCINOL

Fig. 1   Structure of glyceollin I, II, and III and of glyceollin precursors

The glyceollins are substituted pterocarpans with 6aS, 11aS configuration. The EC_{50} against Pmg is 0.17 µmol/ml and the EC_{90}, 0.6 µmol/
ml (4). Accumulation of glyceollins after infection with different
races of Pmg has been studied in soybean hypocotyls and roots. A system
which is closely related to the natural infection process is the inoculation of roots of soybean seedlings with zoospores of different
races of Pmg. The dramatic difference in appearance of the roots between the incompatible and compatible interaction can be seen in Fig.2.

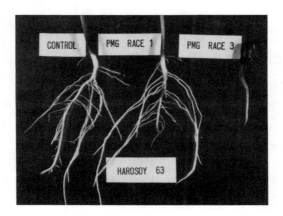

Fig. 2   Soybean roots (cv Harosoy 63) 4 h after inoculation with zoospores of race 1 or race 3 of P.megasperma f.sp. glycinea. Two-day old
seedlings were dip-inoculated with about 10^4 zoospores per 100 µl for
2 h and then planted in sterile vermiculite (from 5).

Accumulation of glyceollin I, the major phytoalexin in soybean
roots, in single whole roots as determined by a radioimmunoassay (6)
is shown in Fig. 3.

At the early times after infection glyceollin accumulates only in
the incompatible interaction, whereas at 28 h after infection the glyceollin content in the compatible interaction was even higher than that
in the compatible reaction.

The sensitivity of the radioimmunoassay and an immunofluorescence
stain for hyphae permitted quantitation of glyceollin I and localization of the fungus in alternate serial cryotome sections from the
same root (5). The results of these investigations, which are not described here, support the assumption that accumulation of glyceollin is
an important early response of soybean roots to infection by P.mega-
sperma, but may not be solely responsible for inhibition of fungal
growth in the resistance response.

How does fungal-plant interaction trigger phytoalexin accumulation?
To answer this question it is first of all important to know how the
plant synthesizes glyceollin.

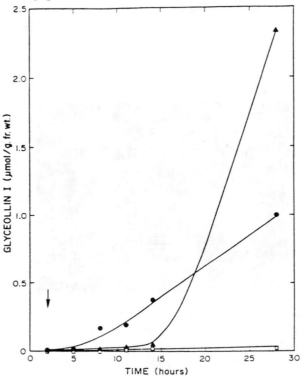

Fig. 3   Glyceollin I accumulation in single roots after inoculation
of zoospores of Pmg race 1 (●) or race 3 (▲) or treatment with water
(□). The arrow indicates the time when the seedlings were transferred
from the zoospore suspension to water (from 5).

2.2 Enzymes of glyceollin biosynthesis

The series of reactions which are known for biosynthesis of the
glyceollin isomers I, II, and III is shown in Fig. 4.

Glyceollin belongs to the group of isoflavonoids which include the
pterocarpanoids. The basic precursors are 4-coumaroyl-CoA, malonyl-CoA,
and dimethylallyl pyrophosphate. 4-Coumaroyl-CoA is formed from L-phenylalanine by the three reactions shown in the top row of Fig. 4, which
are catalysed by the enzymes phenylalanine ammonia-lyase (PAL), cinna-
mate 4-hydroxylase, and 4-coumarate:CoA ligase. Condensation of 4-
coumaroyl-CoA with three molecules of malonyl-CoA leads to the chalcone, which is in enzymatic equilibrium with the (2S)flavanone. So far

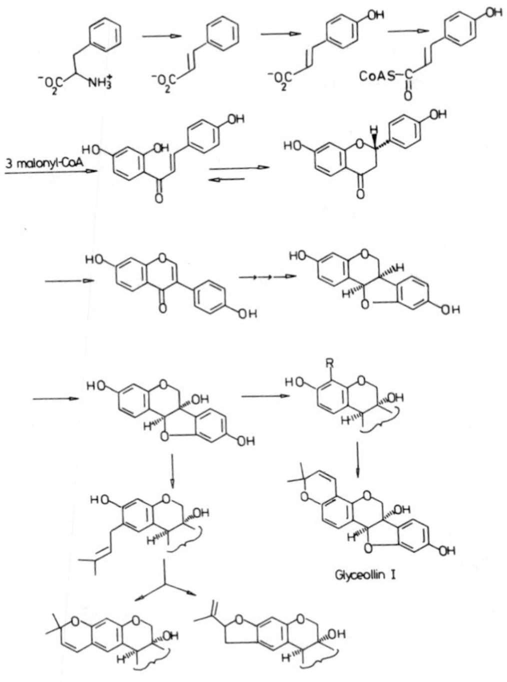

Fig. 4   Reaction sequence for biosynthesis of the glyceollin isomers

only a chalcone synthase leading to the tetrahydroxychalcone (not the
trihydroxychalcone needed for glyceollin) is known. Isomerization of
trihydroxychalcone to (2S)7.4'-dihydroxyflavanone by a specific chalcone isomerase has been described (17). An important step is the rearrangement of (2S)flavanone to isoflavone (daidzein), which involves
a 2,3-aryl migration. A microsomal enzyme system catalyzing this reaction has recently been described by us (7). Unpublished observations
indicate that the reaction proceeds in two steps: an NADPH, O_2 and
cytochrome P-450 dependent rearrangement to a product of as yet unknown structure which is then transformed by a soluble enzyme to isoflavone. According to tracer studies by Dewick (8) in other systems,
the pterocarpan is derived from the isoflavone by reduction to isofla-
vanone, 2'-hydroxylation, reduction of the carbonyl to isoflavanol and
subsequent cyclization to pterocarpan.

Introduction of the angular hydroxyl group at C-6a is catalysed by a microsomal monooxygenase in presence of NADPH and O_2 (9). Optical rotatory dispersion spectra of the 3,6,9-trihydroxypterocarpan formed from racemic 3,9-dihydroxypterocarpan and of the remaining unreacted substrate proved that the product had the natural (6aS, 11aS)-configuration and that hydroxylation proceeds with retention of configuration. A dimethylallyl residue is then introduced into either the 2 or the 4-position of trihydroxypterocarpan by membrane-bound prenyltransferases (10). The fungitoxicity against Cladosporium cucumerinum is considerably increased by introduction of the dimethylallyl substituent. Enzymes for the cyclization of the dimethylallyl compounds to the respective glyceollins are unknown.

About 14 enzymes are involved in the biosynthesis of glyceollin I starting from L-penylalanine, malonyl-CoA and dimethylallylpyrophosphate.

We will now discuss the problem of how accumulation of glyceollins at the infection site is regulated.

2.3   Enzyme induction after infection with P. megasperma f.sp. glycinea

By pulse and pulse-chase experiments with $^{14}CO_2$ it was shown that in soybean seedlings infected with different races of Pmg the level of glyceollin is determined predominantly by its rate of synthesis (11). In healthy seedlings the enzymes involved in biosynthesis of glyceollins are present only in rather low activity or cannot be detected at all. Induction of enzyme activity after infection was first determined in soybean hypocotyls after inoculation with mycelium of race 1 or race 3 of Pmg in a slit wound (12). As an example, changes in PAL activity after inoculation are shown in Fig. 5.

Increases in enzyme activity occurred with an apparent lag phase of about 2,5 h. Significant differences in PAL activity between the incompatible and compatible interaction did not occur until about 14 h after infection. Maximal PAL activity was respectively about 10 and 6 times higher with races 1 and 3 than in the wound controls. Drastic increases of enzyme activity after infection were also found with chalcone synthase. However, in wounded hypocotyls such increases were observed not only for enzymes of the glyceollin pathway but also for glucose 6-phosphate dehydrogenase and glutamate dehydrogenase (12).

Recently we determined changes in PAL activity in soybean roots infected with zoospores of race 1 or race 3. In this more natural infection system the difference in enzyme induction between race 1 and 3 was much more pronounced, as is evident from Fig.6 (A. Bonhoff et al., unpubl.).

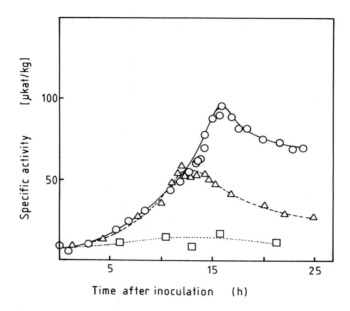

Fig. 5 Changes in PAL activity in soybean hypocotyls (cv. Amsoy 71) after inoculation with Pmg race 1 (incompatible) (o) or race 3 (compatible) (Δ) and in wound controls (□). From (12).

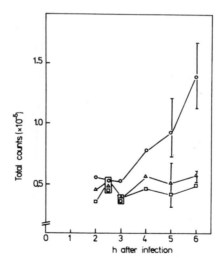

Fig. 6 Changes in PAL activity in soybean roots (cv. Harosoy 63) after infection with zoospores of Pmg race 1 (o) or race 3 (Δ) and in uninfected controls (□).

With race 1 a significantly higher PAL-activity is already seen 4 h after infection, whereas PAL-levels with race 3 are only slightly higher than in controls. This result is in agreement with the hypothesis that in the incompatible interaction a product of the fungus binds to a plant receptor, triggering a defense reaction, whereas in the compatible interaction no such recognition takes place (13). Analysis of other enzymes in the root system is in progress.

In the soybean hypocotyl system as well as in cultured soybean cells treated with a cell-wall preparation (elicitor) from Pmg (section 3), periods of increases in PAL and chalcone synthase activity coincided with high rates of enzyme synthesis, as measured by immunoprecipitation of the in vivo labelled protein (12,14). It was also shown that the induced changes in the rates of enzyme synthesis are associated with corresponding changes in mRNA activity for PAL, chalcone synthase and 4-coumaroyl-CoA ligase (15). Furthermore, with cloned cDNA complementary to chalcone synthase mRNA (16) it was possible to demonstrate that the timing is the same for changes in amount and activity of chalcone synthase mRNA (15). These results, shown in Fig. 7, suggest that glyceollin synthesis is triggered by enhancement of the transcriptional rate of certain genes.

Before addressing the question of what signal could lead to increased transcription, I will describe briefly a model system in which glyceollin synthesis can be induced by a component from the fungal cell wall.

3. Induction of glyceollin synthesis in cultured soybean cells.

Suspension cultured soybean cells were introduced by Ebel et al. (18) as a model system to study the mechanism of action of elicitors. Elicitors are pathogen-synthesized molecules responsible for stimulating accumulation of phytoalexins in their hosts. Cultures of Pmg release an extracellular elicitor into the culture medium which has been characterized as a glucan with $\beta 1 \longrightarrow 3$ and $\beta 1 \longrightarrow 6$ linkages. A heptasaccharide with elicitor activity was isolated and purified from acid-hydrolysed Pmg mycelial walls and was found to have the following primary structure (19):

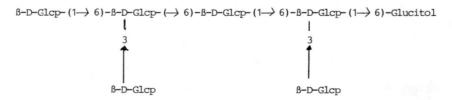

ß-D-Glcp = ß-D-glucopyranosyl

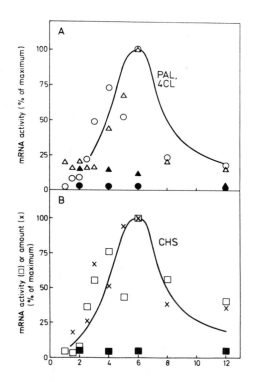

Fig. 7 Time course of mRNA induction in wounded soybean hypocotyls after inoculation with mycelium of Pmg, race 1 (open symbols). Controls closed symbols. (A) Translational activities in vitro of PAL (o,●) and 4-coumarate:CoA ligase (Δ/▲) mRNAs. (B) Translational activity (□,■) and hybridizable amount (x) of chalcone synthase mRNA. From (15).

For most studies crude or partially purified glucans from Pmg have been used as elicitors. All elicitor preparations, while active in inducing glyceollin accumulation, lose their race specificity, e.g. elicitors from race 1 race 3 of Pmg induce glyceollin accumulation in soybean to the same extent. Possible specificity factors and elicitors from other sources are not discussed here.

As already mentioned above, accumulation of glyceollin in soybean cell cultures after elicitor challenge is correlated with activity increases of enzymes of glyceollin biosynthesis including PAL, chalcone synthase, 4-coumarate:CoA ligase, acetyl-CoA carboxylase (14,20), and prenyltransferase (21,27).

Experiments concerning the chain of events between elicitor-plant cell interaction and increase in the transcriptional rate of certain genes are still at the beginning and no clear picture has as yet emered from these studies. Ebel et al. (21) found an enhancement of the elicitor effect on cultured soybean cells by Ca^{2+}ions. Glyceollin accumulation and activities of PAL and chalcone synthase were considerable higher in presence than in absence of Ca^{2+} from the cell culture medium. These results indicate that changes in intracellular Ca^{2+} pools could be involved in signal transduction/transmission, but direct measurements of intracellular $[Ca^{2+}]$ has not yet been accomplished.

Since inositol triphosphate seems to be a second messenger in signal transduction in animal systems (22), we and Ulrich Matern have initiated measurements of inositol phospholipid turnover in soybean and parsley cell cultures after elicitor challenge. In parsley cultures mainly linear furanocoumarines are synthesized in response to Pmg elicitor or to an elicitor from <u>Alternaria</u> <u>carthami</u> (23). By labelling the cells prior to elicitor treatment with $[U-^{14}C]$-myo-inositol, we found in both cell cultures transient increases in the synthesis of phosphatidyl inositol 4-monophosphate and 4,5-bisphosphate within 2-5 min after elicitor challenge, while the level of phosphatidylinositol did not change (unpublished results). Breakdown of polyphosphoinositides in this system has not yet been determined. While these results are rather preliminary, signal transduction via hydrolysis of phosphatidylinositol 4,5-bisphosphate to diacylglycerol and inositol triphosphate is an attractive hypothesis for elicitor action. Diacylglycerol can in presence of Ca^{2+} activate protein kinase C, which is a cyclic nucleotide-independent protein kinase (reviewed in 24). myo-Inositol 1,4,5-triphosphate can mobilize intracellular Ca^{2+}. That Ca^{2+}ions are needed for the elicitor effect is indicated by the results of Ebel mentioned above. We also showed that levels of cyclic AMP monitored by a radioimmunoassay in soybean infected with race 1 of Pmg did not change, while cAMP was not detected at all in the suspension cultured cells (25).

While investigating the question whether the cell wall of cultured soybean cells is needed for elicitor action, H. Mieth and J. Ebel (unpublished) found that in soybean protoplasts glyceollin accumulation is induced by osmotic stress with 0.4 mol$\cdot$l^{-1} mannitol + sorbitol (1:1) to a level which is comparable to that induced by elicitor treatment of cultured soybean cells. This again points to the possible involvement of changes in ion gradients in elicitor action.

Another interesting effect of elicitor treatment is on subcellular phosphate distribution. Matern et al. (26) determined such distribution by ^{31}P-nuclear magnetic resonance spectroscopy of intact parsley cells after challenge with an elicitor from A. carthami. The elicitor caused a temporary increase of vacuolar phosphate at the expense of cytoplasmic phosphate. Concomitantly, the pH of the vacuoles decreased by about 0.5 units within 60 minutes. Whether a transient decrease of phosphate in the cytoplasm could be involved in induction of fungitoxic coumarines in the parsley cells is still a matter of speculation.

Further experiments are necessary to see if any of the various elicitor effects observed are involved in signal transduction. Such investigations will contribute to a better understanding of the regulation of secondary metabolite formation in higher plants. Better knowledge of the biochemical basis of disease resistance could also help to develop new strategies for plant protection against potential pathogens.

Acknowledgement   Our own research was supported by Deutsche Forschungs-gemeinschaft (SFB 206), Fonds der Chemischen Industrie and Badische Anilin und Sodafabrik.

4. References

(1) Bailey, J.A., Mansfield, J.W. (Eds) Phytoalexins (1982), Blackie, Glasgow.

(2) Grisebach, H., Börner, H., Moesta, P.,Ber. Deutsch. Bot. Ges. 95, (1982) 619-642.

(3) Grisebach, H., Ebel, J., Biologie in unserer Zeit 13 (1983) 129-136.

(4) Lazarovits, G., Ward, E.W.B., Phytopathology 72 (1982) 1217-1221.

(5) Hahn, M.G., Bonhoff, A., Grisebach, H., Plant Physiol.77, (1985) 591-601.

(6) Moesta, P., Hahn, M.G., Grisebach, H., Plant Physiol. 73 (1983) 233-237.

(7) Hagmann, M., Grisebach, H., FEBS Letters 175 (1984) 199-202.

(8) Dewick, P.M.,Phytochemistry 16 (1977) 93-97.

(9) Hagmann, M., Grisebach, H., Eur.J.Biochem. 142 (1984) 127-131.

(10) Zähringer, U., Schaller, E., Grisebach, H. Z.Naturforsch. 36c
(1981) 234-241.

(11) Moesta, P., Grisebach, H., Arch. Biochem. Biophys. 212 (1981)
462-467.

(12) Börner, H., Grisebach, H., Arch Biochem. Biophys. 217 (1982)65-71.

(13) Yoshikawa, M. in: (Callow, J.A. ed.) Biochemical Plant Pathology,
J. Wiley & Sons, Chichester 1983, pp 267-298.

(14) Hille, A., Purwin, C., Ebel, J., Plant Cell Rep. 1 (1982)
123-127.

(15) Schmelzer, E., Börner, H., Grisebach, H., Ebel, J., Hahlbrock, K.,
FEBS. Letters 172 (1984) 59-63.

(16) Kreuzaler, F., Ragg, H., Fautz, E., Kuhn, D.N., Hahlbrock, K.,
Proc. Natl. Acad. Sci. USA 80 (1983) 2591-2593.

(17) Boland, M.J., Wong, E., Eur. J. Biochem. 50 (1975) 383-389.

(18) Ebel, J., Ayers, A.R., Albersheim, P., Plant Physiol. 57 (1976)
775-779.

(19) Sharp, J.K., McNeil, M., Albersheim, P., J.biol. Chem. 18 (1984)
11321-11336.

(20) Ebel, J., Schmidt, W.E., Loyal, R., Arch. Biochem. Biophys. 232
(1984) 240-248.

(21) Ebel, J., Stäb, M., Schmidt, W.E. in: (Neumann, K.H. ed.)
Primary and secondary metabolisms. of plant cell cultures (1985)
Springer,Berlin, in press.

(22) Berridge, M.J., Irvine, R.F., Nature 312 (1984) 315-321.

(23) Tietjen, K.G., Hunkler, D., Matern, U., Eur.J.Biochem. 131 (1983)
401-407.

(24) Majerus, P.W., Neufeld, E.J., Wilson, D.B., Cell 37 (1984) 701-703.

(25) Hahn, M.G., Grisebach, H., Z. Naturforsch. 38c (1983) 578-582.

(26) Straßer, H., Tietjen, K.G., Himmelspach, K., Matern, U., Plant Cell Reports 2 (1983) 140-143.

(27) Leube, J., Grisebach, H., Z. Naturforsch. 38c (1983) 730-735.

Current Research on Secondary Metabolism - A General Discussion

summarized by Hans von Döhren

Technical University of Berlin, Institute of Biochemistry and Molecular Biology, Franklinstr. 29, D-1000 Berlin 10 (West)

The general discussion held at the end of this meeting has been fused to discussions following the lectures, and supplemented with a few additional comments. I have rearranged and processed this final message into a summary expressing the contemporary approaches, strategies and scope of the field.

1. Secondary Metabolites

The term secondary metabolite, especially in relation to a microbial growth phase termed idiophase, has been challenged. This approach from the procaryotic side has of course in the meantime been confronted with many contrary examples. John Bu'Lock has given a clear historical introduction to this problem:

> *As someone who had a certain amount to do with introducing this term into chemical microbiology* [1] *.....*
>
> *The object of designating a group of materials as secondary metabolites in the first instance was to indicate that there was a need of special attention, which they were not getting. The problems at that stage turned out to be mainly problems of their origin, so .... over the succeeding years the problems of biosynthesis were largely dealt with. The attention has moved on to the problems of their regulation. And essentially my understanding of the general phenomenon of secondary metabolism is essentially a regulatory problem.... When we have explained the regulatory phenomenon, the term secondary metabolism is no longer necessary. We don't need it because we know what we are talking about, we have got a regulatory mechanism we can discuss ......*

Obviously Martin Luckner, the author and editor of extensive literature on secondary metabolism [2], being familiar with the plant and animal side, has little problems in this respect:

There have been many attempts in recent years to introduce some other terms, but such a term, e.g., idiolite or special product, has some advantages and some disadvantages .... This term secondary metabolite, which was used for one hundred years, introduced again in the 1950s by Paech[3] into plant physiology, is so widespread, that it is useless to discuss whether you can replace it or not ....

The question raised several times to introduce the new term special metabolite was, at least from that point of view, discouraged as a semantic approach.

Although functions have been assigned to some classes of compounds (table 1) as siderophores, sex hormones, germination effectors etc.,

Table 1:   General Functions of Secondary Products   (Luckner)

- detoxication of substances accumulating in primary metabolism
- physiological action
- chemical signals in coordination of metabolism in multicellular organisms
- coordination of activity of organisms of the same species
- mediation of ecological relations

the commercially important compounds still await the elucidation of their microbial function(s). More than 10 years ago Arnold Demain in his essay "How do microorganisms avoid suicide ?"[5] suggested that work should be concentrated onto a single example to obtain at least one solution. The situation did not improve very much, as Juan Martín feels:

It is not clear to me why we have not advanced more, because by now people have been working on antibiotics for more than 20 years .... Many blocked mutants are now available ... and nobody has come out with a clear-cut role for a single product.

Leo Vining questions the physiological role, at least for some secondary metabolites, in this respect:

We have too many examples now of blocked mutants, which we are quite certain have completely lost the ability to produce the secondary metabolite, which function very well, to think that they have a critical role that we are missing somehow, that we are not seeing, because of our inability to understand the organism adequately.

Although he really is convinced that they have a functional role:

> *The role of secondary metabolites must be to increase the fitness of the organism in its natural environment, otherwise I can't believe that they would be there.*

> *I think mutations are so frequent that these pathways undoubtedly would have disappeared ... there has to be a role ..... Assuming a random walk of evolution the opportunities for evolving pathways are many, and once a role is found, the pathway becomes fixed in the genotype. So there may be many pathways according to what the organism happened to come across.*

The right question here, as stated by Heinz Floss, is:

> *do secondary metabolites have an advantage in the evolution of the organism and a particular pathway, without necessarily being important for instant survival.*

Or as Martin Luckner summarizes in his general approach:

> *There are different possibilities as to how secondary products may be used by the producer. I say by the producer and not by the producing cell, that is a big difference.*

Quoting Jacob ("Evolution works like a tinkerer – a tinkerer who does not know exactly what he is going to produce, but uses whatever he finds around him"),

he points out that most animal non-peptide hormones are found in other groups of organisms, too, but don't have a physiological function comparable to the hormone function.

To advance this point of functional role, two approaches have been apparent: to more thoroughly explore the physiology, and to consider the wild type strains and their ecology instead of laboratory strains.

Martin Luckner suggests:

> *If you look for the biological role of an antibiotic you should look in the natural habitat and not at the lab. And nobody asks what may be the role of an antibiotic in a soil, where a lot of other compounds, a lot of other organisms are growing, where the mutants are limited and where wild type strains are living and not the artificial strains we usually have in the laboratory. So, I think this is really an open question, e.g., what is the biological role of antibiotics in nature ?*

In this connection, Udo Gräfe introduced a current speculation on a
signal system: ß-lactam antibiotics $\longrightarrow$ ß lactamases $\longrightarrow$ ß lactama-
se inhibitors, in respect to interactions of micropopulations in soil,
perhaps including gene transfer. This approach clearly differs from the
experimentally more straightforward suggestion by Peter Schindler, who
would rather connect endogenous functions in morphological differentiation of bacteria to ß-lactam compounds. I think it is clear to
everyone, that the field approach to uncover biological functions
involves tremendous experimental problems and difficulties.

Again we are far from understanding in vivo transfer of genes, which
should be a major factor in evolutionary considerations. In the
near future, studies certainly will focus on a deeper understanding
of physiology, and, as will be evident, on the expression of genes.

Two remarks should be added in this general section. Again Peter
Schindler tried to draw some attention to functional roles:

> *let me take an example from the so-called enzyme inhibitor screening ....*
> *amylase inhibitors are produced by streptomycetes only, if we grow the*
> *organism on polysaccharides. So I think there is a clear functional role*
> *which could be to control the glucose flux during the growth.*

And to comment on non-producer mutants, we have to be aware that loss
of a single pathway or effector may be balanced by physiological
responses, perhaps in a complicated network, either by levels of metabolites, or the production of other metabolites. Thus the future experimental aim should be a more thorough approach to physiology, and
need not be a shift to even more complicated systems of interacting
populations, in a heterogeneous surrounding such as soil.

2. Regulatory Phenomena

During the plenary lectures, it became evident through numerous examples
that different signals cause different regulatory events to affect
different steps of primary and secondary metabolism. Again the wealth
of information led Arnold Demain to exclaim:

> *At this point ... one has to find out the intracellular mechanism ...*
> *We have enough descriptive events in   literature already on secondary*
> *metabolism; we don't need any more ... (We have to) understand at least*
> *one of the regulatory effects.*

But before this hopefully is in reach, much more information is needed
on regulatory events. Concerning differences in regulatory principles
of primary and secondary metabolism, there was agreement that

> *the studies of basic mechanisms even in E. coli can lead us to the right*
> *way of looking at things; but as we get closer to our organisms of commercial*
> *significance, we'll learn a lot more ... they very well may be different*
> *(Arnold Demain).*

Leo Vining again points to the missing knowledge of function, and
proposes a sort of general functional approach:

> *Regulation is there for a purpose, and the regulatory (mechanisms) ... are*
> *all functioning in the enterobacteria, because they do something for the*
> *organism. The cAMP system institutes the search for carbon, when the available*
> *carbon supply runs down; this probably means that the function of secondary*
> *metabolism is going to be quite totally related to that regulatory system ...*
> *(If we knew) the purpose of each individual secondary metabolic pathway in*
> *the organisms ... we would have a much better idea of what regulatory con-*
> *trols to look for ... If growth is the primary selective force in the mi-*
> *crobial world, it would make sense that the organism would have an advantage*
> *if it shut off a secondary pathway while it was growing.*

Some observations of the phenomenological descriptive type indicate
different levels and mechanisms of regulation. Juan Martín's group
isolated glucose deregulated mutants in ß-lactam production. These
were found to be deregulated in ß-galactosidase formation, but also
deregulated in ß-lactam cyclase formation. Thus both primary and secondary pathways have been affected. Arnold Demain recalls that carbon
catabolite repression mutants of this type were either of a general
or a specific type, to point to perhaps different mechanisms.

In Braña's lab, glutamine synthetase negative mutants of
S. clavuligerus remained susceptible to ammonium interference in
cephamycin production, while in primary metabolism a marked change in
the nitrogen regulation of urease synthesis was seen. He concludes that

> *we have to take the whole sum ... phosphorylated nucleotides, highly*
> *phosphorylated nucleotides, etc., look ... and not be disappointed if*
> *they do not apply ... We're bound to discover new routes of control*
> *in this area.*

In regard to the general idiophase-productivity relation, Steve
Goulden presented some data on fed batch penicillin fermentations.

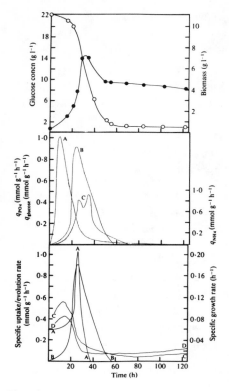

Fig. 1 a:

Batch culture of S. cattleya (7).
Top: Biomass (●) and glucose (○),
Middle: Specific nutrient uptake
rates for phosphate (A), glucose (B),
and ammonium (C).
Bottom: Specific growth rate μ (A),
uptake of glucose (B),
uptake of O_2 (C), and CO_2 (D)

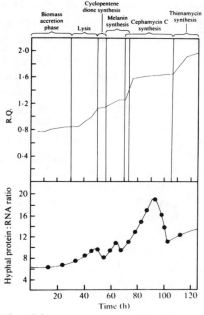

Fig. 1 b:

Batch culture of S. cattleya.
Top: Respiratory quotient (R.Q.) and
different physiological phases.
Bottom: Protein / RNA ratio.

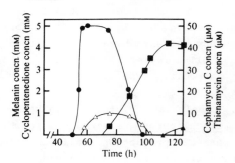

Fig. 1 c:

Extracellular product formation during
batch culture of S. cattleya.
(●)   cyclopentenedione
(△)   melanin
(■)   cephamycin C
(▲)   thienamycin

These data show that penicillin is produced with slow exponential growth, and have specific productivity peaks before growth is finished. In this context, I referred to a study on bacitracin formation by B. licheniformis using different carbon and nitrogen sources to achieve a range of exponential growth rates, and to demonstrate product formation during slow exponential growth [6]. The state of exponentially growing cells certainly has to be differentiated with respect to the growth rate. In many cases an approach correlating idiophase with slow exponential growth may be useful.

The expected diversity of regulatory systems can be well illustrated by work on the S. cattleya fermentation [7] (Fig. 1). The production of melanin, cephamycin C and thienamycin were initiated when glucose, ammonia and phosphate, respectively, became growth limiting. Juan Martín suggested that the structural type of the product may be correlated with the type of effectors operating in the control of pathways. J. Lengeler pointed to the alarmone concept (Bruce Ames), which is well advanced in the enterobacteria. Alarmones, like cAMP and ppGpp, regulate a whole set of metabolic enzymes. Thus, depending on the structural type of metabolite, a specific regulatory system may operate. A relevant example given by J. Betz was the induction of steroid metabolizing enzymes, which could be considered secondary products, in S. hydrogenans. Upon induction, there was the immediate formation of ppGpp and pppGpp together with the formation of more stable mRNA, cellular RNA breakdown, and rise of GTP and ATP [8].

In this context, the use of inhibitors affecting nucleoside phosphates like decoynine should be mentioned. We have seen at this meeting that developmental formation of antibiotics as well as genes may be induced by decoynine (results of Losick et al., and Kleinkauf et al.). Decoynine is a nucleoside analogue that in B. subtilis induces sporulation and causes disappearance of ppGpp [9]. Sets of enzymes under similar control may be coded by groups of genes involved in a distinct physiological change, which also requires a distinct metabolite. As one of the key messages of this discussion, David Hopwood says that

> *the way to find out about regulation of genes, activity of genes, and gene products ... is to study the genes ... This has been true since Jacob and Monod and earlier, in terms of in vivo techniques, and now you have the possibility of isolating the genes.*

And Hans Grisebach stresses the importance to

> *move from phenomenology to the genes, to look for promoter structures ...*
> *Many of the regulatory phenomena can be explained on the basis of regulatory*
> *proteins involved in transcriptional and translational control.*

It is evident that one of the main current approaches is the comparative study of promoter regions. Richard Losick discussed sigma-factor directed binding of RNA polymerase in <u>Bacillus</u> and <u>Streptomyces</u> [10], and overlapping promoter sites. He pointed out that rather than the

> *appearance of (a specific) sigma-factor, the appearance of auxiliary factors,*
> *e.g. regulatory proteins, such as SpoOH, determine the action of sigma.*

Certain homologies of DNA regions can be expected concerning promoters and further extending 5'-regions [11]. These homologies are again related to the structure of the DNA-binding proteins. Mapping of promoter sites or binding sites of regulatory proteins permit an estimation of coordinately induced, but unlinked genes.

These are the first steps in the unraveling of complex developmental processes, like sporulation, and, in the future, will elucidate the mechanism of formation of aerial mycelia, which quite often is a prerequisite of antibiotic formation [12].

Low molecular weight factors, i.e. regulators (or inducers) have been shown in several streptomycetes to initiate formation of aerial mycelia and/or antibiotics; this was reviewed by Udo Gräfe.

3. Genetics

Current approaches based on classical as well as molecular genetics have been the common theme running through all the contributions here. Starting with the recent exciting evidence for silent genes, comments and perspectives on the molecular procedures are summarized.

From the work of George Jones and David Hopwood on actinomycin genes in <u>S</u>. <u>antibioticus</u>, it is clear that genes may be present but not expressed; then activated upon introduction of a certain DNA region [13]. John Bu'Lock concluded from the work of Joan Bennett on aflatoxin production in <u>Aspergillus</u> <u>parasiticus</u> that

> *You can have a non-producing strain in which all the production genes are*
> *present.... actually quite an alarming situation, because this could mean*
> *that these genes are present ... in a permanently silent form ....*

By crossing strains ... you can recover those genes without the
restricted characteristic ... You can put the activator characteristic
back in.

Karl Esser referred to recent work on aflatoxins, relating loss of
extrachromosomal DNA to toxin production reversibly. John Bu'Lock
again pointed out that neither aflatoxin nor zearalenone formation in
Fusarium graminearum are extrachromosomal characteristics. A possible
activation mechanism, however, like A-factor, may well be traced to
plasmid or viral structures. To defect minor differences in the
chromosomes (Hildgund Schrempf) of variants, the experimental procedures have not been of the required sensitivity.

The perspectives of molecular cloning can be grouped into
(1) structural studies of gene products and regulatory region,
(2) the study of regulatory mechanisms, and
(3) the construction of novel metabolites.

Structural studies of gene products will provide some answers to
the many questions of microbial evolution. As John Bu'Lock states:

> *Basically we don't know anything about microbial evolution ... The only*
> *hard knowledge has come in relatively recent years from nucleotide se-*
> *quencing. Now there are many questions ... about secondary metabolic*
> *enzymes. What is the relationship if any between the ß-lactam cyclase*
> *of Cephalosporium and the ß-lactam cyclase of Streptomyes ? ....*
> *We can ask that kind of question until we're blue in the face as long as*
> *all we are only looking at is the structure of the ß-lactam and the chemist'*
> *ideas about the reaction mechanism.... We have in our hands if not today,*
> *then maybe next week,or next year, precisely the kind of sequence data*
> *that will enable us to give a very precise and totally meaningful answer*
> *to that question and to many other questions of that kind.*

And, as Yair Aharonowitz extends,

> *by hydridisation studies to look whether there is a larger distribution,*
> *whether there is any conservation; if there is not, to introduce the trait*
> *to see if there is any effect.*

Expectations from sequence data, in the long run, are relationships
between primary and secondary pathways, rates of mutational modification, rearranging of domains of proteins at the gene level, or

rearrangement of structural genes in the multifunctional enzyme type
for different products.

A direct application, as Arnold Demain reminds us, is to increase the
production of certain enzymes:

> *If we can show that the use of pathway enzymes is practical to make new
> compounds, and to present chemists with new basic structures for modifi-
> cation, large amounts of enzymes are going to be needed.*

And Leo Vining extends this concept to site-specific in vitro mutagenesis:

> *to loosen up the specificity of existing pathways, so that one can modify
> and produce variations of currently successful antibiotics. To think of an
> example ... in the production of cephalosporins, one of the hindrances is
> that a water soluble antibiotic is much more difficult to extract than
> penicillin G. If you could loosen up the substrate requirements of the
> enzyme so that the side chain would become nonpolar, this would*

lead to a considerable process improvement.

In regulatory studies, the introduction of cloned genes into well-
known organisms was strongly encouraged. Concentration of work to the
most well characterized strains, like B. subtilis, S. lividans and
S. coelicolor, and Aspergillus nidulans, would significantly speed
up the analysis of regulatory networks. David Hopwood comments on
these expectations:

> *I think one of the handicaps that Streptomyces genetics has suffered over
> the years is that rather few people have been involved, and people have
> been spreading their efforts over a very large number of strains. Now to
> some extent, that is inevitable because of the fact that antibiotics occur
> in different strains. But there are many aspects of fundamental molecular
> biology that could perfectly well be studied in a common strain.... If the
> development of molecular biology over the last 30 years has told us anything,
> it is that if you concentrate effort on one strain, e.g. E. coli K 12, or
> one phage, or a limited number of phages, you find out a hell of a lot,
> and you are not constantly distracted by differences .....*

This view has been supported by Richard Losick, who reminds us that

> *so little is understood about the fundamental biology and molecular biology
> of Streptomyces that we ought to be paying more attention to that. The only
> way to do that effectively is to make one or two organisms the focal point.*

*General principles will emerge that will be applicable to the other
special hosts. That same viewpoint holds for the fungal system.
Aspergillus nidulans has both excellent classical and molecular
genetic accessibility. What you learn there will have a profound
effect elsewhere.*

Juan Martín questions this approach from the view of point of antibiotic production. He and Steve Goulden emphasized that the current
producer strains have been randomly optimized for metabolite production, and will differ in their regulatory outfit.

J. Lengeler points out that the construction of stable hybrid strains
with artificial metabolic pathways has not been achieved for two main
reasons. Either intermediates are accumulated which turn out to be
toxic, or, if membrane-bound enzymes are involved, amplification
kills the cells, so that selection pressure is on down replication of
plasmids. For academic search, however, the introduction of genes
into other hosts remains a useful technique.

Karl Esser again reminds us that the genetic engineering techniques
are only part of the experimental approaches; they have to be combined with classical genetics and basic biology. Especially in the
field of fungi, fundamental studies are lacking.

To finally summarize our perspective on the construction of new compounds by combination of different steps from different pathways,
Arnold Demain thinks that the chance for useful compounds generally
is small. Leo Vining does not see immediate prospects, when such
hybrids form in a random fashion. David Hopwood raises a more general
point:

*One may well find a significantly different range of compounds by some
serendipitous gene scrambling ... We don't expect to find in nature a
strain that makes an antibiotic which confers no selective advantage in it...
At least no production of disadvantageous material .... In the lab, one
could keep alive a cripple that would not survive in nature... and enable
us to obtain new classes of compounds. At this moment, however, we are
not yet in the position to design useful compounds on the DNA-level that
are products of an enzyme sequence. However, we sure are on the onset of
such developments, which are emerging from the current research presented
at this meeting.*

References

(1)   D. Bu'Lock and A. J. Powell   (1965)   Experientia 21, 55

(2)   M. Luckner, L. Nover and H. Böhm   (1977)   Secondary Metabolism
       and Cell Differentiation, Springer Verlag 1977; M. Luckner (1984)
       Secondary Metabolism in Microorganisms, Plants and Animals.

(3)   K. Paech   (1950)   Biochemie und Physiologie der sekundären
       Pflanzenstoffe, Springer Verlag.

(4)   I. M. Campbell   (1984)   Adv. Microbial Physiol. 25, 1

(5)   A. L. Demain   (1974)   Ann. N. Y. Acad. Sci. 235, 601

(6)   G. W. Hanlon and N. A. Hodges   (1981)   J. Bacteriol. 147, 427
                                    (compare p. 199f of this vol.)

(7)   M. E. Bushell and A. Fryday   (1983)   J. Gen. Microbiol. 129, 1733

(8)   J. W. Betz, B.-H. Schneider and L. Träger   (1977)   Hoppe-Seyler's
       Z. Physiol. Chem. 358, 353

(9)   K. Ikehara, M. Okamoto and K. Sugae   (1982)   J. Biochem. 91, 1089
                                    (compare p.199 of this vol.)

(10)   J. Westpheling, M. Ranes and R. Losick   (1985)   Nature 313, 22
                                    (compare p. 13 of this vol.)

(11)   E. H. Davidson, H. T. Jacob and R. J. Britten   (1983)   Nature 301,
       as one example of the correlation of eucaryotic sequences.

(12)   I. M. Campbell   (1983)   J. Nat. Prod. 46, 60

(13)   G. H. Jones and D. A. Hopwood   (1984)   J. Biol. Chem. 259, 14158

Closing Remarks: Regulation of Secondary Metabolite Formation: Progress and Challenges

Arnold L. Demain

Massachusetts Institute of Technology, Fermentation Microbiology Laboratory, Department of Nutrition and Food Science, Cambridge, Massachusetts 02139, U.S.A.

We are about to conclude three exciting days involving various aspects of regulation of secondary metabolism. The lectures and the discussions following them have been extensive as was the round table discussion just concluded. I now have an opportunity to discuss the thoughts that I shall carry home from this experience.

Among the speakers were a number of distinguished chemists who treated us to their analyses of various biosynthetic pathways. We saw many metabolic pathways and many more chemical structures. We can appreciate the beauty of many of these natural sequences. The question is whether we can put the enzymes to work in a biotechnical sense for the production of novel products. Kleinkauf described the multi-enzyme templates involved in production of small and large peptide antibiotics. A number of speakers dealt with the acyltransferase of penicillin producers. Sir Edward Abraham received many questions after his talk about the specificity of this enzyme especially from commercially-oriented technologists who would love to use such an enzyme to convert the polar side chain of natural cephalosporins (D-α-aminoadipyl) to a non-polar side chain such as phenylacetyl. In this way, cephalosporins could be much more economically recovered from broth. Martín also was questioned on this point. Several speakers, especially Sir Edward, described the difficulty in detecting the activity of the first two enzymes of beta-lactam biosynthesis, namely

L-α-aminoadipyl-L-cysteine synthetase and L-α-aminoadipyl-L-cysteinyl-D-valine (ACV)-synthetase. One wonders whether they are merely unstable or whether we are missing some cofactor or both.

The viridicatin biosynthetic pathways of _Penicillium_ _cyclopium_ was presented by Luckner and those of granaticin and actinorhodin of streptomycetes by Floss. From the latter presentation, I was surprised to find out that in two different species, the "same" enzyme can act in opposite directions. The presentations of Ōmura and Sir Edward (and also my own) pointed out the importance of α-ketogluturate-linked dioxygenases in biosyntheses of antibiotics such as beta-lactams and macrolides. Since the α-ketogluturate is lost in the reaction, I wonder whether the unexplained stimulation by organic acids of certain antibiotic processes could be due to replenishment of this keto-acid. The glyceollins, which Grisebach explained are phytoalexins of soybean, were both strange and intriguing to many of us strictly involved with microorganisms. He was pressed somewhat on the function of these compounds which appear to be induced in the plant to combat fungal infections. It appears strange to me that the scientific public is much more agreeable to the idea that phytoalexins are weapons in the competitive war between biological species than it is to accept a similar function for antibiotics.

It is my hope that all of the above presentations on pathways and structures have stimulated the Hoechst chemists in the audience to carefully examine the enzymes involved for the purpose of producing novel biodynamic compounds. One such enzyme is isopenicillin N synthetase (which I affectionately call "cyclase") which Sir Edward described. He mentioned the studies of Baldwin at Oxford in which analog penams containing the five-membered thiazolidine ring can be made by conversion of ACV analogs. However Baldwin has also discovered the ability of cyclase to make novel structures containing six-membered rings (e.g., cephams) and even seven-membered rings (e.g., homocephams). Indeed some fifteen new unnatural structures are known to be produced by cyclase. When one is dealing with structures as commercially important as beta-lactams with an annual market in the billions of dollars, it certainly should pay to examine such novel structures to determine whether they can be modified into new and useful chemotherapeutic compounds.

The main purpose of our workshop was to examine regulation and we certainly did spend much time discussing this topic. I come away with renewed confidence that regulation exists in secondary metabolism –

no doubt about it ! For example, Martin talked about glucose regulation in Penicillium of ACV synthesis, perhaps by affecting the
levels of internal free amino acids. He also described his studies on
Nocardia lactamdurans and showed that glucose negatively affects ACV
synthesis and represses desacetoxy-cephalosporin synthetase ("expandase"), that ammonium interferes with ACV synthesis and represses
cyclase, epimerase and expandase, and that inorganic phosphate,
glucose-6-phosphate and fructose-1,6-diphosphate inhibits expandase.
I presented Braña's studies on the ammonium repression of cyclase
and expandase (but not epimerase) in Streptomyces clavuligerus, Keller
discussed nitrogen control of alkaloid synthesis in Claviceps, Běhal,
the phosphate repression of anhydrotetracycline oxygenase in Streptomyces aureofaciens and Ōmura, the repression of valine dehydrogenase
by ammonium and phosphate in Streptomyces fradiae.

All of the above reports make it evident that there exists strong
nutritional regulation of secondary metabolism. The fact that we do
not understand the underlying mechanisms or the possibility that such
regulation involves intracellular signals different from those affecting primary metabolism does not decrease the significance of the control. It is there: it is not going to go away; and we must get smarter
about solving the mechanisms involved. Let me comment about a point
Luckner brought up during the round table discussion, i.e., that many
of the strains with which we work are highly mutated. I would not
want anyone in the audience to go away thinking that one should not
study such strains. Indeed, both the wild strain and the highly modified strain should be examined and compared. In the wild strain, we
will see control mechanisms which have been eliminated in the highly
productive strain. By such comparisons, we can learn about the most
important regulatory controls which had to be removed before production became significant for commercial operation.

In certain cases, the regulation is exerted on the supply of precursors rather than on the synthetases themselves. Aharonowitz
described the importance of deregulating aspartokinase to feedback
inhibition by threonine plus lysine in production of cephamycins by
Streptomyces clavuligerus, such inhibition restricting the formation
of the cephamycin precursor, α-aminoadipate. By such mutational deregulation, antibiotic production was increased six to eight-fold.

Gräfe discussed the very exciting phenomenon of induction of secondary metabolism by endogenous molecules ("autoregulators") which
also effect structural differentiation (e.g., production of aerial

mycelium in streptomycetes). His discussion included the original discovery of A-factor by Khokhlov and his own studies on similar inducers of anthracycline biosynthesis. It is interesting that 75% of Streptomyces griseus isolates produce A-factor but amazing to hear that 40% of all streptomycetes do so. It was also interesting to hear that cobalt increases A-factor synthesis. I know of many antibiotic processes which require cobalt but this has usually been attributed to an effect on methylation; perhaps it is more relevant to autoregulator production. Luckner described P-factor in Penicillium cyclopium which is involved in both sporulation and benzodiazapene alkaloid production, thus indicating that autoregulation is also important in fungi.

Vining appeared pessimistic about control in his chloramphenicol-producing streptomycete. However, his data certainly supported the existence of such control e.g., the repressing effect of nitrate. I feel that nitrate could be the key to nitrogen regulation of chloramphenicol synthesis and merits more attention. Nothing is known about the ability of the organism to make nitrate from different amino acids and the more repressive ones could be merely supplying nitrate. A number of years ago, we[1] reported that nitrate is the main repressive nitrogen source of aflatoxin production in Aspergillus parasiticus. Vining's chemostat data were of interest since two runs at the same growth rate but with different media resulted in a marked difference (six to seven-fold) in ammonium levels. Although he correctly concluded that growth rate was not important, the large difference in free ammonium (and possibly nitrate) could have caused the difference in chloramphenicol synthesis. Vining also pointed out that glucose effects its control via growth rate modification and that chloramphenicol represses arylamine synthetase, the first enzyme unique to the chloramphenicol pathway. He also correctly pointed out that competition between primary and secondary metabolism always has to be considered; i.e., sometimes one gets a positive effect on antibiotic synthesis by inhibition of cell wall or protein formation and vice versa. Yes, regulation exists in streptomycetes making chloramphenicol but it probably is unlike anything previously encountered in well behaved organisms such as Escherichia coli. This poses a real challenge to us to delve further into the genetics and molecular biology of our antibiotic-producing strains and this applies to researchers in industry as well as academia. We should not expect all organisms to behave like E. coli. As pointed out by Losick, Bacillus does not; neither does Pseudomonas, where clustering of genes occurs to a much lesser extent than in E. coli and certain biosynthetic genes are inducible. Fungal regulation is also very

different from that in E. coli. We must of course be very knowledgable
about data obtained with E. coli but not obsessed by it. We also should
not be frustrated by our slow rate of progress in elucidating the mechanisms of control in fermentation organisms. Masses of scientists
worked for thirty years to bring E. coli knowledge to where it is
today whereas in the field of secondary metabolism we have a few in-
vestigators involved in fundamental studies and each one is working on
a different process ! Indeed it may take a hundred years to understand secondary metabolism to the extent that we understand primary
metabolism in E. coli. Keep in mind that A-factor would have never been
discovered if Khokhlov only studied E. coli.

I would like to make a point concerning complex media. It was stated
during one of the presentations that since antibiotic production
occured in complex medium in the laboratory, there probably was no
nutritional control being exerted on the process. This is an incorrect
concept since there are balanced complex media and unbalanced complex
media, just like balanced and unbalanced defined media. Forget the
term "rich media" and think "balanced or unbalanced". Just because a
medium is complex does not mean it is loaded with repressive compounds;
instead it could contain stimulatory compounds and limiting levels of
phosphate or glucose.

An intriguing question arose in my mind throughout this workshop.
What is the effect of the supply of carbon, nitrogen and phosphorus
nutrients on the time of appearance and/or the concentration of
A-factor ? I doubt that anyone has examined this question.

I was very interested in Luckner's data showing that enzymes of
secondary metabolism can be produced days before they act and then
be turned on by formation of a "master" protein. Can this be explained by compartmentation, e.g., can the master protein be a specific enzyme breaking down the envelope of the organelle containing
the enzyme ? He also put forth the concept of stable messenger RNA
for synthetases of secondary metabolism but isn't it possible that we
are dealing with continuous transcription rather than stable messages ?

I have some words for the engineers in the audience. Please don't
go home from Ōmura's presentation feeling that you must put soil or
clay in your fermentors to carry out an optimum process. I hope you
realize that such "tricks" are used by the microbiologists working in
small flasks to approach the performance of the engineers' computers

and feeding equipment in order to limit repressive nutrients. I might add that his discovery of three new antibiotics when such natural materials were added to the flasks should be of great interest to those interested in antibiotic discovery.

Let me shift to genetics. Bu'Lock's presentation in this area indicated that heterokaryons between a parent strain and a restricted (i.e., domesticated) non-producing strain can yield increased product titers. This should be examined further in industrial strain-improvement programs. Esser told us about the use of mitochondrial DNA for the construction of vectors useful for filamentous fungi. Developments in this field are sorely needed in view of the important products made by fungi, e.g., penicillins, cephalosporins, cyclosporin, alkaloids, zearelanone. Also of interest was Esser's statement that no changes in mitochondrial DNA were evident between his low-cephalosporin producer and a high producer developed by the Eli Lilly company. Thus the multiplicity of mutations involved in the development of the superior strain did not involve modification of mitochondrial DNA.

A number of presentations showed data indicating that high producing strains have higher levels of pathway enzymes. Martin dealt with cyclase in Penicillium, Běhal with anhydrotetracycline oxygenase and tetracycline dehydrogenase in Streptomyces aureofaciens and Keller with the D-lysergic activating enzyme in Claviceps. This should be kept in mind as possibly an easier way to screen for superior mutants than is the antibiotic production process itself.

Another message is that deregulated mutants make higher levels of antibiotic. Thus Aharonowitz increased cephamycin production by desensitizing aspartokinase to feedback inhibition by threonine plus lysine and Běhal improved tetracycline production by deregulating anhydrotetracycline oxygenase to phosphate repression.

Filamentous microorganisms often are difficult to improve by mutagenesis due to the lack of single cells. Keller showed that a useful technique is to mutagenize hyphae and then to obtain single units by protoplasting. Indeed one clone showed an eight-fold increase in alkaloid production !

Those of us interested in new antibiotics were intrigued by Okami's discovery of indolizomycin by a novel protoplast fusion technique. The fusion products from two parents were selected for simultaneous resistance to both parental antibiotics. One such resistant clone pro-

duced the new antibiotic. Of great interest was the combined work of
Hopwood, Floss and Ōmura in producing new antibiotics by recombinant
DNA technology. Kleinkauf reported on the cloning in E. coli of one
of the amino acid-activating enzymes of the gramicidin S synthetase
complex from Bacillus brevis. This is a significant advance in the
area of Bacillus peptide antibiotics.

The clustering of biosynthetic genes on streptomycete chromosomes
was mentioned a number of times, e.g., by Vining (chloramphenicol)
and Hopwood (actinorhodin). This is a fortunate situation for the
cloning of such pathways. Hopwood's report that one single extra
copy of an operon resulted in a thirty-fold increase in antibiotic
production is remarkable, since this means that one does not have to
depend completely on high copy number vectors which may have deleterious side effects. Also of interest was Hopwood's finding that a
regulatory gene (an activator gene) was mapped in the midst of the
actinorhodin structural genes whereas in the methylenomycin A case,
the regulatory gene was at the end of the operon but a resistance
gene was in the midst of the cluster. We obviously must learn what
these regulatory genes are doing if we want to fully exploit control
in streptomycetes.

It appears possible from the above that one could use cloning of
antibiotics resistance as a means of introducing multiple copies of
structural and regulatory genes into a recipient culture, thus increasing production. Certainly hybrid antibiotics are now a reality
and awaiting further exploitation. Hopwood states that streptomycete
recombinant DNA technology is ready for industrial application. I
would hope that Esser and others bring the filamentous fungal system
up to a similar level in a few years although problems seem more difficult here.

The greatest challenge facing us is to find ways to apply the techniques and results of the geneticists, especially those described by
Losick in Bacillus subtilis. There appear to be almost too many points
of control for easy exploitation. For example, there appear to be
different regulons associated with the switching on and switching off,
at different times, of synthesis of various products and structures;
the expression of one sporulation gene (spoVG) depends on the expression of three other spo genes; expression is also dependent on
particular sigma factors of which there are some seven or eight (compared to one in E. coli) to allow the organism to transcribe different
parts of the genome at different times during development. It is

hoped that within a short time, the molecular biologists will be able to relate their time of appearance with specific functions in secondary metabolism. Losick also discussed promoters, two of which were thought to overlap, the importance of their "minus 35" and "minus 10" regions, and another region upstream ("activator") which had a major effect on operon expression. I wonder what effects simple factors like carbon, nitrogen and phosphorus nutrition might have on the production and time of appearance of sigma factors; indeed, does it matter how much of a sigma factor is made ?

   The big question is how to use genetics to unravel the mysteries of secondary metabolism. Three possibilities come to mind.
(1) Those of you in industry should develop genetic systems in the organism of major commercial interest.
(2) Some of us in academia should center our attention on one particular species as a model organism, rather than each of us working on different species.
(3) We should study regulation of secondary metabolism in organisms whose genetics is already well-known such as Bacillus subtilis.

   In this regard, we might even use E. coli to study control of aerobactin synthesis. This iron-transport factor, discussed by Kleinkauf, could be a good model; we should not forget that many of these siderophores also have antibiotic activity. Well, if even some of the above challenges are met, we shall have lots of progress to discuss at the next Hoechst Workshop on the Regulation of Secondary Metabolite Formation.

   Although this sixteenth Workshop Conference is the first in the area of microbiology, let's hope that it is not too many years until Hoechst AG invites us back again to Schloß Gracht.

Reference

Kachholz, T. and A.L. Demain. 1983. Nitrate Repression of averufin and aflatoxin biosynthesis. J. Nat. Prods. 46: 499-506.

Index